OXFORD MEDICAL PUBLICATIONS

Doctors' Decisions

Ethical Conflicts in Medical Practice

Doctors' Decisions

Ethical Conflicts in Medical Practice

Edited by

G. R. DUNSTAN

Emeritus Professor of Moral and Social Theology, University of London

and

E. A. SHINEBOURNE

Consultant Paediatric Cardiologist, Brompton Hospital, London

Oxford New York Tokyo

OXFORD UNIVERSITY PRESS

1989

Oxford University Press, Walton Street, Oxford OX2 6DP
Oxford New York Toronto
Delhi Bombay Calcutta Madras Karachi
Petaling Jaya Singapore Hong Kong Tokyo
Nairobi Dar-es-Salaam Cape Town
Melbourne Auckland
and associated companies in
Berlin Ibadan

Oxford is a trade mark of Oxford University Press

Published in the United States
by Oxford University Press, New York

British Library Cataloguing in Publication Data
Doctors decide : ethical conflicts in medical practice
1. Medicine. Ethical aspects
I. Dunstan, G. R. (Gordon Reginald).
II. Shinebourne, Elliot A.
174'.2
ISBN 0–19–261631–5

Library of Congress Cataloging in Publication Data
Doctors' decisions.
(Oxford medical publications)
Includes index.
1. Medical ethics. I. Dunstan, G. R. (Gordon Reginald)
II. Shinebourne, Elliot A. III. Series.
[DNLM: 1. Ethics, Medical. W 50 D6367]
R724.D63 1989 174'.2 88–31264
ISBN 0–19–261631–5

Set by Pentacor Ltd, High Wycombe, Bucks
Printed in Great Britain
at Bookcraft Ltd, Bath

Preface

The origin of this book is simply described. One of the editors was invited by Oxford University Press to write a book on medical ethics. He declined, because he is not a doctor. He offered instead to invite a medical friend to join him in editing a volume in which the majority of chapters would be written by doctors. Perspectives from the Jewish and Christian traditions would be drawn in, and a moral philosopher would survey the whole range at the end.

So it came about. We have covered a fair range of specialties, narrow as it must seem when all those that might have been covered are considered. We are indebted to our friends for consenting to write for us, and for all the work to which that initial consent committed them. We would also thank the staff of Oxford University Press for their initiative, for their patience, and for much help.

1988

G. R. D.
E. A. S.

Contents

Contributors

Michael Baum, Professor of Surgery, King's College School of Medicine and Dentistry, London.

Rabbi J. David Bleich, Herbert and Florence Tenzer Professor of Jewish Law and Ethics, Benjamin N. Cardozo School of Law, Yeshiva University, New York.

Sidney Bloch, Consultant Psychotherapist, Warneford Hospital, and Clinical Lecturer in Psychiatry, University of Oxford.

Margaret A. Branthwaite, Consultant Physician and Anaesthetist, Brompton Hospital, London.

Peter R. Braude, Clinical Director of the Embryo and Gamete Research Group and Hon. Consultant in Obstetrics and Gynaecology, University of Cambridge Clinical School.

Peter Byrne, Lecturer in the Philosophy of Religion; a Director of the Centre of Medical Law and Ethics, King's College London.

A. G. M. Campbell, Professor of Child Health, University of Aberdeen; Hon. Consultant Paediatrician, Grampian Health Board.

Brian W. Cromie, Director, Cambridge Applied Nutrition, Toxicology, and Biosciences Group.

E. J. Dunstan, Consultant Geriatrician, Selly Oak Hospital, South Birmingham Health Authority.

G. R. Dunstan, Emeritus Professor of Moral and Social Theology, University of London; Hon. Research Fellow, University of Exeter.

Malcolm A. Ferguson-Smith, Professor of Pathology, University of Cambridge.

Marie E. Ferguson-Smith, Cambridge University Centre for Medical Genetics, Addenbrooke's Hospital, Cambridge.

Peter L. Freedman, Medical Director, Cambridge Applied Nutrition, Toxicology and Biosciences Group; Hon. Senior Clinical Fellow Department of Medicine, Addenbrooke's Hospital, Cambridge.

John W. Funder, Medical Research Centre, Prince Henry's Hospital, Melbourne, Australia.

Raanan Gillon, Director, Imperial College Health Service, University of London; Editor, *Journal of Medical Ethics.*

M. J. Hare, Consultant Gynaecologist, Huntingdon Health Authority; Senior Member and Former Fellow, Hughes Hall, Cambridge.

Contributors

Terence Larkin, Consultant Psychiatrist, St John of God's Hospital, Dublin.

Michael Linnett, General Practitioner, London.

Maurice Lipsedge, Consultant Psychiatrist, Guy's Hospital, London.

A. Mindel, Academic Department of Genito-Urinary Medicine, The Middlesex Hospital Medical School.

Lady Oppenheimer, Philosophical Theologian, Jersey.

Elliot A. Shinebourne, Consultant Paediatric Cardiologist, Brompton Hospital, London.

Stephen Spiro, Consultant Physician, University College Hospital and Brompton Hospital, London.

Jeremy Wilde, Consultant in Obstetrics and Gynaecology, Odstock Hospital, Salisbury.

Eric Wilkes, Emeritus Professor of Community Care and General Practice, University of Sheffield; Co-Chairman, Help the Hospices.

1

The doctor as the responsible moral agent

G. R. DUNSTAN

I

The purpose of this book is to enable doctors to expound for themselves the ethics of their practice. Upon reflection, this purpose may not prove as naïve as it may appear to be. In the mounting tide of publications on medical ethics, few books are written by doctors. Most are written by philosophers or by other non-medical adherents to a new speciality of 'ethicists' or 'bio-ethicists'. Theologians add to the number, some out of a tradition of moral theology, others not. In the USA, ethicists have established a career structure attached to medical schools and hospitals. Together with lawyers they dominate the discussion of medical ethics and even ethical decision. Consultancies are available to advise doctors, for a fee, how to exercise their profession: a precautionary response, perhaps, to the complex of social theories, economic pressures, and legal hazards prevailing in that society.

The plan of this book embodies a conviction that doctors are themselves the responsible moral agents in their respective areas of practice. Inherent in the concept of a profession is the element of moral obligation, the belief that the relevant experience, knowledge, and skill ought to be used 'ethically', that is, in pursuit of ends reckoned altruistic and good and in the avoidance of ends reckoned inordinately self-regarding and bad. What ends are good and what bad, both in general and in particular cases, is, of course, open to discussion. The doctor is properly a party to that discussion, not an arbiter. But, having consulted and listened as he must, he is professionally, that is morally, responsible for clinical decisions relating to his own patients. The responsibility is entrenched in the practice of medicine as it has been received in the traditions of the West: Greek, Arab, and European. This book was planned on the supposition that to erode that responsibility, to devolve it on others singly or in committee, would not be for the good of medicine, that is, for the benefit that medicine can render to patients and to society. Rather, it were better to reaffirm the responsibility of doctors as moral agents in their practice, to enhance their competence in its discharge, to hold them accountable, and to restore a presumption of trust in their favour.

II

The exercise of such responsibility presupposes authority, the intrinsic authority attaching to knowledge, experience, and skill, socially validated in the medical role. This is evident in Hippocrates, tempered by a high respect for the patient and for the art. It is defensible still today—though the defence carries with it its own admonition and submission to audit, as was emphasized in the recent Rock Carling monograph on clinical freedom (Hoffenberg 1987). It is not coincident with social status, for doctors have ranked, at different times and in different cultures, from slaves to the confidants of kings. It is brought under question in our own time, and not only by those who distort its features with such pejorative terms as 'authoritarianism' and 'paternalism'.

The intrinsic ground of the authority changes as the knowledge-base changes. A new medical science, developed over two or three professional generations, has required the formulation of a new medical ethics to accompany it (Welbourn and Dunstan 1981). But the pursuit of this new science, and its application in new medical technology, are both group or team activities: the medical practitioner is no longer the sole repository of the one nor the sole executant of the other. The change gives the practitioner more information to be taken into account, and more colleagues to be consulted, in making his decision; it does not remove his responsibility for decision. Rather, it strengthens it: one mind has to synthesize the inputs from so many sources, and that must be the mind of the clinician, be he consultant or general practitioner, responsible for the patient.

Some of this knowledge, being common to the biological and some physical sciences, is widely comprehensible outside medicine in a generation educated in these things. Television and intelligent journalism extend awareness more widely, even if they sometimes distort significance in so doing. (Television may in fact encourage an unhealthy, voyeuristic preoccupation with high-technology medicine, just as chatty radio discussion may over-simplify issues or get them out of proportion: not all medical decisions are 'agonizing' or 'life and death' decisions; most are routine, about improving bodily functioning or palliating ills.) Medicine is, therefore, no longer the mystery it used to be in the sense of an arcane art, the secret of its practitioners. But it is still, when properly practiced, a mystery in the older sense of an art, a craft, an office or ministry of a skill.

Social, economic, and political change have also made their mark. Medicine, for long a profession whose corporate identity was expressed in small collegiate, faculty, or society structures (medical faculties in the universities, physicians, barber-surgeons, apothecaries) and for a time in local medical societies, is now organized nationally in Britain and for the most part incorporated into a National Health Service covering both general practice and hospital care. Although the doctor–patient relationship remains at the heart of medical practice, medical ethics cannot be reduced to it. The doctor exercises his clinical responsibility under new restraints, inherent in the structure of the organized service, and imposed episodically by financial limitation. General practitioners must prescribe for their National Health Service patients the medicines judged best for them but, in some categories, chosen from a Limited List restricted to what the NHS will pay for—a restriction recognized to cause no great harm in practice because, afer initial fumbling, the list was drawn with consent. Surgeons may admit to operation only the number of patients for which beds and nurses can be provided or for which, in the private sector, patients will pay. Their decisions therefore extend from how to treat to whom to treat, and the grounds of decision cannot always be unequivocally clinical.

The statutes which created the National Health Service conferred on patients certain rights: the right to consult a general practitioner; and a right to the hospital and other services, clinically indicated, to which he should introduce them. These statutory rights, in a generation bombarded with the rhetoric of rights, can easily be extended in imagination into a 'right' to whatever service or remedy the patient desires or is persuaded would be good for him. So we hear of the 'right' of an infertile woman to bear a child—because advances in the treatment of infertility make it possible for some few to do so; of the 'right' of a couple to know the sex of a fetus, ascertained incidentally from chorionic villus sampling or amniocentesis, even when no sex-linked disorder has been diagnosed—and even to abort a fetus of the unwanted sex; of the 'right' to deliver a child in the place and manner of choice; of the 'right' to read one's own medical records; of the 'right' to choose, to live, to die; and so on.

The clinician has therefore to decide, not only what are genuine rights and legitimate interests matched by corresponding duties, but also what wishes or interests are being presented in the language of rights, and how far he should go to serve them, if serve them he should. Readers of the chapters which follow will see how some of the authors decide these questions. The inflation of the language of rights can only do harm to medicine because it is bound to polarize as adversaries—even to the point of expensive lawsuits in pursuit of damages in the Courts—those, doctor and patient, who can work together properly only in a relationship of trust. Observers point to the threat of this in the litigious spirit now endemic in the USA; but it is evident in Britain also.

The polarization is worsened when, as now happens, the initiative in formulating the discussion of medical ethics is taken by philosophers, lawyers, and 'ethicists', and not by doctors themselves. The terms of a discussion are set by the words used to initiate it. Words, used at first with controlled meaning, tend to gain an independent momentum, becoming slogans to which absolute command is attached. So patients' 'rights' are justified by appeal to patients' 'autonomy'. Doctors rear up in defence with 'clinical autonomy'. So we have two autonomies, the one ranged against the other. Patients may demand a service which a doctor in conscience cannot provide—examples occur in the chapters which follow; or a doctor or a nurse may refuse, on grounds of conscience, a service to which a patient is morally and lawfully entitled.

Autonomy cannot be absolute in a human world. The word is a recent import from the sphere of politics into the personal and medical spheres. The Greek work *autonomia* means 'living by one's own laws': a principle dear to the self-governing Greek city-states, but something of a hindrance to them when combination was required to meet a common foe or invader. Our word for it in politics is sovereignty. Within our own sovereign states room has been found for self-governing, autonomous corporations, like chartered boroughs or companies, colleges, the Inns of Court, the Church. But absolute autonomy none could enjoy. The English Reformation was in fact a successful challenge by a sovereign nation to the absolute autonomy or sovereignty claimed by the Roman Catholic Church

In the early nineteenth century autonomy came to be used of personal freedom, and as such it has a legitimate usage today. It stands, in the medical context, for a recognized claim to remain inviolate: not to be treated or operated on without consent. And the fine judgements required by respect for this principle in clinical decisions are well illustrated in the chapters which follow. But autonomy as now rhetorically used stands for more: for freedom to order one's life as one will; to assume an unfettered capacity for choice and to claim paramount, indisputable value for that choice, even to enforce it on others. This claim, whether made by patient or doctor, cannot be defended in theory nor admitted in practice. It may not be invoked by patients to override conscience or professional obligation. It may not be invoked by doctors to justify continuance in a medical or surgical practice either not validated by adequately controlled trials, or regardless of cost.

There are other principles, too, implicit in the traditional pragmatic conscience of medicine, which are distorted by exaggeration in contempory debate. The duty to respect confidences, not to reveal secrets, is inflated into an abstraction called 'confidentiality'. The word can be used as an impediment, not simply to a serious discussion of duty in sensitive areas (by assuming a strict or absolute duty which has yet to be proved), but also to co-operative action when such is required for the better service or protection of a patient.

'Consent' waited a long time for articulation as a principle governing medical intervention (Polani 1983); though it was clearly stated as an axiom—and proxy consent also—in relation to surgery by St Thomas Aquinas in the thirteenth century (*Summa Theologica*, 2a, 2ae, 65.1). Today 'informed consent' is held to be a *sine qua non* of medical action. The English courts have striven to preserve the application of the principle, consistently with the interest of patients, from the extremes to which it has been driven elsewhere (House of Lords 1985). But the dogmatic insistence urged by ethicists on the patient's 'right to information'—to be told everything—is one which clinicians, pragmatically concerned with their patient's interests, are bound to question and, sometimes, to resist. Inherent in the moral agency is a duty of discretion, of reserve; a duty to measure the amount of information given in such a way as will enable the patient to decide whether to accept the treatment proposed for him, and, if he consents, to co-operate in it. The doctor is not under a duty, in obedience to some dogma or ideology imposed on him, to impose all knowledge of everything upon a patient, regardless of the patient's interest or his capacity to assimilate and to live with it.

Some doctors are still too reserved. Either because they underestimate the mental and reflective capacities of the patient, or because they are personally unskilled in such communication, or for sheer pressure of time, they tell their patients less than they could or should. For lack of information—why this question or that is asked, or this course of action or that is advised—a patient may be less able to co-operate with the doctor either in his assessment of the patient—a necessary prerequisite of effective treatment—or in the treatment itself.

III

The tension between practitioners and those whom they have sometimes called sophists is as old as medicine itself. It is evident in Hippocrates and Galen, to look no further. It is not of necessity an adversarial tension. For centuries Arab culture held in high respect the philosopher-physician (indeed, western science and philosophy are deeply in its debt); and post-scholastic Renaissance Europe aspired to the same ideal. Thomas Vicary, resident surgeon-governor of St Bartholomew's Hospital in the mid-sixteenth century, described Galen (mistakenly, as it happens) as 'the Lanterne of all Chirurgions' and 'the Prince of Philosophers' (Dunstan 1986). The tension should not be exaggerated today. R. Gillon, trained in philosophy as well as medicine, writes Chapter 10 as a physician; although at the end he would seem to justify his ethical stance by its conformity with the 'four prima-facie principles' set out in a well-known text book of medical ethics.

The gravamen in Hippocrates and Galen was that the sophists marked out a web of theory to which the practice of medicine must be stretched to conform, whereas the practitioners believed that practice must be directed by observation and the nature of the art. The sophists' habit of mind is still evident in the writings of some ethicists in the literature of medical ethics. Principles are stated; practice is then judged, prospectively and retrospectively, in accordance with them, sometimes as though they had absolute force, admitting of no discretion. In this book the principles themselves are put under trial: what place have concepts like 'autonomy', 'condidentiality', and 'informed consent' in clinical decision? Have they absolute command? Or have they strong presumptive force, claiming respect always, but subject to discretion in the service of the patient's own and other commanding interests?

The defence of moral agency—of the capacity and duty to decide—is not a defence of naked autocracy, of clinical absolutism set up against the absolutism attached to principles. Decision is the culmination of a corporate process in which information and assessment are shared. This appears again and again in the chapters below: decision is taken but consideration is shared; the family is to be listened to, but the decision is the doctor's. Accountability requires this. As each participant—nurse, laboratory scientist, junior doctor, social worker—is responsible for information or assessment professionally offered, so the consultant or general practitioner accepts responsibility for the conclusion, the resultant decision, and is accountable for it. Accountability requires honest and accurate record keeping, and that records should remain secret unless disclosure is required by a competent authority.

Accountability has prospective force as well as retrospective application. A clinician is not always at liberty to comply with a patient's wishes, or even to serve his supposed interests, regardless of social consequence. Uncertainty there must be in the earliest attempts at innovative treatment—requiring the discipline of controlled trials for its resolution. Uncertainty heightens the duty of prudence in clinical management, particularly when the possibility of ill-consequence is foreseeable. Treatments for infertility which, either for lack of strict monitoring or because of the unrestricted transfer of gametes or embryos, result in a high multiple birth, can have dire consequences, not only for the mother and her tiny premature babies, but also for a neighbourhood denied access to a neonatal unit preoccupied with the multiple birth. The transplanting of organs from a newly born anencephalic child, to whom the normal criteria of brain-stem death cannot be applied, can revive old fears and controversies about established cadaveric transplant surgery with the resultant decline in the availability of organs for patients who need them. Enthusiasm for the transplanting of fetal tissue before all the considerations are weighed rouses legitimate fears about interests imperilled or rights overriden in pursuit of theoretical but as yet hypothetical benefits (McCullagh 1987). Management given in the name of clinical freedom which professional opinion treats with reserve and which a reflective public judges to be bizarre creates a prejudice against any innovative therapy from which both the legitimate discipline and patients may suffer.

IV

The location of clinical decision in one identifiable individual, the doctor who accepts responsibility for the patient, has a basis in belief as well as the warrant of tradition and pragmatic justification. The belief—a datum of Christian theology—is that human personality is rational and social, disposed towards the just and the good though capable of turning away from both, and endowed with the faculty of moral judgement with which to discern the good and the just from the evil and the unjust. Medicine is one of the professions in which these characteristics are incorporated and recognized institutionally, entrusted with social function, and for this rewarded (Emmet 1966).

Doctors are no more immune than members of other professions to temptation which might skew judgement. When angioplasty or hysterectomy operations, for instance, or haemodialysis or delivery by Caesarium section, in the private sector significantly outnumber those in the public sector in its different national forms, the reason may not lie in a shortage of funds in the public sector preventing necessary operations; it may be that a fee for service system, linked with insurance and entrepreneurial medical facilities, results in more unnecessary operations (Hoffenberg 1987, pp 29–31). The ethical conduct of clinical trials requires that the reward to investigators be not disproportionate to the work involved or given in such a way as to influence prescribing or other practice adverse to the best interest of patients (Royal College of Physicians 1986*a*). It must also be tempting, sometimes, simply to dodge decision; to 'leave it to the patient' because decision is difficult, even painful and wearing; or to fall into routine when the particulars are not routine.

When conscience succumbs to pressure there must be safeguards of the public good. The profession itself is and should be the first line of defence and agent of redress (Royal College of Physicians 1986*b*). Research ethics committees (called institutional review boards in some countries), each with articulate non-medical members, oversee research in hospitals, medical schools and research institutes, and in general practice (Royal College of Physicians 1984; Nicholson 1986). Clinical practice is less vigilantly scrutinized, except by informal peer review. Should the professional safeguard fail, resort must regrettably be had either to statutory authority in the General Medical Council or to the Courts in civil action for redress or in prosecution for offences against the criminal law. The rising frequency of litigation, notably in the USA but increasingly in Britain also, and the rising scale of the damages awarded, while they represent an attempt to do justice to individuals, also result in harm. Litigation and insurance against the risk are notoriously expensive; damages awarded against Health Authorities divert precious funds from their intended purpose. More pertinent to this book is their ethical impact. The intimidated mind resorts to defensive medicine: legitimate expedients are not attempted for fear of ill-consequence and expense; unnecessary tests and investigations are imposed for fear of the imputation of negligence. The very language and structure of ethics are distorted: questions of moral obligation too quickly become questions of legal obligation; 'what I ought to do' becomes 'what I may safely do'. The boundaries of freedom are narrowed and the benefits of freedom are in jeopardy.

V

Clinical decisions become ethical decisions when there is in them an element of choice and where the questions are posed, implicitly or explicitly, in terms such as 'ought' or 'should'. It is the work primarily of philosophers and theologians to analyse the concept and sources of moral obligation, and not only in medicine. It is for lawyers, similarly, to relate moral obligation to law. Philosophers, theologians, and lawyers have an ancillary function when invited by clinicians to help in the elucidation of moral perplexities when they attend clinical decision. They have other functions also when professional action or inaction threatens or conflicts with the rights of persons or with the interests and order of society. Lack of vigilance in the past, when notorious wrongs were done, has done much to determine, in reaction, the aggressive factors in medical ethics today. But that is not the subject of this book.

The faculty for moral reasoning on which the clinician relies is personal to himself. Yet it partakes also of a corporate conscience, that of his profession, moulded by his induction into the profession and by association with colleagues in his specialty. The corporate conscience, too, can benefit from the stimulation, even the stiffening, of adjuvant philosophy, theology, and law. The professional conscience, personal and corporate, may falter. It can become sluggish, complacent, and insensitive to human liberties and claims—though less insensitive, probably, than those of pressure groups which would forbid any deviation from the absolutist moral stances professed by themselves alone. Yet when the alternatives are considered—decision by committee or tribunal, for instance, or regulated in detail by the criminal law—it may seem preferable to leave moral agency where it is, with the person medically identified with the care and interests of the patient. It remains for us to assure that the doctor is morally equipped for the task.

REFERENCES

Dunstan, G. R. (1986). Religion, philosophy, and ethics in relation to medicine. In *The Oxford Companion to Medicine* (ed. J. Walton, P. S. Beeson, and R. Bodley Scott), pp. 1227–45. Oxford University Press.

Emmet, D. (1966). *Rules, Roles and Relations*. Macmillan, London.

Hoffenberg, R. (1987). *Clinical Freedom*. Rock Carling Lecture 1987. Nuffield Provincial Hospitals Trust, London.

House of Lords (1985). Sidaway v. Bethlem Royal Hospital and the Maudsley Hospital Authority and others. *The Times* Law Report, 22 February 1985.

McCullagh, P. (1987). *The Foetus as Transplant Donor: Scientific, Social and Ethical Perspectives*. John Wiley, Chichester.

Nicholson, R. H. (1986). *Medical Research with Children: Ethics, Law, and Practice*. Oxford University Press.

Polani, P. E. (1983). The development of the concept and practice of patient consent. In *Consent in Medicine* (ed. G. R. Dunstan and Mary M. Seller), pp. 57–84. King's Fund Publishing, London.

Royal College of Physicians (1984). *Guidelines on the Practice of Ethics Committees in Medical Research*.

Royal College of Physicians (1986*a*). *The Relationship between Physicians and the Pharmaceutical Industry*.

Royal College of Physicians (1986*b*). *Research on Healthy Volunteers*.

Welbourn, R. B. and Dunstan, G. R. (1981) Medical Science and Medical Ethics. In *Dictionary of Medical Ethics* 2nd edition. (ed. A. S. Duncan, G. R. Dunstan, and R. B. Welbourn) pp. xviii–xxvii and xxviii–xxxi. Darton, Longman, and Todd, London.

2

Experiments on animals in medical research

JOHN W. FUNDER

This is a personal account, by a medical research worker who uses thousands of experimental animals per year. At the end of their time under study the animals, with very few exceptions, are killed. As a biologist, I am used to studying phenomena with some degree of variation between individual organisms, and thus to making observations on populations; the notion of a personal statement on experiments on animals, of an $n=1$, is thus not a particularly comfortable one. Clearly, in terms of what medical research workers think in the area of animal ethics, it would be very much preferable for the range of issues deemed important to be factored into a well-designed, computer-compatible questionnaire, and for this to be appropriately administered and analysed. My justification for an n of 1 is that of Eric Newby or Patrick Leigh Fermor, in that I have been there; what I am writing is a traveller's tale, with no claim to speak for or be representative of others working in this area.

I began experimenting on animals in 1967, as a Ph.D. student in physiology at the Howard Florey Institute in Melbourne, having completed a medical degree and an internship. As an intern, I found the pace with which my mentors approached clinical medicine a problem. Patients died, patients got better; to me, and it seemed, to them, there was no time to ask why one died and another recovered. No time to think, to reflect; obviously an intellectual snob, probably a trouble-maker, the boy would be better off in research. For three and a half years, then, I worked on sheep. The studies involved a lot of surgery, including constricting the renal artery supplying blood to the kidney; placing fine plastic tubes in the renal artery to infuse hormones; and transplanting the adrenal gland from just above the kidney to a pouch prepared in the dewlap, the abundant folds of neck skin in the Merino, where the blood going to and from the gland could be altered, or sampled, by tubes in the carotid artery and jugular vein. All of these surgical procedures were done with the sheep under general anaesthetic, initially under the guidance of an expert surgeon, in an operating theatre which was better equipped than those in all but the largest hospitals in Melbourne. Post-operatively, the sheep were closely monitored in a dedicated recovery room, but were not given any analgesia. They were used for days or weeks (renal artery cannulae), for many months (renal artery constriction), or for many years (adrenal transplants), in studies on blood pressure and adrenal steroid hormone production.

The studies done on these animals would normally be considered a solid contribution. They were published in good international journals, and did not include any screaming 'breakthroughs'. Like so much of any science, they represented individual tiles in the mosaic, the size, shape, or contribution of any one of which is difficult to justify taken out of the context of, say, San Marco. Since that time—in San Francisco, Paris, and now back in Melbourne—I have always used rats, sometimes sheep, and occasionally guinea pigs and mice as experimental animals; in addition, I have undertaken basic scientific (non-therapeutic) experiments on normal human volunteers and patients, and have been involved in a number of cell- and tissue-culture studies. More tiles, no screaming breakthroughs, and San Marco still not in sight.

At the time of my Ph.D. studies I was (and remain) more concerned about human bioethics in general than the particular area of the ethics of animal experiments. Like many of that generation educated in Catholic schools, I enjoyed a thorough grounding in apologetics, some of which was defensive, but much more a basic primer in ethics. Perhaps predictably, for me then the issues were contraception, abortion, euthanasia—all in the context of a democratic, pluralist society; now (for comparison) they are resource allocation, informed consent, embryo experiments, and the power of single-issue groups in democratic, pluralist societies.

This may be thought rather grandiose, and perhaps slightly too comfortable; a dyed-in-the-wool animal experimenter, blind to the ethical issues involved in his day-to-day work, finding justification in being concerned about areas like informed consent or embryo experiments in which he does not have to make decisions. There may well be some truth in this; it may represent a defence, a mechanism of guilt-deflection, given the thousands of rats and hundreds of sheep that I currently use each year. On the other hand, I think that it is more than merely defence, or guilt deflection. At base, I think that ethics is fascinating, in a sense in proportion to the complexity of the action. Informed consent involves two actors, doctor and patient; embryo experiments four—gamete donors, scientist, developing embryo. Animal experiments involve one actor, the research worker; the animals have no responsibilities, are incapable of moral or immoral, ethical or unethical action. For this reason—as well as a defence, or a deflection—I think that what is loosely termed animal ethics is *per se* less challenging than various other areas.

That said, I should like to re-emphasize that the ethics of animal experiments are a part of human bioethics. Animals have patterns of behaviour, within and between species, which are characterized by terms also used to describe human behaviour (e.g. caring, aggressive); it is commonplace to use ethical terms about animal behaviour ('good dog' for waiting for the signal to eat, 'bad dog' for worrying sheep). This is, in fact, monstrous anthropomorphism; and, in the ethological sense, truly unethical behaviour. Naturally, dogs bolt their food and worry sheep, and the lion lies down outside the lamb. Nobody can gainsay the usage 'good dog', 'bad dog'—but it is important to see it for what it is, and to stop short of ascribing the status of moral agents to animals, however we may categorize their behaviour in response to our commands or prejudices.

Currently, the experiments in which I am involved cover a range of areas including endocrinology, neuro-endocrinology, circulatory control, and behavioural science; the human disease categories to which these areas correspond are stress, high blood pressure, infertility, learning, and memory. Most of the studies use sheep, often after complicated neurosurgery on the base of the brain and pituitary gland, and rats in a variety of ways. Most of the rats are operated on under anaesthetic, for removal of their adrenal glands, ovaries, or testes, and are treated through their drinking water or by injection for days or weeks; they are then killed, and their tissues taken for analysis. In the case of both sheep and rats, control (unoperated and/or untreated) groups are used for blood and tissue samples. Occasionally I use guinea-pigs and mice; very often, I go to the abattoir to collect tissues (usually offal), to obviate the need and expense of purpose-killing an animal. Control animals—from which particular tissues are taken and analysed as a baseline upon which to judge the effects of treatment—very often also serve as tissue sources for other, unrelated experiments. In the words of the Chicago stockyards, we try to use everything but the squeak.

Going to the abattoir, using everything but the squeak, is evidence of frugality, given that animals often comprise a significant amount of research budgets; it is also evidence of what I might term ethical parsimony. If several experiments can harvest various tissues from the same group of control animals, then fewer laboratory rats will need to be bred and killed.

Most animal experimenters have a very real concern for life; some, myself included, are very much inclined to emphasize the importance of life over pain. A number of my experiments involve swimming naive rats, not to exhaustion, but for 15 and then 5 minutes in a plastic jar containing water at 25°C (midsummer swimming-pool temperature). For me, the ethical question is not whether or not I should swim the rats, which is a mild-to-moderate stress by a number of indices; the real question is how I can justify killing perfectly healthy rats, after a total of 20 minutes swimming on two occasions 24 hours apart. This concern may betray a background in the physical rather than the behavioural sciences, inasmuch as I see using kidneys and liver and brain and blood as justification for killing a rat, whereas studying the effects of hormones and neurotransmitters on learning and memory is no such justification. But the central reason for my concern is ethical parsimony; the rat could go on living its normal 2–3 years after the behavioural experiment, but only a dead rat can provide kidney and liver and brains and blood for analysis.

The swimming rat studies provide an insight into the often idiosyncratic thinking underlying decisions taken by institutional ethics committes. In these studies, the animal is given an injection, placed in the water for 15 minutes on one day, removed, dried, fed, and watered; next day it is retested in the water for 5 minutes. When I took my proposed studies to the ethics committee, the Professor of Surgery (who worked on dogs) was of the opinion that the studies were ethically marginal; rats were perhaps all right, but there was no way that similar studies could be done on dogs, for instance. When I asked if I could do them, again just for example, on medical students, the surgeon had absolutely no qualms.

I think that there are two points to be made here, one about species of animals/vertebrates/life-forms, the other about ethics committees. As we get to know more and more about biology, the commonality of life-forms becomes clearer and clearer; for example, one of the basic proteins which cover DNA in the nucleus (histone IV) has 98 per cent identity in the human and the sweet-pea. Most biologists are privileged to spend at least part of their time in awe, faced with the wonderful world of living things; that this wonder is not confined to biologists is evidenced by the success of David Attenborough's '*Life on Earth*' programmes. Without pretending to be a Jain, I believe that this awe and wonder need to be accorded the tree and the ant, as well as the laboratory toad, the companion dog, or the chimpanzee in the zoo.

Or, indeed, the human being: and if you cut down trees to build houses, or kill sheep to eat or to do experiments on, do you object to killing people for food, or for study? If so, given the continuum you have sketched in terms of life-forms, how can you justify this distinction? I do object to killing people for food, or for study, or indeed for any reason (capital punishment and the 'just' war included); the reason I distinguish people from other life-forms is, in a nutshell, because *Animal liberation* was written by Peter Singer, and not by a chimpanzee; because the RSPCA is staffed by people, not dolphins; because I am in awe and wonder at particular human individuals (family members, Mozart, etc.), but not individual rats. Individual is perhaps a key word; substantive for people, adjective for rats.

The second point to be made post-swimming rats is about animal ethics committees. Such committees have come into particular prominence since the late 1970s; for a number of years for example, all applications for research funding to the National Health and Medical Research Council (NHMRC) of Australia have to include documentary evidence of having been submitted to and approved by the appropriate (university, hospital, whatever) institutional ethics committee. In addition, an NHMRC Animal Ethics subcommittee monitors all grant applications, and flags potentially sensitive areas for detailed scrutiny. Such institutional ethics committess include veterinarians, representatives of the RSPCA, and lay people with no other institutional connection, as well as medical and scientific personnel; they are commonly hard-working and, in a public sense, very successful.

They are not without their problems, however. Principal among the problems faced by such committees is that their present constitution and status largely reflect pressure from variously styled 'animal rights' or 'animal liberation' groups. By dedication, tireless publicity, arguments from worst-case examples, and occasional violence, these groups have very effectively lobbied the legislators, and to a large extent, cowed the animal experimenters. Currently, for example, in this state a hospital is required by law to air condition its animal house, but not its wards.

A second problem is that only a minority of the members of institutional animal ethics committees have any background in research, as opposed to animal care, clinical medicine, or laboratory science. I apply for approval to experiment on a certain number of rats and sheep per year, describing in detail the various surgical and experimental procedures proposed, anaesthesia, means of disposal, etc. I am constantly told that I should really be seeking individual approval for each experiment, so that the committee can be satisifed that they know exactly what procedures are being done to *each animal*.

My reply is that this is doctrinaire and unworkable. It betrays total ignorance of how research works, on a day-by-day basis. I cannot know whether we will need more rats to be adrenalectomized than ovariectomized, next week or next month; it depends on what we find today and tomorrow. If you are worried about my using too many rats, take consolation in their cost and the frugal nature of research budgets for consumables. If I want to do new and different procedures on rats or sheep, then I routinely put them before the committee for approval (or rejection) before I begin. In terms of individual rats, however, the committee—and the community that funds biomedical research—will ultimately have to trust the experimenters, that they are not spiriting animals off to voodoo ceremonies, or in any other way transgressing the published and accepted Code of Practice in Animal Experimentation.

Part and parcel of the animal lobby-inspired level of surveillance is that the committees feel constrained to take the part of the experimental animals, rather than considering the effects of the proposed experiments on those who are to carry them out. When a code of practice speaks of humane treatment of animals it is to the experimenters that 'humane' refers, not the animals. What the ethics committee should be is expert, in terms of biology and experimental design (as well as containing community representatives); its principal role is to ensure that the procedures proposed do not demean the experimenters by allowing them to trivialize animals.

Finally, in this context, animals ethics committees appear preoccupied with pain, rather than life. I do not for a moment dispute that there are circumstances in which life—human or other animal— may be deemed not worth continuing, due to the presence and certain prospect of unrelieved pain. On the other hand, most people suffer mild to severe pain, often not without complaint, but without thinking they would rather be dead. The crucial factor is probably the consciousness of the future, the prospect of relief; rats can certainly be unconscious, but to what extent they are conscious—of the future, in particular—is open to speculation.

This is perhaps the implicit rationale behind 'putting animals down', i.e., killing them when they are in severe pain—or simply unwanted, like stray cats or dogs. Rats can make choices, but perhaps not at the level of death now, or death some weeks away after an operation under anaesthetic and a series of injections, for instance. For this reason, for example, I cannot agree with those (sometimes successful) lobbyists who argue that stray cats and dogs should be killed 'humanely' rather than used as experimental animals. There are few activities more truly 'humane' than trying to understand living things, and merely to kill the offending creature seems to be a prodigal waste of animal life.

All this said, there can be no question that public funding bodies, such as the Medical Research Council (MRC), National Institute of Health (NIH), or the NHMRC, can appropriately demand adherence to a code of practice in animal ethics. Research, of its nature, is a triad of hypothesis, testing, and publication; in this sense, then, there is no such thing as 'private research', so that the community has a very real stake in ensuring that its funds are not being spent in activities that cause animals undue suffering, that trivialize their lives, or that demean the humanity of the experimenter. What is important for the community to realize—and in particular its policy-givers and law-makers—is that inevitably there are trade-offs. Few of us want a particular fur coat so badly that we face with equanimity the prospect of stunned baby seals skinned alive on ice floes; on the other hand, most of us use toiletries screened by the much-publicized Draize test, and if we are to proscribe the test we will need to find other methods for quality control of existing products, and for testing the next breakthrough in shampoos. Similarly, if we are going to have medical (and veterinary) practice based on science, rather than credo and prejudice, then we need experiments: on human subjects, including control subjects; on primates, and dogs and cats, and rats and mice; on cells in tissue culture; on bacteria and viruses—in short, on the whole gamut of life-forms.

The medical research workers, whom the community supports to do experiments including animal studies, have often been slow to point out this trade-off, and defensive in the face of the animal rights/liberation lobby; the practising doctor, increasingly fortified by a scientific base to his or her knowledge, has been curiously silent. I believe that the defensiveness of the medical research workers—who for the very large part would much rather not offend anybody—has served to focus the attentions of the animal lobbyists on hospital and university laboratories; they know that they would get much shorter shrift in an abbatoir, or among racehorse trainers, or from housewives trying to train a puppy to conform with our current notions of a companion animal.

If, on the other hand, the animal rights/liberation groups are able to persuade a majority of the community that scientific medicine and biological knowledge are not worth the candle, we have a problem on several levels. First, the majority of the community does not engage in private, consenting homosexual activity; currently, mercifully this is not proscribed by law in most pluralist, democratic countries. The fact that a majority approves or disapproves of something—rather than participates in the activity, be it animal experiments or homosexuality—similarly does not necessarily make it appropriate for the attentions of the law.

On the other hand, it might be argued that there are fairly generally accepted canons of behaviour involving animals, often on a national basis, and to some extent sanctified by tradition. For example, bear-baiting and cock-fighting are illegal in the UK. It is important, however, to remember that they are proscribed as spectator sports; if two roosters chance their arm unobserved in a rustic barnyard, the law is unconcerned—its focus, very properly, is on the effects on the people involved, as partisans or spectators. In southern France, and Spain, the societal judgement is that bull-fighting does not trivialize the bull, or brutalize the spectators; such judgements may vary between Nîmes and Nottingham, Boston and Barcelona, *pace* football crowds and ice hockey *versus* the bull run at Pamplona. What should be the same, in Europe, America, or wherever, are the criteria on which the judgement is based—those of parsimony and non-trivial use of animals, and of the possibility of dehumanizing effects on the people involved.

To conclude, I should add that I strongly support clinical research as well as animal experiments. Such clinical research needs to be both on normal volunteers, and on patients even if there is no immediate therapeutic benefit. The crucial determinant of whether or not such research is ethical is whether informed consent has been freely and unambiguously given. The extent to which the procedures proposed are painful may well influence whether or not consent is given; they do not, *per se*, determine whether the research is ethical. People run marathons of their own free will, and some women choose to have more than one baby.

Secondly, I make an absolute distinction in ethical terms between people and other animals, a distinction which is much less clear in biological terms. Explicit or implicit, this is probably a crucial distinction for any animal experimenter to make, against nightmares of becoming Herod the Great or Josef Mengele. This distinction is based on intuition, and is supported by arguments which I find convincing; others, perhaps, find them less so. I respect their right not to eat meat, wear leather shoes, or do experiments involving animals. In a democratic, pluralist society, I would hope that the leaders of the animal rights/liberation groups would explicitly undertake to respect the informed judgements of the rest of the community to eat meat or wear leather, and my right to do research involving experiments—both on consenting humans and on other animals.

This essay began on a personal note, and thus perhaps not inappropriately might end on one. Apart from man's vileness towards his fellow man, what I most mourn is the loss of species. Plant and animal, they have taken millions of years to reach their present state, and are then snuffed out. We are blurring the canvas of evolution, for whalebone stays or dubious aphrodisiacs, and it is the only canvas we have. Whether or not this process can be slowed is moot; perhaps the single most effective way would be for the prodigious energies of the animal rights/liberation groups to be refocused, from individual animals to species; ultimately, disappearing DNA is more of a disaster than the Draize test.

3

Relationships between patient, clinician, and scientist in prenatal diagnosis

MALCOLM A. FERGUSON-SMITH and MARIE E. FERGUSON-SMITH

INTRODUCTION

Until recent times, the living fetus inside the mother's womb has been comparatively inaccessible to the diagnostic skills of clinical medicine and most fetal abnormalities were unrecognized before birth. It is true that the position of the fetus could be determined by palpation, its heart rate monitored by a stethoscope, and gross abnormalities detected by X-ray, but these observations were made mostly in late pregnancy with the aim of avoiding complications of delivery.

During the past 20 years much has been learnt about the developing fetus from studying the amniotic fluid surrounding it *in utero*, from the development of real time ultrasound which allows the fetal body, limbs, and organs to be visualized and measured, and from more invasive techniques including fetoscopy and fetal blood sampling. These techniques have brought modern laboratory diagnosis direct to the living fetus and thus the potential to practise medicine *in utero*.

The first fetal disorders to be detected by these methods were naturally those that produced the grossest changes in fetal morphology or the most obvious chromosomal or biochemical defects in cultured amniotic fluid cells. Anencephaly, gross spina bifida, Down's syndrome, and severe metabolic disorders are incurable, and so the only benefit that prenatal diagnosis at 16–20 weeks can offer to the pregnant woman and her husband is the knowledge of the condition of the fetus and the option of termination of pregnancy. The development of prenatal diagnosis has led more recently to the ability to detect an ever-increasing range of lethal and non-lethal fetal disorders much earlier in pregnancy and occasionally even before implantation. For some of the less severe conditions, fetal therapies are now being developed, and diagnosis which leads to improvements in treatment and management of fetal disease is universally welcomed and uncontroversial. For some developmental malformations, prenatal diagnosis forewarns the surgeon and allows arrangements to be made for delivery in a unit with facilities for prompt surgical correction. However, for the majority of fetal abnormalities, intervention is still a matter of deciding about selective termination of pregnancy, or making preparation for the care of a handicapped child. Such decisions on the destruction of fetal life are greatly influenced by ethical and moral opinions. These involve not only the patient but also the medical, scientific, and religious communities and, beyond them, a variety of political and social agencies.

In this chapter we discuss a number of dilemmas about prenatal diagnosis which confront patients and which the scientist and clinician have to face in the service they seek to provide. It looks at ways in which these dilemmas may be resolved and suggests how the various responsibilities relating to prenatal diagnostic services may be apportioned among some of those concerned, namely the scientist, the clinician, and the Minister of Health. But first it would seem appropriate to consider briefly the types of fetal disorder under discussion, the arrangements for advising parents about them, and the procedures used for diagnosis. Sources for more detailed descriptions of the techniques of prenatal diagnosis and of fetal disorders are given in the list of references: Connor and Ferguson-Smith 1987; Ferguson-Smith 1983; Hamerton and Ferguson-Smith 1984; Liu *et al.* 1987.

FETAL ABNORMALITY AND GENETIC COUNSELLING

Genetic disorders and fetal malformations occur in approximately 5 per cent of all livebirths. This consists of 0.5 per cent for unbalanced chromosome aberrations (such as Down's syndrome and trisomies of chromosomes 13 and 18), 1 per cent for single gene defects (such as cystic fibrosis, muscular dystrophy, and Huntington's chorea), and 3.5 per cent malformations. Among the latter, spina bifida and related disorders (2 per 1000), congenital heart disease (6–8 per 1000), limb abnormalities (2 per 1000), and kidney disorders (4 per 1000) are the most prominent. There is no evidence that any of these disorders are becoming more frequent at birth, but, with improved medical and nursing care in the developed and developing countries, an increasing proportion of such infants are surviving to lead lives of variable handicap. In the past most of these infants would have succumbed shortly after birth and would therefore place no continuing burden on families and the community.

During pregnancy and pre-pregnancy counselling it is helpful to ensure that mothers appreciate not only the 5 per cent empiric risk of abnormality or genetic disorder among livebirths, but also that there is a 15 per cent fetal loss by spontaneous miscarriage among all recognized pregnancies. In over half of these miscarriages an unbalanced chromosome abnormality is the cause and in a proportion of the remainder a developmental malformation of the embryo can be identified; in others a dominant lethal mutation may be responsible. The high proportion of miscarriages in which a definitive cause can be found indicates that miscarriage is nature's usual response to serious fetal abnormality and thus the most important factor in limiting serious handicap among livebirths. Parents who appreciate these facts are able to understand that prenatal diagnosis identifies pregnancies affected with severe fetal abnormality which escape spontaneous miscarriage. Selective termination of affected pregnancies often appears more acceptable to parents when considered against this background of natural selection.

Some mothers are at greater risk of fetal abnormality or genetic disease in their offspring than others. For autosomal dominant conditions, such as Huntington's chorea, myotonic dystrophy or neurofibromatosis, the children of an affected parent have each a one in two risk of developing the disease. For autosomal recessive conditions, like cystic fibrosis and thalassaemia, the risk of recurrence in families is one in four. The same risk is found in the offspring of female carriers of X-linked recessive conditions, such as haemophilia and Duchenne muscular dystrophy; however as only sons are normally affected, the risk of disease in sons is one in two, whereas daughters have a one in two risk of being unaffected carriers. Familial chromosome abnormalities may also be associated with comparatively high rates of abnormality in offspring, the risks varying widely and depending on the exact nature of the chromosomal rearrangement.

Most mothers know of the increased risk of these abnormalities only because they have previously given birth to an affected child. Having had the experience of caring for a severely-handicapped child, few mothers will contemplate having further children without the option of prenatal diagnosis and termination should the fetus prove to be similarly affected. Other mothers may learn of their increased risk because a more remote relative is affected or because the fetal abnormality was detected fortuitously during an ultrasound scan. Older mothers often know that the risk of Down's syndrome and other chromosome trisomies increases with their age and will seek advice about the level of risk. Carrier detection programmes in populations where a genetic abnormality is particularly common, for example thalassaemia in Sardinia or Cyprus, have been very important in ensuring that prenatal diagnosis is offered to mothers at high risk. Maternal serum alphafetoprotein screening for neural tube defects and chromosome abnormalities is being used increasingly to identify the high risk pregnancy (see below).

PROCEDURES FOR PRENATAL DIAGNOSIS

Amniocentesis, which is the withdrawal of fluid from the amniotic cavity, has been used for over 20 years for the prenatal diagnosis of fetal chromosome abnormalities, metabolic defects, neural tube defects, and a number of other disorders. It is usually performed when the patient is 16–18 weeks advanced in pregnancy which means that if termination is indicated by an abnormal result this cannot usually be done before 19–20 weeks gestation. At that time an induction of labour is required to achieve an abortion. Some 25 000–30 000 amniocenteses are undertaken each year in Britain, mostly for fetal chromosome analysis in mothers aged 35 years or over, and the technology is well established among obstetricians and cytogeneticists. As the laboratory techniques depend for the most part on culturing the viable amniotic fluid cells which are shed by the fetus and membranes into the amniotic fluid, there is usually a delay of at least three weeks between the time of amniocentesis and the time the result is reported. This delay often occasions considerable anxiety in the mother who would like an earlier and more rapid diagnosis. This has led to the establishment of first trimester chorionic villus sampling (CVS) between the eighth and twelfth week of pregnancy. At that time the trophoblast lining the chorionic villi of the developing placenta is actively dividing and contains many cells in mitosis. The chromosomes of these dividing cells can be examined directly under the microscope without culture, and a chromosomal diagnosis can be available within 24 hours. Confirmation of the direct result can be available after ten days by growing fibroblasts from the chorionic villus mesenchyme. The chorion villus sample can be obtained by a plastic catheter introduced through the uterine cervix, but this method is now being replaced by transabdominal CVS using a rigid needle under ultrasound guidance.

The main hazard of both amniocentesis and CVS is the risk of inducing abortion. Amniocentesis carries a 1 per cent risk and CVS a 2–3 per cent risk in experienced hands. Randomized trials are in progress to determine the risks of these and other complications more precisely.

Among the less commonly used invasive techniques for prenatal diagnosis are fetal blood sampling and fetoscopy. The former involves venepuncture of the umbilical cord or the placental bed under direct ultrasound visualization and is usually not undertaken before 18 weeks gestation. It is used for the diagnosis of a number of rare blood disorders, for rapid fetal chromosome analysis at advanced gestations, for confirming equivocal CVS and amniocentesis results, in pregnancies at risk for the fragile X syndrome of mental retardation, and in pregnancies in which ultrasound scanning has revealed physical features suggestive of a chromosomal syndrome. Fetoscopy (also after 18 weeks gestation) involves direct observation of fetal parts through an endoscope and is sometimes indicated for the diagnosis of dysmorphic syndromes or for obtaining fetal skin or liver biopsies. Even in experienced hands the risk of miscarriage after fetoscopy is in the order of 3–4 per cent.

Ultrasound examination of the fetus is non-invasive and without risk to the fetus or mother; it has been recommended by some as the method of choice for screening for fetal abnormalities in all pregnancies. Some severe fetal abnormalities (such as anencephaly) may be detected by ultrasound as early as 12–14 weeks gestation, but most fetal defects cannot be seen before 16–18 weeks. An adequate ultrasound scan at that time cannot usually be completed in under 20 minutes and few antenatal clinics have sufficient numbers of experienced ultrasonographers to provide this as a routine service. Ultrasound scanning is therefore generally restricted to cases in which there is a substantial risk of a dysmorphic condition, or where the maternal serum AFP result is abnormally high. For some recurrent conditions notably hydrocephaly and microcephaly the abnormality may not become apparent until 24 weeks or later in pregnancy, and serial measurements are important in achieving a diagnosis. As the critical time for diagnosis of fetal abnormality by ultrasound is between 18 and 24 weeks gestation it it important that future legislation allows parents the option of termination in such cases. Any reduction in the legal limit, for example to 18 weeks gestation, would force mothers to carry a seriously handicapped fetus to term or alternatively to seek an illegal abortion.

This brief summary of prenatal diagnostic procedures would be incomplete without mentioning maternal serum screening for neural tube defects and chromosome abnormalities. This is a voluntary screening test which is widely used in Britain and has been effective in reducing the birth incidence of spina bifida and related conditions. A small sample of clotted blood is taken from the patient at approximately 17 weeks gestation and tested for the level of alphafetoprotein (AFP). This is the predominant blood protein in the fetus at this stage and normally only small amounts pass into the maternal circulation. However, in spina bifida and some other disorders, fetal blood from the fetal defect passes into the amniotic fluid and from there reaches the maternal circulation. The elevated serum AFP is detected by the screening test, and this acts as a signal for further diagnostic tests including ultrasonography and amniocentesis. False positive tests commonly occur in twin pregnancies or where the gestation has been underestimated. These difficulties can be resolved easily by ultrasound examination. In regions that offer serum AFP screening the utilization rate among pregnant women is between 70 and 80 per cent. Together with ultrasound scanning, some 75 per cent of all neural tube defect pregnancies (i.e. including those not screened) are detected.

While *elevated* serum AFP results indicate pregnancies at risk of neural tube defects, *low* serum AFP results have been found in pregnancies affected with Down's syndrome and other chromosome abnormalities. Up to 40 per cent of Down's syndrome pregnancies can be detected by taking account of the AFP risk factor and the maternal age risk. More recently, it has been found that Down's syndrome pregnancies are associated also with low levels of unconjugated oestriol and high levels of chorionic gonadotrophin in the maternal serum. It is estimated that a combination of all these predictors might lead to the detection of over 60 per cent of affected pregnancies and this is the subject of considerable current research.

Those involved in the introduction of new procedures for prenatal diagnosis have a major responsibility to ensure that they are as safe and as effective as existing procedures. In fact many regard as unethical the introduction of new procedures without randomized testing. Thus a number of trials are currently in progress on the safety and diagnostic reliability of CVS by following the outcome of pregnancy in patients randomly assigned to CVS and amniocentesis. Other trials compare transcervical and transabdominal CVS. Similar care should be exercised in the case of early amniocentesis which has recently been advocated at 12–14 weeks gestation. However the need for this particular procedure is uncertain in view of the attendent risks to the pregnancy and current success with transabdominal CVS.

DILEMMAS EXPERIENCED BY THE PATIENTS

It is not difficult to appreciate that the mother who has already experienced the birth of a handicapped child is more prepared to consider prenatal diagnosis that one who has just been told by her doctor that she is at risk because of her age, or serum AFP result, or the findings of a recent ultrasound examination. The former knows better than anyone else the degree of disability of her affected child, her ability to look after the child, how much time she has for the rest of the family, and the degree of help she can expect from social services. She will have discussed with her husband and others in the family the possibility of trying for a healthy child and in many cases a decision will have been taken to have no more children. In other families the desire for children and the possibility that the handicapped child may not survive will lead to a decision either to risk a recurrence or to seek prenatal diagnosis and selective termination. It is the experience of most clinical geneticists that a decision to take the risk is extremely rare and that almost all couples who have a seriously handicapped child and want to have another pregnancy will do so only if prenatal diagnosis is available to them. Very occasionally, parents will ask for prenatal diagnosis, not for selective termination, but to allow them to prepare for the birth of a handicapped child. With this exception, the couple's answer to the question 'Are you prepared to take the risk of having a second affected child?' is invariably 'No'. It is a common misapprehension to interpret the negative answer to the question 'Do you wish that you had been offered prenatal diagnosis and termination during the pregnancy of your affected child?' as a desire not to have prenatal diagnosis in subsequent pregnancies. This question can be interpreted by parents as a suggestion that they may not love and care for their affected child, which causes considerable resentment. Those who ask it often have moral objections to selective abortion for fetal abnormality and claim that the answer indicates that mothers are content to have handicapped children. Perhaps there would be a greater chance for this to be true if mothers could rely on society to give them the resources and assistance needed to provide proper care and supervision of their affected children. The truth is that society does not give the amount of assistance needed and continues to expect individual families to shoulder the burden.

The dilemmas facing the mother who has previously had no idea that her child would be anything other than perfectly healthy, and learns for the first time that a test during pregnancy indicated that something may be wrong, are very different. She is totally unprepared for the various options presented to her. Unlike the other mother, she has no experience of the abnormality and does not know what to expect. She resents the suggestion that her baby may be abnormal and may blame her attendants for the abnormality, for not diagnosing it earlier, and for not giving her proper care. She worries in case the diagnosis is mistaken and may seek a second opinion. She is inclined to resent her dependence on the doctors for information and is angry at them for forcing her to make decisions about whether or not to continue the pregnancy.

To some extent these problems can be avoided if care is taken early in pregnancy to mention to all expectant mothers the risk of fetal abnormality and to ensure that the mother understands why ultrasonography is being done, why her blood is being assayed for AFP, and why fetal chromosome analysis is indicated because of her age. She needs to know what is meant by Down's syndrome and spina bifida, and that the tests cannot detect all abnormalities and sometimes fail to work.

Occasionally the mother is presented with the fortuitous finding of an unexpected abnormality. For example, when Down's syndrome is excluded, fetal chromosome analysis may reveal a sex chromosome abnormality such as XXY Klinefelter's syndrome or an XYY male. The disability associated with these disorders is usually comparatively mild and the patient is faced with the dilemma of deciding whether or not the pregnancy should continue. The usual view is that the prognosis of the disorder should be fully explained to the patient and her husband and the option discussed. Decisions are thus greatly influenced by the doctor's conception of the disability and in practice about half of the pregnancies affected with the XXY and XYY sydromes are terminated.

There is evidence that parents' views about the indications for prenatal diagnosis are changing. Thus ten years ago, when cystic fibrosis families were asked if there was a need for prenatal diagnosis, this was widely denied. Now that accurate prenatal diagnosis by DNA analysis is available, large numbers of families are coming forward to be tested. Similarly, for treatable conditions such as phenylketonuria and haemophilia, the demand for prenatal diagnosis seems to be increasing. For phenylketonuria, parents wish to avoid the constant reliance on hospital monitoring, the dietary restriction, and the risk their affected daughters have of producing offspring seriously damaged by the maternal metabolic disturbance. For haemophilia the risk of contracting AIDS from therapy with donor blood products is now becoming a factor in increasing the demand for prenatal diagnosis.

The development of the powerful techniques of DNA diagnosis has brought with it new dilemmas for the patient. For some important disorders such as Huntington's chorea, it is possible to offer to a young parent who has a one in two chance of developing the disease later in life the opportunity of excluding this possibility in future children. If, for example, the father is at risk, prenatal exclusion is achieved when it can be demonstrated that the paternal chromosome transmitted to the fetus is the one that the father received from his *unaffected* parent. If the fetus receives the paternal chromosome transmitted from the father's *affected* parent, the fetus has the same one in two risk as the father. The parents have then to decide whether they wish to terminate the pregnancy on the basis that the risk of developing the disease is identical to the father's risk. Many parents will consider that this is the only way to prevent the transmission of a serious disease to subsequent generations, but all find the decision a difficult one.

The mother known to be at risk of transmitting a serious genetic disorder, for example because she is a carrier of X-linked muscular dystrophy, has a series of dilemmas throughout her life about disclosing this information. Should she inform her partner before marriage? Has she a responsibility to inform other relatives who might also be at risk? What does she say to her children when she attends hospital for prenatal diagnosis and afterwards returns without the baby? If she decides against termination, how should she prepare the family for the handicapped baby? The anxieties created by these dilemmas sometimes influence patients' decisions concerning marriage and childbearing, and during pregnancy about whether or not to have prenatal diagnosis. Only the most complete information about these matters, and the knowledge that the mother is not alone in facing these decisions, can help. The introduction of first trimester CVS has also helped greatly by providing privacy to mothers who contemplate prenatal diagnosis. The test can be done at 8–12 weeks when only the mother and husband need know about the pregnancy. Diagnosis tends to be quicker and termination simpler than during the second trimester. It is therefore important to ensure that facilities are available and that arrangements for antenatal care take account of this need. At present because of the limitation of the NHS system most mothers in Britain have their first antenatal clinic appointment too late for first trimester CVS.

The increasing use of drugs to treat infertility by induction of ovulation, and the development of *in vitro* fertilization, now result in the increasing occurrence of multiple pregnancies with four or more embryos. The chance of survival of any of these fetuses is greatly reduced and approaches nil when the number is more than five. In order to achieve a successful outcome in such pregnancies the practice of 'embryo reduction' has been introduced. This involves the selective destruction of all but two of the embryos by injection at an early stage in the pregnancy. The concept is highly distateful to parents who have to make a difficult decision. Clearly the solution is to avoid such multiple pregnancies in the first place, by more careful control of drug therapy and by limiting the number of pre-embryos implanted after *in vitro* fertilization. Selective destruction of the fetus later in pregnancy (feticide) has been used in twin pregnancies where one of the twins has a fetal abnormality and the other is normal. Parents have less difficulty in accepting the procedure in these circumstances.

DILEMMAS EXPERIENCED BY THE CLINICIAN

Interruption of pregnancy poses the most difficult dilemma for the physician, as it appears to run counter to the medical obligation to treat disease and preserve life. Many doctors find it difficult to allow any exception to this rule, while others would accept termination of pregnancy for fetal abnormality in early pregnancy but not later. Recent discussions on possible amendments to the Abortion Act reveal that there are different views about the acceptable limit for termination.

However, an increasing number of doctors see selective termination for fetal abnormality as an extension of the process of natural selection which so successfully achieves the elimination by spontaneous miscarriage of the majority of the serious disorders of development due to genetic and other causes. They are impressed by the considered decision of many parents who have had the experience of caring for a handicapped child and who feel themselves unable to shoulder the burden and responsibility of further affected children. Such families and their doctors look at the large number of abortions of normal fetuses which are carried out for less pressing social reasons and ask the question 'If it is acceptable for these reasons why should it not be acceptable for the prevention of handicap?' Other doctors believe that it may be more compassionate and humane to allow selective termination than to consign an individual to a life of distress and handicap. Society has responded to these concerns by legislating for abortion under certain conditions, including where there is a substantial risk that the fetus will be born handicapped. As a result many thousands of women have been able to proceed to have healthy children when, without prenatal diagnosis, they would not have felt able to start another pregnancy.

Clinicians and scientists have undoubtedly been strengthened in their resolve to provide improved prenatal diagnosis by the needs of these thousands of families who look to the procedure as the only acceptable approach to having a family. It is accepted that those doctors who have a conscientious objection to prenatal diagnosis and selective termination have a moral duty to refer their patients who request such advice to other doctors who are prepared to help.

Having accepted that there is a case for prenatal diagnosis, the next dilemma which faces the clinician is the question of who should decide whether the fetal disorder is serious enough to warrant diagnosis and termination. Does he take the decision, does he leave it to the parents and should he restrict his role to advising them of the disorder? In cases where there is high risk of severe fetal abnormality or disease there is usually no problem. Even if the clinician has little experience of the disorder, the patient may have no hesitation. It is in cases where the risk of abnormality is comparatively low, such as the risk of trisomic Down's syndrome at a maternal age of 34 years or where the disorder is treatable, such as with haemophilia, that difficulties arise. There is a tendency for the clinician to be more restrictive when prenatal diagnosis is provided by the State. The argument of health service priorities in the light of limited resources, the risk of inducing an abortion by CVS or amniocentesis compared with the risk of fetal abnormality, and the danger of inducing excessive anxiety in the mother, are all cited as components in the decision. If prenatal diagnosis is being provided in the private sector, economic considerations are not so important, and the patient may be granted greater freedom of choice. The fact that prenatal diagnosis for maternal anxiety and for women under 35 years of age seems to be more common in the private sector points to the importance of a financial component in these decisions.

The clinician is in more difficulty when the patient asks for prenatal diagnosis and selective termination on grounds that seem reasonable to the patient but do not involve abnormality of the fetus. In cases of rape by an assailant, the pregnant woman may find it difficult to continue the pregnancy if the assailant and not her partner is the father. She may request prenatal diagnosis and DNA fingerprinting of her fetus and then ask for termination of the pregnancy if it can be shown that the assailant is the father. The indication for abortion is social and not medical, and society is sympathetic to the pregnant woman. It is therefore usual in such cases to follow the wishes of the patient and her family. However, it is much more difficult to accede to a request for fetal paternity testing in order to allow the pregnant woman to choose the most acceptable father from a series of partners. Such cases have been reported and clearly not many clinicians would feel able to condone destruction of a normal fetus on these grounds.

Similar concerns arise about requests for selective abortion in order to allow parents to choose the sex of their offspring. Gender choice appears to be relatively infrequent in Western cultures but is currently the most frequent indication for prenatal diagnosis in Asian countries. In India it is understood that, although not permitted by law, the current charge for this service is 3000 rupees (£120). In China the practice is also prohibited by law, although the pressures to choose the gender of the child in a single child family must be considerable. Various subterfuges may be used to evade legal strictures, the most common practice being for the family to claim that state-subsidized contraception has failed; the expectant mother will not then insist on a termination if it can be shown that the fetus is male.

A small number of cases are known in Britain where prenatal diagnosis was requested on grounds of maternal age or maternal anxiety and the pregnancy terminated in a different hospital for social reasons when the fetal sex was not that desired by the parents. These occurrences have led some scientists routinely to withhold the fetal sex in their reports of fetal chromosome analysis and simply state that 'the fetus has an apparently normal karyotype'. These concerns stem from the ethics of equality between men and women, in a world where this is still not universally accepted.

A recent questionnaire sent to medical geneticists in 18 nations has revealed some surprising information about gender selection (Fletcher *et al.; Wertz et al.*, 1989). Of all those who answered 42 per cent said they would perform prenatal diagnosis for sex choice alone (or would refer the mother elsewhere for this), but there were major differences between countries. The percentages in favour were 47 per cent for Canada, 60 per cent for Hungary, 52 per cent for India, and 62 per cent for the United States. A number of countries showed a different consensus namely 4 per cent for the Federal Republic of Germany, 6 per cent for Japan, 17 per cent for Australia and Norway, 18 per cent for Italy, 13 per cent for France, and 24 per cent for the United Kingdom. It is not possible to do more than speculate on the factors responsible for these major differences. The autonomy of the individual in making such decisions might be a major factor in the United States, while economic, cultural, and religious factors all contribute to a varying degree in other countries.

In the light of such experience it appears that clinicians see the aims of prenatal diagnosis in a number of different ways. A majority would agree that the aim is to help mothers avoid the birth of severely handicapped children. Others would see the aim in a wider perspective, namely to reduce the burden of handicap in the community. And clearly some would see prenatal diagnosis as giving parents control over the quality of life and sex of their children. Clinicians currently have a role in drawing the line between what is regarded as acceptable practice and what is unacceptable, and their major partners in making such decisions must be the mothers and fathers of handicapped children, for they have the necessary experience to give informed advice to the rest of society.

DILEMMAS EXPERIENCED BY THE SCIENTIST

It is doubtful if any branch of laboratory medicine is associated with more responsibility than the prenatal diagnosis laboratory. The scientist knows that the life of a fetus may depend on the result of every test she or he undertakes. This burden of responsibility can create considerable strains within the laboratory and this has led to the development of a particular relationship between scientist and clinician in the medical genetics department, so that both share responsibility for providing the correct advice to the pregnant patient. The obstetrical team, including the obstetrician and his junior staff, the ultrasonographer, the antenatal clinic sister, and the clinic receptionist, is in the line of communication between the patient and the scientist. The scientist frequently has anxieties about the safe transfer of information from the laboratory to the patient through these 'middlemen', each of whom may require advice on the interpretation and significance of the laboratory findings. Failure of correct interpretation may mean the abortion of a healthy fetus or the continuation of an affected pregnancy, in just the same way as would a laboratory error.

The particular responsibilities of the scientist are to ensure meticulous and accurate handling of samples and patient information so that each patient receives the correct report. Tests must be run with adequate internal and external quality assurance; in the case of fetal chromosome analysis this means that every result is checked by two people. The results of prenatal diagnostic tests must be checked for reliability against the outcome of pregnancy. If this is a normal birth, it may be necessary to test a cord blood sample from the newborn infant. All terminations must be tested to confirm the prenatal result, in order to monitor the reliability of the laboratory. The maintenance of the highest possible standards not only reassures those who make use of the service, but also reassures the scientist that he is discharging his responsibilities correctly.

A common dilemma which faces the scientist is that posed by an inadequate sample which gives an inconclusive result. Many of the errors made in the early days of prenatal diagnosis were the result of drawing false conclusions from an inadequate sample. Naturally, there is resistance from the clinical team to repeating the amniocentesis and subjecting the patient to unnecessary risk. Consequently, there is pressure on the scientist to give an opinion when this is scarcely possible. With experience, an inadequate sample is readily recognized and such problems seldom if ever occur. The same might be said for delay in diagnosis, due to poor growth of cells in culture. With the advent of CVS and fetal blood sampling as alternatives to amniocentesis, failures due to delay in amniotic fluid cell cultures seldom lead to failure to give a result. The hazard of growing maternal instead of fetal cells, always a rare problem, is now becoming of less importance with experience. Chromosomal variation allows fetal cells to be distinguished from maternal cells and so comparison with a maternal blood sample can usually provide the answer. The scientist strives to achieve the best service for the patient by the establishment of high standards in the laboratory and the development of improved techniques. Advances in technology in recent years have led to first trimester diagnosis, to a reduction in reporting time after amniocentesis, and to the diagnosis of an increasing number of genetic disorders by DNA analysis of chorion villus samples.

None of these developments have helped the scientist with one major dilemma in the interpretation of results. This stems from the occurrence of chromosomal mosaicism for abnormal and normal cells arising in extraembryonic fetal tissues. Mosaicism can be observed in both amniotic fluid cell cultures and chorion villus samples but is much more frequent in the latter. It is the major cause of false negative and false positive results in prenatal diagnosis by CVS, estimated to occur in 1 in

5500 and 1 in 1800 prenatal diagnoses respectively in a recent analysis of 11 000 cases (Mikkelsen 1988). Chromosomal mosaicism involves numerical chromosome aberrations much more frequently than structural chromosome aberrations. It appears that these arise as somatic mutations in the early pre-embryo so that a proportion of the embryonic cells may have an extra chromosome, while the remainder have a normal complement. The abnormal cells may be confined by chance to a proportion of the extraembryonic tissue, or to a proportion of the embryo itself, or be present in both. In the first case a chromosomal analysis of a CVS or amniotic fluid leads to the diagnosis of chromosomal mosaicism although only normal cells will be found in the fetus at termination or in the child at delivery. In the second case, mosaicism will *not* be apparent on prenatal diagnosis, and the child may be found to be a mosaic on delivery. In the third instance, mosaicism will be identified both by prenatal diagnosis and afterwards in tissue from the fetus or child.

What is the significance of such mosaicism? Certain guidelines are now becoming apparent.

1. If the trisomic cell line represents a chromosomal abnormality which is *not* known to affect live-born children it is likely to be confined to the fetal membranes (e.g. trisomy 20 mosaicism).
2. If the trisomic cell line is known in livebirths (e.g. mosaic trisomy 21) it *may* be associated with fetal abnormality. However the chance of disability is much less than in livebirths. This is because ascertainment bias results in livebirths with abnormality being detected more readily than livebirths without abnormality. Thus 90 per cent of prenatal diagnosis of 45, X/46, XY mosaicism continue to the delivery of normal boys without abnormality. This form of mosaicism is recognized only *after* birth if it is associated with infertility or ambiguity of the external genitalia. The current practice is to allow pregnancies with 45,X/46,XY mosaicism to continue, whereas pregnancies with trisomy 21 mosaicism are usually terminated.
3. Some types of trisomy are viable only when present in mosaic form, e.g. trisomy 8 and trisomy 9. Thus the prenatal diagnosis of mosaicism must be confirmed either by amniocentesis or fetal blood sampling, to reduce the chance that the somatic cells of the fetus are affected.

In the past the finding of mosaicism has led to uncertainty about the correct form of management. When this indecision has been transmitted to the parents, the majority have responded by requesting termination of pregnancy. This is unfortunate for it has undoubtedly led to the abortion of many normal fetuses. This can often be avoided by close consultation between the scientist and clinician whenever mosaicism is found.

The scientist also shares with the clinician the responsibility of maintaining confidentiality. This is not difficult with prenatal diagnosis records, except in cases where extended family studies are required to make a diagnosis by DNA analysis using genetic linkage. For example, in the process of excluding a fetus as carrying the gene for Huntington's chorea, the scientist may acquire the information that one of the parents is a definite carrier. This information may be unwelcome to the carrier parent and can, of course, only be divulged to other family members with the consent of the individual involved. Apart from the knowledge that he carries the gene for an unpleasant and fatal illness, the carrier parent may be disadvantaged in many other ways by having this information. He may be obliged to divulge details about his condition by the terms of contract with his employer, insurance company, mortgage society, and driving authority and as a result may fail to get employment, be refused insurance, or banned from driving. Clearly the question of passing information to relatives poses many dilemmas to the scientist and clinician and may inhibit the patient from carrier detection tests and from requesting prenatal diagnosis in future pregnancies.

DILEMMAS EXPERIENCED BY SOCIETY

It will be apparent to anyone who has followed this account of the dilemmas facing those involved in decisions about prenatal diagnosis that the questions raised are not simple ones, readily dealt with by legislators and by the judiciary. Who therefore is to advise society and how are we to proceed? We believe that the concern expressed by society as reported in the media, by debates in Parliament and on television, may be in part due to doctors and scientists failing to take sufficient responsibility for informing the public about the techniques available and the options open to those at risk of having handicapped children. The reticence of the medical profession to discuss such matters in public is understandable in view of the medical ethic that doctors preserve rather than destroy life; any other attitude might mean losing the confidence of their patients. In addition, the public remain ignorant because they do not hear the views of parents of and carers for handicapped children, nor do they hear dispassionate argument in which the handicapped are recognized as worthwhile. Only those with extremist views seem to be heard. In the hope of being constructive we suggest that there are certain responsibilities to be taken by those providing prenatal diagnostic services.

Responsibilities of the scientist

In addition to the responsibility for maintaining a high standard of laboratory service (including the development of fast and more reliable diagnostic testing) the scientist has a responsibility for providing the public with an up-to-date account of current technology. This could be in the form of a summary document regularly up-dated by the profession, and made widely available. Such a document would include information on the safety, reliability, and benefits of the various procedures, together with a proper evaluation of new procedures based on appropriate clinical trials.

Responsibilities of the clinician

The clinician, whether family doctor, medical geneticist, or obstetrician, has a responsibility to ensure that individual patients are informed about the availability of prenatal diagnosis and screening tests in good time. The best time is clearly before a pregnancy is planned, but it is important that the matter is raised again at the time a pregnancy is confirmed. For many conditions, the specialist advice of neurologists, ophthalmologists, dermatologists, and other experts must be sought. Where the genetic aspects are complex, the medical geneticist will be involved in counselling the family about the genetic risks. Mobilization of the necessary expertise is very much a matter of team work and in Britain this is the responsibility of the Regional Genetics Services.

Responsibilities of the Minister of Health

We look to the Minister of Health as the person in our adminstration charged, among his other duties, with the responsibility to make provision for the prevention of handicap and the care of the handicapped in the community. We suggest that if he is to understand the needs of the public in these matters, he should first seek the advice of the parents of the handicapped and then ask his medical advisers about the scale of the need for prenatal diagnostic services and how these services should best be supplied. From the parents of the handicapped he will hear harrowing accounts of how they first learnt of the disorder in their child and how hard it was for them to obtain the specialist advice that they needed. Often he will be told about the resentment parents feel at learning too late that the birth of a seriously disabled child could have been avoided; of the long period of anxiety mothers have to suffer before they receive the result of the prenatal diagnostic test in the second trimester of pregnancy, when a simpler test in the first trimester could have yielded a prompt result. He will discover that only a minority of mothers at risk of bearing handicapped children receive any genetic advice before starting a family.

The consequence of this widespread ignorance is that many severely disabled children are born to families who, if given the opportunity and advice, would have elected to avoid such a occurrence. If the Minister is concerned about the financial costs of helping such families, he should consult the evidence in the literature on the costs and benefits of prevention of genetic disease. He will find that the lifetime cost of caring for two or three of the severely disabled is more than the lifetime salary of a clinician who advises hundreds of families at risk each year.

To give some idea of the deficiencies of the service to families with genetically-determined disease, it should be appreciated that in Britain there is in post less that one Consultant Medical Geneticist per million population. In each Regional Health Authority this means that there are on average between one and two medical geneticists; one region has none. It is no wonder that only a small proportion of the community at need ever receive adequate advice. Despite their small number, medical geneticists and their scientist colleagues have built up a regional network of services throughout the country which, given the necessary manpower, could form the foundation of a most effective service for the counselling of families, the prevention of genetic disease and the reduction of handicap. With the introduction of DNA techniques for prenatal diagnosis and carrier detection the opportunities for progress in this area of preventive medicine have never been greater. The time seems ripe for more informed debate on the issues involved so that decisions can be taken about providing the service so many families need but fail to receive.

REFERENCES

Connor, J. M. and Ferguson-Smith, M. A. (1987). *Essential medical genetics*, second edition. Blackwell Scientific Publications, Oxford.

Ferguson-Smith, M. A. (1983). Early Prenatal Diagnosis. *British Medical Bulletin*, **39**, No. 4, 301–408.

Fletcher, J. C., Wertz, D. C., Sorensen, J. R., and Berg, K. (1987). Ethics and human genetics: a cross cultural study in 17 nations. *Proceedings of the 7th International Congress of Human Genetics*, (ed. F. Vogel and K. Sperling). Springer-Verlag, Berlin. pp. 657–72.

Hamerton, J. L. and Ferguson-Smith, M. A. (1984). Collaborative studies in prenatal diagnosis of chromosome aberrations. *Prenatal Diagnosis*, **4**, 11–162 (Special issue).

Liu, D. T. Y., Symonds, F. M., and Golbus, M. S. (1987). *Chorion villus sampling*. Chapman & Hall, London.

Mikkelsen, M. (1989). Proceedings of the 4th International Conference on Chorion Villus Sampling and Early Prenatal Diagnosis (in preparation).

Wertz, D. C. and Fletcher, J. C. (1989). Ethical problems in prenatal diagnosis: a cross-cultural survey of medical geneticists in 18 nations. *Prenatal Diagnosis* **8, 9**, 145–58.

4

Research on early human embryos *in vitro*

PETER BRAUDE

The birth of the first 'test-tube baby' in 1978 drew many people's attention for the first time to the ramifications of this revolutionary treatment for infertility (Edwards and Steptoe 1980). Not surprisingly, the ability to fertilize eggs *in vitro*, and thus generate 'human life' in the laboratory at will, frightened many people. Visions of men in white coats creating Frankenstein-like monsters, and of Huxley's *Brave new world*, seemed to be realized. It is probably fears of this sort more than specific ethical concern that has made research on human embryos such a controversial and highly emotive issue for some members of the public. As a scientist and a clinician I shall try to lay out simply the nature and purpose of the proposed research and some of the ethical dilemmas raised by it. I hope that a basic understanding of the biology of the early embryo and an appreciation of the intentions of the medical scientist will help to allay some of these fears.

What is meant by research

The definition and limits of research with reference to experiments on human embryos were addressed by the Committee of Inquiry into Human Fertilisation and Embryology and published in its Report (DHSS, 1984; Warnock 1985). The Inquiry attempted to define two types of research: pure research 'aimed at increasing knowledge of the very early stages of the human embryo', and applied research, which was defined as 'research with direct diagnostic or therapeutic aims for the human embryo; or for the alleviation of infertility in general'. Although we may arbitrarily divide research on embryos into 'pure' and 'applied', there is little to choose between them in respect of their value to society, for they have the same ultimate goal; it is merely the routes by which that goal is achieved that differ. Whereas 'applied' research is embarked upon with the aim of finding a practical solution to a particular problem (technological advancement), 'pure' research sets out to answer more fundamental questions about events and mechanisms in the system under study without necessarily looking at immediate practical applications. This is not to say that 'pure research' is not directed; this type of investigation provides the framework upon which technological advance can be made.

In a peculiar lapse of logic, the Warnock Committee excluded from the concept of research 'new and untried treatment, undertaken during the attempt to alleviate the infertility of a particular patient'. If we regard research as 'the endeavour to discover new facts by scientific study' (which includes the gathering of information by controlled observation as well as by designed experiment), then clinical research surely must be included. For new techniques and treatments are constantly introduced in medicine which means that many patients (with or without their informed consent) will be part of this ongoing research process (Vere 1988). However, there is a formal path which is normally followed before any new technique is introduced into therapeutic practice. It is generally expected that tests of safety and efficacy have been performed on 'non-persons' (animals or cells *in vitro*) before application to patients in controlled clinical trials. Progress in the application of infertility treatment and in the development of techniques for prenatal diagnosis should be no different. However, since direct extrapolation of results from animal embryos *in vitro* to the human can be misleading, and since human embryos can now be cultured *in vitro*, the question that must be asked is whether it is ethical to use human embryos *in vitro* in making this transition from animal experiments to clinical application.

IS THERE A NEED FOR RESEARCH USING HUMAN EMBRYOS?

Male infertility

Subfertility owing to male factors probably accounts for about 40 per cent of all infertility. In a few cases the cause will be a coital one such as impotence or retrograde ejaculation. This type of infertility may be treatable by some form of artificial insemination with husband's (AIH) or donor's (AID) sperm. However, the vast preponderance of male infertility is caused by a problem with spermatogenesis which manifests as a detectable defect in semen quality. A reduction in the number of spermatozoa in an ejaculate is accompanied invariably by a defect in the motility and in the morphology of the spermatozoa. Although we know that low sperm numbers are associated strongly with subfertility, many men with quite severely depleted numbers of spermatozoa will father children if their partner is fertile. It is thus of practical importance to be able to tell which men with defective spermatogenesis retain fertility.

However, we have little knowledge about the functional relationship between the usual parameters measured in a routine semen analysis (count, motility, and morphology), and fertilizing capacity. Thus the 'pure' science question to be posed in this context is 'What is a fertile spermatozoon?'. At present the best laboratory assessment of sperm function utilizes hamster oocytes which, when specially prepared by removing the outer coating of the egg (the *zona pellucida*), will allow penetration by fertile human spermatozoa (Yanagimachi *et al.* 1976). However, it is becoming increasingly clear that fertilization of human eggs can be achieved with spermatozoa that fail to penetrate hamster oocytes. It would thus be of great importance to try to devise some more objective parameters of fertilizing capacity (Braude *et al.* 1986). For example, the patterns of motility, enzyme activities, and levels of free radicals of the spermatozoa have been suggested, but not yet proved, as valid parameters for the examination of sperm function. Proof (or otherwise) requires a direct and reliable bioassay for sperm function which must be the ability to initiate development of a human oocyte. Human oocytes are therefore still required to validate less direct assays of sperm function and the end point of the tests will often be the creation of a human embryo *in vitro*.

In contrast to this 'pure' research approach which endeavours to provide information about the nature of sperm defects, the technological or 'applied' research question is: 'Can we overcome a lack of sperm numbers or the inability to penetrate the egg's coverings by removing those coverings or by injecting single spermatozoa directly into the egg?' Animal models are now being used to develop these techniques but the application to clinical problems requires the use of human material. Here there is a choice. Either spare or donated eggs, which are not destined to be replaced into the uterus should fertilization be successful, can be used, or alternatively the experiments can be performed on eggs from couples hoping to become pregnant should the fertilization technique succeed. In the latter case, it is clear that the experimental subject ceases to be the egg or the embryo, but becomes the person into whom the cleaving embryo is to be replaced. It would therefore seem reasonable that the former option is chosen in the early stages of research, so that doctors can be cautiously confident of the normality of the injected zygote before therapeutic replacement is attempted. Thus the Warnock Committee suggested that 'no embryo that has been used for research should be replaced in the uterus of a woman'. However this common sense conclusion is not shared by the opponents of embryo experiments. In Australia, the Senate Committee on Human Embryo Experimentation has forbidden any research on embryos where there is not the intention to replace the embryos into the uterus (Australian

Senate Select Committee 1986). It seems extraordinary that the Australian Senate Committee would expect human adults together with the replaced treated embryos to be the subject of clinical experiment before any potential hazards have been first eliminated by laboratory research restricted to small groups of embryonic cells.

Improvement of IVF techniques

It is now clear that the chance of establishing a pregnancy by the transfer of one human embryo to the patient's uterus after IVF is about 10 per cent (Osborn and Moor 1985). The scientific question to be answered is: 'Why do so many embryos fail in culture or fail to implant after transfer?' The technological question to be answered is: 'Can we improve the success rate by increasing the number of embryos replaced, or by changing the stage of replacement?' It is clear that the common object of these questions is to endeavour to improve the success of the treatment of infertility. In the first approach, early embryos not required for transfer to the uterus can be used in controlled *in vitro* culture experiments, whereas the second approach requires that again the patient becomes the subject of the experiment until satisfactory answers are achieved by trial and error.

Prenatal diagnosis

Perhaps the most exciting and new area of embryo research is in the field of prenatal diagnosis. The newer techniques of molecular biology such as *in situ* hybridization and enzyme micro-assays could be applied to preimplantation human embryos in attempts to diagnose inherited genetic diseases in those groups of individuals who are at substantial risk of transmitting the defect (McLaren 1987). Fertilization *in vitro* and replacement of unaffected embryos is a preferable alternative to multiple therapeutic abortions after diagnosis by amniocentesis or chorionic villus biopsy. However, preimplantation diagnosis will only be a realistic alternative if (a) sufficient material can be obtained by biopsy from the developing conceptus for the test to be performed without jeopardizing the survival of the rest of the conceptus, and (b) the rest of the conceptus can be stored successfully at low temperatures until the results of the test are available, or preferably, the test can be performed rapidly and an answer obtained prior to the normal time for embryo replacement. Although animal oocytes and embryos will be needed to develop these techniques, eventually human embryos will have to be used and the techniques evaluated *in vitro* before the first therapeutic attempts are made. Already, the feasibility of the concept of preimplantation diagnosis has been shown using a mouse model in the case of the Lesch–Nyhan syndrome. This syndrome is characterized by a deficiency of the enzyme hypoxanthine phosporibosyl transferase (HPRT); children born with this affliction are severely mentally retarded and exhibit self-mutilation. Marylin Monk and her colleagues have been able to remove a single blastomere from an 8-cell mouse embryo or a small fragment from a blastocyst and type the biopsy for the presence or absence of the enzyme (Monk *et al.* 1987; 1988). The remaining portions of the biopsied embryos were transferred to the uteri of foster mothers and examination of the newborn mice confirmed the accuracy and feasibility of the technique.

SOURCES OF EMBRYOS FOR RESEARCH

Embryos for research derive from two sources. Either they are 'spare' to therapeutic procedures or they are deliberately generated from donated oocytes from women undergoing diagnostic laparoscopies or laparoscopic sterilizations (Braude *et al.* 1984; Braude 1987). Is there a moral difference between the use of 'spare' embryos for research and the use of those created specially for that purpose? This distinction was made in the Warnock report where four members of the committee objected specifically to research being 'permitted on embryos brought into existence for that purpose, or coming into existence as a result of other research'. However the majority view was that there was no difference, concluding that the moral right or wrong rested solely on whether the early human conceptus should be the subject of experiment at all. If one believes that it is morally acceptable to perform research on the human conceptus then this is true irrespective of the origin of that conceptus.

There is however a major *practical* dilemma to be faced by the use of 'spare' embryos for research. Spare embryos themselves can come from two sources. In order to minimize the chance of large multiple pregnancies it has been recommended that only three embryos are replaced into the uterus after IVF, and similarly only three eggs should be placed down the fallopian tubes at a GIFT (Gamete Intra-Fallopian Transfer) procedure (VLA report 1987). Thus there may be 'spare' embryos from IVF, or 'spare' eggs from GIFT which may be fertilized *in vitro* and result in 'spare' embryos. Is it ethical to use these 'spare' embryos for research purposes, or should they be frozen and stored for the patient's own future use? While the latter might seem to be the more ethical alternative, it amounts in effect to a 'research' procedure itself, for the processes of freezing and thawing human embryos and eggs are still in their infancy, and each embryo that is subjected to the cryopreservation process is still part of an ongoing experiment (Trounson 1986). New cryoprotectants, rates of cooling, rates of thawing, stages of replacement, are all being tried in the hope that one of the methods might improve the present poor rate of pregnancy after transfer of thawed embryos. Unfortunately it is all too easy for an IVF centre to offer 'freezing facilities' without the necessary expertise or experience to offer a viable thawed product. Can we be certain that this type of research, for that is what it is, is any more ethical or fruitful than the use of the embryos in experiments specifically designed to improve the chances of successful pregnancy by developing better culture conditions or by improving the present, rather crude criteria used for selecting which eggs or embryos should be replaced in a GIFT or IVF procedure? Thus, the decision to be made is not *whether* spare embryos should be the subject of experiment but *which experiment* should be undertaken.

LEGAL PROTECTION OF THE CONCEPTUS

There is a body strongly of the opinion that the human embryo should be protected by law from the time of fertilization, since from this moment onwards a new human life, a genetically unique person, comes into existence. Has this view any scientific foundation, and is it consistent with current legal and social practice?

Although penetration of the egg membrane by the spermatozoon can be defined precisely, the genetic contributions from the spermatozoon and the egg do not fuse until some 27 hours later. Prior to this time the paternal and maternal contributions are still entirely separate, such that it is still possible experimentally to remove one or another of these pronuclei (Surani *et al.* 1984). Thus the genetic make-up of the embryo is not established until after the pronuclear fusion occurs, the developmental stage that has been adopted by the state of Victoria in Australia as the time from which the human conceptus is deserving of protection in law.

Does fusion of the pronuclei establish an 'embryo'? By about five days of development the cells derived from cleavage of the fertilized egg usually differentiate into two major kinds of tissue, those destined to contribute exclusively to the embryo and those that will form only extra-embryonic tissues (which include placenta and membranes) (McLaren 1986). However, in some conceptuses the embryonic component does not form and only the extraembryonic portion survives as a trophectodermal vesicle. This manifests in humans as the well recognized syndrome of 'missed abortion' where the patient experiences all the symptoms of a pregnancy due to the production of the hCG hormone from the trophoblast but the embryonic sac contains no embryo. Thus despite being a product of fertilization and pronuclear fusion, there is no potential for a fetus to form.

There is yet a third possible outcome of fertilization which does not result in a 'new life'. For reasons as yet unknown, the male genetic material may duplicate and develop preferentially at the expense of the female genetic material. If animal models are correct, then cleavage apparently occurs normally and a blastocyst forms, but the further developments of embryonic precursor cells are severely deficient (Surani *et al.* 1984). However, the extraembryonic contribution proliferates in an exaggerated manner and eventually results in a tumour of placental tissue, the hydatidiform mole. In about 10 per cent of cases the hydatidiform mole will become malignant and without modern chemotherapy would result in the rapid demise of the woman. Here we have unequivocal fertilization but the outcome is not a fetus but a cancer. Thus 'a new life' is neither the inevitable nor the only outcome of the fertilization process.

Does genetic uniqueness provide grounds for protection of the human embryo as a person? Both placenta and embryo are derived from differentiation of the cells within the blastocyst and thus have an identical genetic make-up. Moreover, should the embryonic component of the blastocyst split in two during early development, genetically identical twins may result. Once the twins are born they are both regarded as deserving of respect despite their not being unique. Furthermore although the placental tissue shares with the twins their human genetic 'uniqueness', discarding it causes no moral dilemma. Thus genetic uniqueness does not confer personhood and is irrelevant in deciding on protection of the conceptus in law.

If we do decide to protect the embryo *in vitro* by law, will this have any repercussions on current social and medical practice? At present, the embryo *in vitro* has no legal rights but does enjoy protection under the Infant Life Preservation Act (1929) if it is capable of being born alive. It is also protected even before this stage by the Offences Against the Person Act (1861). These limitations apply only to the implanted embryo. But what of the fertilized egg or the non-implanted human blastocyst *in vivo*? Many accepted forms of contraception are effective because they prevent implantation of the conceptus by mechanical means (the intra-uterine contraceptive device) or chemical means (oestrogens for post-coital contraception) which result in the destruction of the early embryo. Although the Roman Catholic church is consistent in its teaching on the need to protect 'potential new life' by prohibiting all forms of contraception, there are people who avail themselves of the above forms of family planning but will not countenance embryo research or even the practice of IVF in case some fertilized eggs might have to be destroyed *in vitro*. To be consistent, protection of the egg from the moment of fertilization in order to protect the embryo *in vitro* would also necessitate a ban on all the above forms of contraception.

PROTECTION OF THE PUBLIC INTEREST

Decisions about allowing research on human embryos are difficult. For some the dilemma centres on how to reconcile religious teaching with scientific observation, as it has faced society on many occasions (e.g. evolution, movement of the planets, contraception). For others it is the fear of the slippery slope; that once research on human embryos is allowed then experiments on neonates and children will follow. This fear is not supported by the many examples of arbitrary yet clearly drawn rules to which the medical and scientific professions adhere (e.g. the time of legal abortion).

Nevertheless the public has a right to demand some form of assurance that their worst fears will not be realized. The suggestion by the Warnock Committee that embryos *in vitro* should receive some form of protection in law, but that experiments on early embryos should be allowd up to 14 days only under license of a Statutory Licensing Authority, is one solution which has been favoured by legislators, scientists, doctors, and much of the general public (DHSS 1987). However, drafting of clear legislation is not easy and will raise many new dilemmas. Should the law apply only to the whole embryo or should it also apply to parts of an embryo? Embryonic biopsy (i.e. removing one or more cells from the early cleaving embryo) for the purposes of diagnosis of genetic disease is acceptable to many for whom embryo experiments are repugnant. Since it is possible to produce identical lambs by splitting an early cleaving four-cell sheep embryo into its four constituent totipotential cells (Fehilly and Willasden 1986), it becomes necessary to clarify whether a cell removed for the purpose of diagnosis is a biopsy or whether it should be regarded as another embryo. Under the suggested legislation may a sheet of cells (a cell line), derived from a single cell biopsy from an embryo, be cultured *in vitro* for longer than the 14 day limit? Furthermore, since in the mouse it is possible to activate *in vitro* cleavage of an egg in the absence of spermatozoon by simple changes to the chemical constituents of the growth media, it may be possible to achieve this with a human egg. Should such an *in vitro* derived parthenogenetic 'embryo' be governed by the same rules as a normally cleaving embryo derived from fertilization?

The instinctive reaction of many is to avoid addressing these difficult questions and simply request a blanket ban on all forms of embryo research. It would be irrational and unwise to stop all embryo research on such grounds, for the development of many practical and safe gains for a large minority within our society would be precluded. We must hope that informed dialogue between doctors, medical scientists, philosophers, theologians, and lawyers will enable politicians to enact legislation that will protect the public interest while allowing regulated scientific advancement within the moral framework of contemporary society.

REFERENCES

Australian Senate Select Committee on The Human Embryo Experimentation Bill 1985 (1986). *Human Embryo Experimentation in Australia.* Australian Govt. Publishing Service, Canberra.

Braude, P. R., Bolton, V. N., and Johnson, M. H. (1986). The use of human pre-embryos for infertility research. In *Human embryo research: yes or no?* (ed. G. Bock and M. O'Connor), pp. 63–82. The Ciba Foundation, Tavistock Publications, London.

Braude, P. R., Bright, M. V., Douglas, C. P., Milton, P. J., Robinson, R. E., Williamson, J. G., and Hutchinson, J. (1984). A regimen for obtaining mature human oocytes from donors for research into human fertilization in vitro. *Fertility and Sterility*, **42**, 34–8.

Braude, P. R. (1987). Fertilization of human oocytes and culture of human pre-implantation embryos in vitro. In *Mammalian development—a practical approach*, (ed. M. Monk), pp. 281–306, IRL Press, Oxford.

Department of Health and Social Security (1984). *Report of the Committee of Enquiry into Human Fertilization and Embryology.* Cmnd 9314. HMS0, London.

Department of Health and Social Security (1987). *White paper on human fertilization and embryology: A framework for legislation.* [Leaflet, obtainable from: Her Majesty's Stationery Office.]

Edwards, R. G. and Steptoe, P. C. (1980). *A matter of life.* Hutchinson, London.

Fehilly, C. B. and Willasden, S. M. (1986). Embryo manipulation in farm animals. In *Oxford reviews of reproductive biology*, vol 8, (ed. J. Clarke), pp. 379–413. Clarendon Press, Oxford.

McLaren, A. (1986). Prelude to embryogenesis. In *Human Embryo Research: Yes or No?*, (ed. G. Bock and M. O'Connor), pp. 5–23. The Ciba Foundation, Tavistock Publications, London.

McLaren, A. (1987). Can we diagnose genetic disease in pre-embryos? *New Scientist*, 10th December, 1987, 42–7.

Monk, M. Handyside, A., Hardy, K., and Whittingham, D. (1987). Preimplantation diagnosis of deficiency of HPRT in a mouse model for Lesch–Nyhan syndrome. *Lancet*, ii, 423–6.

Monk, M., Muggleton-Harris, A., Rawlings, E. L., and Whittingham, D. (1988). Pre-implantation diagnosis of HPRT deficient male and carrier female mouse embryos by trophectoderm biopsy. *Human Reproduction* 3, 377–81.

Osborn, J. C. and Moor, R. M. (1985). Oocyte maturation and developmental competence. In *In vitro fertilization and donor insemination*, (ed. W. Thompson, D. N. Joyce, and J. R. Newton), pp. 101–21, RCOG, London.

Surani, M. A. H., Barton, S. C., and Norris, M. L. (1984). Development of reconstituted mouse eggs suggests imprinting of the genome during gameteogenesis. *Nature*, **308**, 548–50.

Trounson, A. (1986) Preservation of human eggs and embryos. *Fertility and Sterility*, **46**, 1–12.

Vere, D. W. (1988). The ethics of adverse drug reactions. *Adverse Drug Reaction Bulletin*, **128**, 480–3.

Voluntary Licensing Authority (1987). *The second report of the Voluntary Licensing Authority for human* in vitro *fertilisation and embryology* 1987. [Leaflet, obtainable from: The VLA Secretariat, The Medical Research Council, 20 Park Crescent, London W1N 4AL.]

Warnock, M. (1985). *A question of life*. Blackwell, Oxford.

Yanagimachi, R., Yanagimachi, H., and Rogers, B. J. (1976). The use of zona-free animal ova as a test system for the assessment of the fertilizing capacity of human spermatozoa. *Biology of Reproduction*, **15**, 471–6.

5

Caesarean section: whose choice and for whom?

JEREMY WILDE

The intrapartum care of women has had to adjust to their individual needs; however the way that this care is given has also been moulded by the opinions of society. From the earliest times it was assumed that the principal objective of a pregnant woman was to provide a child who would be the son and heir to his father. The emphasis was very much male dominated and the role of the mother was subservient to the wishes of the father.

An early example of this attitude is that shown during the delivery of Jane Seymour (Dewhurst 1980). After what sounds like a lengthy and difficult labour, the physician went to King Henry VIII and asked him whether his wife or his son should be saved. We presume from this that the Prince was presenting by the breech. The response from the King was that the Prince should be saved. The obstetricians then set to work in some surgical fashion and the Prince was duly delivered. The actual surgical procedure is not described but could have been either the first recorded Caesarean section on a live mother in Renaissance England, or may have been a symphysiotomy where the ligament joining the mother's pelvic bones was divided. In that Jane Seymour is recorded to have attended the christening of the Prince a few days later it is more likely that the latter procedure was employed. The Queen sadly died of sepsis a short time afterwards.

The life of the Queen was effectively seen to be subordinate to that of her son and the father's wishes were paramount. We have no record of the Queen's opinion and indeed she may have felt that she was serving King and country in allowing a surgical delivery which would have been well known to be life-threatening. Alternatively, her clinical condition may have been so demonstrably weak and exhausted that consent to operate was sought from her next of kin. This view cannot be sustained in the light of the King's choice that his wife should undergo a procedure almost certainly detrimental to her wellbeing and that the undelivered child should take precedence over its mother. It is more likely that Jane's opinion was of no importance in coming to a decision. At that time the imperious will of a monarch was paramount. Furthermore, Henry VIII's wish for a son was desperate and indeed the English reformation turned on it. The concept of freely given and informed consent by the patient (the Queen) does not ring true in these circumstances.

As medical care gradually improved the doctrine which came to prevail was that the life of the mother was the all-important commodity and should be preserved at all cost. She would then be able to look after existing children and would probably be able to have another attempt at childbirth at a later date if the current pregnancy did not result in a live birth. The effects of better nutrition and the alleviation of terrible social deprivation contributed to a fall in the maternal mortality rate. Medical care of the pregnant mother also slowly improved. The role of the obstetrician as a specialist in preventive medicine gradually evolved as it was appreciated that many of the conditions which were most destructive to pregnant women could not only be identified earlier, but by intervention were often avoidable or amenable to treatment, thus preventing maternal death. For example the maternal mortality rate per 100 000 total births fell from 98.9 in 1951 to 8.9 in 1981 (DHSS Report on Confidential Enquiries 1986). The rate prior to this had been very much higher and even in 1935 the figure would have been 420 maternal deaths per 100 000 total births.

It has thus become uncommon in the United Kingdom for a woman to die in childbirth or as a result of pregnancy. In 1981, 57 women died out of 639 000 total births in England and Wales. Along with this fall in maternal mortality rate there has been a substantial decline in the perinatal mortality rate. The latter is the sum of those babies who are stillborn or who die in the first week of life. In most obstetric units in this country the perinatal mortality rate is falling year by year and is now approximately 10 per 1000 total births.

It is against this backdrop of a low maternal mortality rate and relatively few baby deaths that contemporary pregnant mothers view their prospects of successful childbirth. It is conceded that the risks to an individual mother and her baby of death or damage are small. The role of the obstetrician is therefore one of defensive, preventive medicine rather than the more usual doctor–patient relationship where the patients recognize that they are ill and seek help from the doctor to have their illness treated. As such it is difficult to stipulate what the professional relationship is between an obstetrician and the healthy pregnant woman who is to be delivered by her midwife. The doctor takes on a supervisor's responsibility and serves to assist the midwife if the clinical case deviates from the normal course. It is really only when these abnormal circumstances occur that one can say that the pregnant woman is truly a patient of the doctor. The doctor checks his patient for the normal progress of her labour and also for the signs of onset of exhaustion. It is also his role to watch for evidence of fetal distress. As such he takes on a role of guardian for the health and welfare of this baby and adopts a position of defence for the baby so that harmful complications may be avoided. It is easy to see that in his attempts to protect or treat either of his charges he may well be at odds with the wishes or needs of the other party.

At this stage it is necessary to cite some simple examples of these differences so that we may develop the scenario of conflicting needs at a more complicated level, but along the same principled framework. Also at this stage I shall apologize to those who may feel offended when I refer to the obstetrician as a male doctor. This makes for clearer text and regrettably reflects the current staffing situation in the National Health Service.

For our first example of conflict I should like to use a case where the labouring mother requires analgesia for the pain of contractions. If she receives such a large dose of opiate that analgesic requirements are totally met then the likelihood is that the baby may be born with heavy respiratory depression and thus need resuscitation. In practical terms the mother's analgesic needs are not fully met but a smaller dose of opiate is given so that the baby does not need ventilation. There is thus a trade-off between the mother's wishes and the possible harmful effects on the baby if her request were to be followed to the letter. One of the functions of the education classes offered to pregnant mothers is to explain these difficulties and to highlight where a mother could be putting her baby at risk. Most mothers have only the interests of their baby at heart and go out of their way to conduct their lives in a fashion most advantageous to the baby, e.g. by curtailing consumption of alcohol and cigarettes.

The conflict is, in most instances, tolerable and tolerated by both partners in the above maternal–fetal trade-off. However if one or other partner puts up an excess or unreasonable demand then the trade-off does not work and there is consequential suffering or death by the losing party. In this context I should like to discuss fetal distress.

Here the baby is showing signs that all is not well in its environment and that unless the conditions causing the distress are reversed or removed it will be affected by cerebral anoxia (lack of oxygen) and may develop irreversible damage which is most often cerebral. The condition of the mother may well be unaffected and indeed she may be in perfect health. However if the labour is not sufficently advanced to allow immediate delivery by natural means then the requirement is for the mother to undergo a surgical delivery by forceps or Caesarean section. Either of these procedures causes her pain and distress, and also, by employing general anaesthesia in labour, she is put at increased risk of losing her own life in addition to the risk of the procedure itself. Needless to say, most mothers would not think twice about exposing themselves to such a risk if it meant that their babies would be born healthy and without brain damage.

It is difficult however to weigh up to what extent the obligation to obtain informed consent has been met. The labouring mother may be in real pain, she may have received injections of analgesics which confuse her cognition, and the consent may be obtained in such a rapid fashion that she has no time to reflect, discuss, or question. The fact that she is told that her baby is starting to develop possible brain damange may be seen to equate more with coercion and duress than it does with purely factual information. This paternalistic attitude of the attending obstetrician would be more acceptable if we were able to claim that our diagnosis of fetal distress was particularly accurate (Leveno *et al.* 1986). All of us have seen the most alarming cardiotocograph tracing of severe fetal distress only to deliver a baby a few minutes later which is in perfect health and screaming volubly. This does not inspire confidence in our methods of diagnosis but these very methods have led us to adopt a very defensive form of medicine in which the interests of the fetus are all important and the morbidity of the mother has been put as a necessary payment for the health of her child. It hardly seems necessary to say that these attitudes have led to opposition from a group of mothers who see themselves as not being ill, not requesting help from the doctor, and certainly not expecting that the very person who should be supporting them is in fact trying to enforce on them the very type of intervention which they are trying to avoid. The argument that the intervention is on behalf of their baby may well not be accepted, particularly if the advice is based on observations that in themselves may be fallable or inaccurate. To put it more simply, the paternalistic attitudes of the obstetrician have been rumbled by those whom he chooses to call his patients but who see themselves as no such thing. The situation in our modern labour wards has become one of conflict and in many circumstances one of dissatisfaction. One would be tempted to ascribe the dissatisfaction entirely to the long-suffering mothers; but I feel it is now true to say that many obstetricians are beginning to see that the paternalistic and heavy-handed approach to their mothers in labour is not one to be continued or recommended.

It then follows that the only course left open is one of continued detailed accurate information transmitted to the patient, from which she may make sensible decisions about what is best for her and her baby. The avoidance of such conflicts of interest serve all concerned much better than attempts to battle it out.

We are, however, left with the case in which the mother chooses to ignore the advice of the obstetrician who we assume has been able to identify a very real set of dangers for the fetus in this labour. It is at this juncture that the ethical decision is at its most difficult. Should the doctor ignore the mother's legitimate claims for her autonomy to be respected and allow her to refuse the proposed treatment to save her baby, or may he invoke an argument that any caring mother would wish the best for her baby and that by refusing such help she is not acting responsibly, and therefore should not be treated as a fully responsible person? By so doing he is then able to dispense with respect for her autonomy.

I have already highlighted the difficulties surrounding how consent is obtained from the labouring mother. She is most often not in a condition in which we could claim that the consent was obtained freely and without any hint of duress, from a patient who has understood fully all the implications of the information provided, and from whom an assessment of comprehension of this information has also been obtained as a test of informed consent. The problem is often aggravated by the views of the father who may act as a go-between. As a result the information which the mother receives is often also biased or accentuated by the views of her husband or boyfriend. Obviously the ultimate example of this is where the father is acting as interpreter. The obstetrician offering advice and suggesting intervention on behalf of the baby is never sure whether the labouring mother is in fact receiving this information in a fashion which is not distorted by the interpreting father's own view. It is also augmented by the fact that the parents may have a totally different set of values in their own culture (e.g. Pakistani) and feel that the imposition of Caesarean section is so great and so degrading to the mother that it were better that the baby should die rather than be born by such means.

We are left in the end with the greatest ethical problem with which to deal. In our final analysis we must consider the problem that arises where a mother has been fully acquainted with the facts regarding the risks which her unborn is undergoing but where she chooses to ignore the advice that she is given. She refuses the intervention which her baby requires to prevent subsequent brain damage. All the tests of comprehension have been valid and we are satisfied that the mother in labour has understood what she has been told regarding the risks which her unborn baby is suffering; but she is adamant that she will not undergo surgical intervention to deliver the baby.

Our ethical problem is to discover whether or not she has the right to subject another person to injury and a life of unfulfilment and lost capacity. A definition of the limits of autonomy has suggested they lie where 'my fist meets your nose'. We accept that people have the right or freedom to act in the manner that they desire so long as this does not interfere with the similar right of others. In our example above, the labouring mother is clearly transgressing this boundary.

Interestingly, the situation changes abruptly once the baby has been born. Should a mother neglect or injure her baby, then there is clear legal power in the United Kingdom whereby the baby is taken into care so that further injury is avoided. Should the baby also show signs of physical damage, the parents may also face criminal proceedings for child abuse. However the same type of injury before birth carries no such stigmata and there is no requirement in law for the mother to co-operate for the good of her baby. To legislate in such a way would make the mother subordinate to her fetus and remove her freedom of action. We are therefore left with the most difficult of ethical voids. The only solution in practical terms is to attempt to avoid the occasion of conflict in labour. Our only hope of so doing is via an educational route. This educational process is not, however, restricted to the mother-to-be; a large element of it must be directed at the obstetric practitioners who see a fully monitored 'high-tech' labour as the only safe form of delivery. They are deceiving themselves into a belief that such monitoring systems are either foolproof or are particularly accurate in their prediction of which baby will be damaged in the long term. This is not the world in which we now work. The reality is that the tools of our obstetric trade are as yet ill-refined and are generally blunt. The fall in the maternal and fetal mortality rates has been won at the expense of patients' autonomy and they, as a consumer group, are currently rebelling against the iron hand of authoritarian obstetricians. It is surely not necessary to go back to a higher mortality rate to convince everyone that co-operation and avoidance of conflict are essential if a successful outcome of undamaged mothers and babies is to be achieved. We are presently facing one of the most difficult of ethical dilemmas, that is, who has the greater claims—the mother or the baby? The least appropriate place to be discussing this ethical problem, however, is in the busy labour ward where a battleground of conflict has already supervened.

REFERENCES

Dewhurst, J. (1980). *Royal Confinements*, p. 7. Weidenfeld and Nicholson, London.

Leveno, K., Cunningham, F., Nelson, S., Roark, M., Williams, M., Guzick, D., Dowling, S., Rosenfeld, C., and Buckley, A. (1986). A prospective comparison of selective and universal electronic fetal monitoring in 34 995 pregnancies. *New England Journal of Medicine*, **315**, No. 10, 615–19.

Department of Health and Social Security (1986). Report on confidential enquiries into maternal deaths in England and Wales 1979–1981. *Report on Health and Social Subjects*, **29**. Her Majesty's Stationary Office, London.

6
Some ethical issues in neonatal care

A. G. M. CAMPBELL

INTRODUCTION

Recent advances in medicine have brought many benefits to patients and have given doctors enormous power. The 'miracles' of modern medicine receive regular media attention and acclaim. Public expectations for success in conquering disease and disability have never been higher. Anything, or almost anything, now seems possible. Unfortunately there is a darker side to this exciting scenario. In some circumstances all treatments and all technologies must eventually fail. Patients may be left no better off or perhaps even worse. Coping with failure leaves emotions in turmoil and may result in family resentment and chronic sorrow. Trust between doctor and patient (or doctor and parents in the case of children) may be eroded particularly as the 'personal doctor' of old becomes replaced by multidisciplinary teams. In concentrating on the technical aspects of treatment each doctor may leave contact and communications with families to others. Unless there is strong medical leadership by one doctor primarily responsible for care and main-enance of sensitive communication with families (listening as well as talking), disillusionment and anger may result in a legacy of bitterness that will last for years (Stinson and Stinson 1981).

In using new skills and technologies responsibly, doctors are increasingly faced with troubling moral and legal questions for which there are no obvious or easy solutions. The most difficult of these dilemmas are concerned with issues of life and death, and perhaps nowhere are they more poignant than at the beginning of life; at birth and in the newborn intensive care nursery.

LIFE, DEATH, AND INTENSIVE CARE

Doctors have a clear commitment to respect and preserve life. Nowhere has this been more evident than at birth and in the early weeks of post-natal life. Almost a hundred years ago Pierre Budin, the French obstetrician, demonstrated the benefits of what we now call 'newborn special care', and showed that merely by keeping premature babies warm he could achieve a remarkable improvement in survival (Budin 1907). Modern perinatal intensive care, in conjunction with improvements in maternal health and socio-economic circumstances, have led to perinatal and infant death rates that are a fraction of what they were last century. But even Pierre Budin recognized that there were limits: 'We shall not discuss infants of less than 1000g, they are seldom saved and only very rarely shall I need to allude to them.'

It is only relatively recently that the salvage of all infants born alive has been seen by some to be a desirable social goal (Silverman 1981). In the pre- and post-Christian era newborn infants, especially those with abnormalities, were accorded less status and therefore less protection than older children to whom full familial and community commitments were made (Ferngren 1987). Until the 1950s the high mortality among premature and abnormal infants was accepted with an 'it's probably just as well' attitude that reflected not just the inadequacies of contemporary treatment but also concern about the future health and quality of life and in the privacy of the home, and even in the hospital delivery room, death may have been hastened to avoid more prolonged 'suffering'. Parents grieved for their loss but most were able to celebrate the birth of a healthy infant or infants in subsequent years.

Fortunately, most infants treated in a modern intensive care nursery grow up to be healthy or to suffer from only minor disability. A few survive with handicaps sufficiently severe to affect their lives disastrously and to have major implications for their families. In treating these infants today, many difficult questions must be faced. What kinds of infants are likely to survive with severe handicaps? How can we recognize them? Can future 'quality of life' be predicted with sufficient accuracy to justify its use as a criterion for life or death decisions, or should all infants *routinely* be given intensive care and other treatments to prolong their lives to the best of our abilities? Can it ever be right to withhold or withdraw treatment in the knowledge that death will result? Should death be hastened to avoid pain or distress when further treatment seems futile? Who should be involved in these decisions? Are they too important and too complex to be left to doctors? Should others be involved? What about the parents—apart from the child, surely they are the ones most affected? Should the State (Government) have any role in these decisions which affect its newly born citizens?

Infants can be divided into three prognostic groups:

1. Those for whom available treatment is usually successful. Their treatment poses few difficult moral questions. They are treated aggressively from birth with every expectation of success.

2. Those for whom available treatment is of doubtful benefit. Decisions about the appropriate use of various treatments to save or prolong life are particularly difficult. They are the subject of detailed discussion in this chapter.

3. Those for whom all treatments are likely to be futile. As these infants are likely to die within a short time in any case, treatment decisions are less controversial. Nevertheless their continuing need for care while dying will pose moral and legal dilemmas that will be particularly difficult and troubling for parents and staff alike.

Thus decisions about infants who are expected to recover and be healthy are relatively easy and present few problems. Decisions about the severely disabled and dying are problematic and have been the subject of continuing debate in recent years (Duff and Campbell 1980). Arguments about the appropriate care for infants in groups 2 and 3 above are focused on three broad options.

First, there is a moral obligation to respect and preserve life to the utmost. The Hippocratic Oath suggests a pledge *not* to practise euthanasia. This can be interpreted by doctors as a commitment to treat all infants equally without regard to their condition or quality of life. It follows therefore that efforts should be directed towards providing all necessary and available treatments to save or prolong life including the surgical correction, when feasible, of life threatening congenital abnormalities. This view is expressed by individuals and organizations promoting a 'sanctity of life ethic' and is reflected in the 'Baby Doe' legislation recently introduced in the United States (Annas 1984).

Secondly, where infants have suffered from severe damage or disability, particularly to the brain, and where there is a high likelihood of resulting life-long handicap, various treatments, apart from those necessary to relieve pain or distress, may be withheld or withdrawn after discussion with the parents and preferably with their agreement. In other words, these infants should be 'allowed to die' as usually would have happened before the introduction of modern aggressive intensive care. This option, or variations of it, is favoured by most paediatricians, is supported by parents who have experienced these tragedies and so far as can be judged, by the general public. It is the option that most closely reflects current practice in the United Kingdom (British Medical Journal 1981).

Thirdly, some philosophers but probably very few paediatricians consider that 'allowing to die' is morally no different from 'killing'. They argue that killing quickly and painlessly, though at present illegal, is more humane, and morally more defensible than allowing to die, perhaps slowly and painfully (Rachels 1975).

Doctors who experience these dilemmas soon realize how our traditional codes of ethics have failed to keep pace with changes in medical practice and contemporary society.

'The old answers will not do any longer; they were made for other times and for other places. There are no authoritative answers. The Law, one kind of authority, is a mess and is unhelpful here. Ethicism based on religion deluges us with cut-and-dried precepts based on outmoded, almost mediaeval concepts . . . ' (Ladd 1980).

In discussing the 'rights and wrongs' of medical decision it must be emphasized that paediatricians, like others, will view these issues in different ways. In questions of morality we all tend to 'draw lines' at what are acceptable or not acceptable to us as individuals. At the same time we must acknowledge the ethical standards of our profession and of the society in which we live, and be aware of the laws of the land. There may also be incongruity between morals and laws. An action such as euthanasia may be viewed as morally correct although illegal, while another like abortion may be legal but morally unacceptable.

Infants of very low birthweight

Like Pierre Budin, we used to consider 28 weeks gestation age (term = 37–42 weeks) as the limit of viability for an infant born prematurely. Nowadays infants born between 24–28 weeks have a good chance of survival and occasional 'successes' have been reported with infants born under 24 weeks. Unfortunately while the prospects are good for the larger and more mature babies (over 28 weeks or 1000g), for infants under 26 weeks (under 800g) the risks of severe disabling complications and future handicap increase significantly (Sell 1986). We must ask if it is sensible to rescue all infants born alive to the best of our abilities and without regard to the consequences for the child and family; or should a line be drawn somewhere? As the limits of post-natal viability are extended further and further into the second trimester of pregnancy it is worth reflecting that we may overlap with the upper limit for therapeutic abortion as it is not always easy to date a pregnancy accurately. Elsewhere I have suggested a 'cut-off' birth weight of 750g, below which the likely outcome and future implications, with or without treatment, should be discussed with the parents before various resuscitative and intensive care procedures to maintain life are continued or introduced. Obviously, using a 'cut-off' weight only makes sense if it remains flexible and is used as only one of a number of criteria that should be considered before coming to such a fundamental decision (Campbell 1982). Some neonatal units use these or similar criteria; but others, because of different or conflicting moral views, or perhaps because of anxiety about 'moral busybodies' and the law, continue to treat all infants aggressively from birth, even those weighing as little as 500g or less. In practice, most doctors will initiate maximum treatment, including intubation and assisted ventilation if necessary for all infants who seem potentially viable, to give them a 'trial of life'. If further developments or later assessments indicate that there is a high likelihood of extensive brain damage, treatment will be stopped and the infant allowed to die. What part parents play in reaching these various decisions is difficult to assess but from published accounts, paediatricians seem increasingly willing to discuss the options for care fully and frankly with them and to seek their views before making any final decision (Young 1984). New developments in knowledge, skill, and technology, along with careful follow-up studies of the survivors, will dictate continuing changes in criteria for the care of these infants. It has to be acknowledged that criteria will vary from country to country and nursery to nursery according to the resources available, and increasing pressure to modify criteria acccording to resources will become a fact of life even in advanced societies. Doctors cannot ignore these constraints but must ensure, so far as they can, that the interests of individual patients are kept as their first priority.

The severely damaged or malformed infant

The second category where doctors will be faced with dilemmas about starting, stopping, or continuing treatment is with infants who have been damaged before, during, or after birth, or who have congenital malformations that seriously jeopardize their chances of a normal life. Even with the shock of abnormal birth, parents have some understanding of what brain damage means for their child's future health, happiness, education, relationships, and future independence—what Rachels calls 'having a life' as opposed to merely 'being alive' (Rachels 1986). This is undoubtedly one of the major factors influencing paediatricians when advising parents about the wisdom of withdrawing or continuing life support. Specific examples of conditions with a risk of brain damage include severe perinatal asphyxia, congenital virus infection, and certain forms of intracranial haemorrhage. There are also a number of chromosomal disorders with multiple abnormalities that are almost invariably associated with severe mental handicap. In some of these, (e.g. trisomy 13) the infants are so grossly deformed that anything like what parents would view as an acceptable life for their child is impossible and early death is likely in any case. On the other hand Down's Syndrome (trisomy 21), the best known of the chromosomal disorders, is in a very different category and has been the subject of many ethical and legal controversies (Shepperdson 1983). These children have a wide spectrum of abnormalities and intelligence and they may survive for many years. Although most require special schooling and remain dependent, an increasing number are able to start mainstream education and achieve a certain measure of independence provided that they receive appropriate stimulation and support. Within a loving family it would be ridiculous to suggest that they have an unacceptable quality of life. Decision to withhold or withdraw treatment from certain of these infants should remain the responsibility of doctors and parents who are familiar with the unique circumstances of each child and family, but the current climate of opinion in this country is that they should be treated like normal infants. Ethical and legal difficulties are likely to arise only when an infant is rejected by parents or they refuse permission for a life-saving operation. Lasting rejection because of Down's Syndrome alone is unusual but in my experience parents will occasionally reject a life-saving operation, e.g. to correct intestinal atresia or a major heart defect because they believe sincerely that it is in their infant's own interests not to survive. Whatever the cynics might say, inconvenience, the effect on the rest of the family, or the potential drain on family finances, are seldom uppermost in their minds. Nevertheless any decision to withhold life-saving surgery from an infant with Down's Syndrome is now liable to be contested by someone and it is unlikely that the courts would find in favour of the parents with or without the support of their doctors. Many parents remain extremely concerned about who will care for these children if they, the parents, become ill or should die first. They may continue to view their child's early death as a preferable alternative to sudden incarceration in an institution. These anxieties may continue to influence them in accepting or rejecting medical or surgical treatment for their child.

Killing and allowing to die

Most doctors reject an absolute adherence to the sanctity of life as inhumane vitalism that takes no account of tragic errors in development or the realities of disease and human suffering. On the other hand they are wary of suggestions that the swift, painless putting-to-death of deformed or brain-damaged infants would be more humane and should be sanctioned by law. Paediatricians generally prefer an intermediate position which recognizes that there are occasions when withholding or withdrawing life-preserving treatments and allowing an infant to die is best for the child and the family and is probably best for society. There may be no *moral* distinction between 'killing' and 'allowing to die' but I believe that there is a powerful *psychological* distinction which is important particularly to parents and to the staff of intensive care nurseries. Although the end result is the same, to them there is a big difference between not using a respirator to keep an infant of 600g alive, and giving a lethal injection.

Within this intermediate position or 'grey area', there will be considerable variations in individual moral reasoning which make a treatment or a no-treatment decision acceptable or unacceptable. It must be remembered that the parents who (apart from the child) are most affected may also take different positions. Doctors must be careful not to impose unwelcome choices on families through feelings of moral superiority, worries about the views of colleagues, or excessive timidity about the law; yet they may have to guide parents towards what is acceptable not only medically but morally and socially, and what is within the law. Thus much latitude in decision is to be expected and should be tolerated. Occasionally the parents' understanding of the medical realities and their views on the options available may be so faulty that agreement on a course of action will be impossible and it will be necessary to seek court assistance in order to proceed with urgent treatment. Parents will sometimes ask the doctor to 'do something' to hasten death in an infant whose prolonged dying is causing great anguish. While such an action might be viewed as morally correct, the parents must understand that it would be illegal and that there might be legal consequences for them as well as for the doctor.

Withdrawing or withholding treatment: taking the decision

For a number of years it has been my view that the main burden of decision must continue to be borne by the doctor or doctors primarily responsible for the infant's care in conjunction with the family, primarily the parents (Duff and Campbell 1973). Both doctors and parents will seek advice from others. The doctor will consult with specialists and other colleagues and employ all available technologies to ensure accuracy of diagnosis and prognosis—good ethical decisions begin with good facts (Fost 1981). The doctor should discuss the issues with the general practitioner who may know the family well and with the nurses who provide the consistent hour-to-hour care and often come to know the parents intimately at the cot-side; and with others such as a social worker who function as part of the intensive care team. The parents may seek the views of grandparents, clergymen, friends, and perhaps many others. As reflected in national and cultural differences, some parents will still prefer to leave much or all of the decision to doctors, trusting them to act in their baby's best interests. This pattern of decision has been called 'family-centred' because families are most aware of their own strengths, weaknesses, and resources and must bear the consequences of any decision (Duff and Campbell 1976). Lawyers have attacked the lack of 'due process' in such a policy and have pointed out the legal dangers to paediatricians (Robertson and Fost 1976). Up to a point this criticism is valid, but the problems of individual infants interacting with individual family circumstances may lead to complex and almost unique situations for which only general guidelines can be provided, and it can be argued that the medical diagnosis and prognosis should not necessarily be the only determinants of care. In discussion there must be some consideration of values cherished by individual families—personal, religious, and cultural. I and others have been resistant to interference by outsiders in these tragic and intensely private affairs unless there are clear abuses of trust and harm is being done to someone. Death is not always a harm, just as life is not always a good (Kohl 1987). The decisions should be made openly and documented so that doctors are seen to be accountable for their actions. They should be prepared to defend them in court if necessary. Committees can provide valuable objective analyses of the issues and can suggest policy guidelines but, like armchair ethicists, philosophers, and lawyers, they can only be peripheral to the individual tragedies. The admitted less than 100 per cent certainty about prognosis, judgements about quality of life, and loose interpretations of the law may be upsetting for them but moral imperatives, lofty philosophical concepts, and rigid legal definitions seem less important in the heat of an intensive care unit. 'As there are few atheists in fox-holes there tend to be few absolutists at the bedside' (Ingelfinger 1973). Caring persons are likely to make caring decisions when faced with tragic choices. The more remote the decision-makers, the more remote the decision from infant and family realities.

Rhoden (1986) calls the family-centred approach an 'individual prognostic strategy', and believes that it is 'most consistent with a clinical practice sensitive to the parents' role and unconstrained either by an over-simplistic vitalism, excessive fear of legal liability, or an emotionally appealing but ethically untenable distinction between withholding and withdrawing treatment. This strategy both recognizes and reflects the complex nature of these dilemmas. It is not without flaws—but it is probably the best that doctors, parents, and society can do'.

Withdrawing or withholding treatment: what happens next?

Once the decision is taken to withhold or withdraw various treatments like assisted ventilation, the care given subsequently may cause considerable argument and tension within the intensive care nursery. It has been a frequent subject for armchair debate by philosophers and other ethicists. My view is a fairly simple one. Once a decision has been made to allow an infant to die it is illogical and pointlessly cruel to do *anything* that prolongs the infant's life unnecessarily. In debating the justification of omitting or continuing certain treatments, terms like 'ordinary', or 'extraordinary' are often used, a distinction that is recognized by the Roman Catholic Church and has become established in ethical reasoning. 'Ordinary' is usually taken to mean a treatment that is normal or routine while 'extraordinary' suggests a treatment that is unusual and beyond what is necessary or normal. Some have taken 'ordinary' care to mean obligatory or mandatory care while 'extra-ordinary' care can be considered as optional, hence the justification in denying it in certain circumstances. Much more detailed definitions have been suggested by Father Gerald Kelly (Kelly 1950). He defines 'ordinary' as 'all medicines, treatments and operations which offer a reasonable hope of benefit for the patients and which can be obtained and used without excessive expense, pain and other inconvenience' while 'extraordinary' is defined as 'all those medicines, treatments and operations which cannot be obtained without excessive expense, pain or other inconvenience or which if used would not offer a reasonable hope of benefit'.

All these definitions can be interpreted variously to the point of absurdity. A treatment considered 'extraordinary' a decade ago may be very ordinary today and what is extraordinary in some circumstances may be very ordinary in others. Surely the important point is whether or not it is a good thing for life to be prolonged? Does prolonging this life offer a reasonable hope of benefit to the individual concerned? If so then 'ordinary' *and* 'extraordinary' treatments may be appropriate. If not, then both 'ordinary' and 'extraordinary' treatments may be inappropriate with the exception of those treatments, usually ordinary, that are necessary to relieve distress.

There is general agreement that infants should receive loving human contact (cherishing), adequate warmth, air, oral liquids as tolerated, and be ensured freedom from pain or distress even if it is necessary to use analgesics or sedative drugs to the extent of a 'double effect' of shortening life. It has also been suggested that feeding milk to maintain nourishment is every infant's 'right' regardless of circumstances, even when 'life' as we like to think of it has long since ceased to exist. In some circumstances, such as the persistent vegetative state, 'life' can be prolonged almost indefinitely by tube feeding to maintain nutrition, and antibiotics to control infection. Once a decision has been made that death is preferable to continued life of this kind I believe that anything, including feeding, that prolongs this artificial existence is wrong for the infant, wrong for the family, and wrong for society (Campbell 1984). Doctors have a duty to use treatment responsibly and must protect patients from such pointless exercises. At the same time they must take the lead in providing support for the grieving parents who should have been involved in any decisions to stop treatment. Arrangements should be made to allow the family to keep close contact and continue to participate in the infant's care until death. If given the opportunity, and appropriate support especially from their general practitioner and health visitor, the parents may derive comfort from having their baby at home. Dying may be prolonged and will be an exacting time emotionally but its manner can provide some comfort to bereaved parents. There must be opportunities for reflection, review of earlier decisions based on progress, and a willingness to consider a change of management if that seems appropriate.

Government involvement in non-treatment decisions ('Baby Doe')

Since May 1982 the US Department of Health and Human Services (DHHS) has attempted to outlaw 'quality of life' criteria in determining care. These efforts at legislation have come to be known as the Baby Doe Rules after a controversial and widely publicized Indiana decision to withhold life-saving surgery from an infant with Down's Syndrome. (In the US, male and female infants whose identities are protected are known to the public as John Doe and Jane Doe respectively). These 'ill-considered' proposals were attacked by many individuals and medical organizations including the American Academy of Pediatrics (AAP) and, in their original form under the Rehabilitation Act of 1973, have been rejected in numerous courts as 'invalid, unlawful, and without statutory authority'. Nevertheless the champions of this legislation including various 'pro-life' groups and, significantly, the US Surgeon General, a distinguished ex-paediatric surgeon who is himself a 'right-to-life' advocate, did not concede defeat. They defined 'withholding of medically indicated treatment' as 'medical neglect' and brought it within the already existing legislation on child abuse, a move that families and doctors acting sincerely in infants' best interests found particularly offensive. The amendment to the Child Abuse Prevention and Treatment Act came into effect in October 1984 and required individual States to set up their own procedures for dealing with reports of failure to provide treatment. The amendment defines this as all treatments likely to be effective in ameliorating life-threatening conditions except:

1. When the infant is 'chronically and irreversibly comatose'.
2. When the provision of treatment would:
   (a) merely prolong dying;
   (b) not be effective in ameliorating or correcting all of the infant's life-threatening conditions; or
   (c) otherwise be futile in terms of the survival of the infant.
3. When the provision of such treatment would be virtually futile in terms of the survival of the infant and the treatment itself under such circumstances would be inhumane.

One important result of the AAP opposition to the Baby Doe Rules was an agreement that hospitals might set up their own ethics committees (now known as Infant Care Review Committees) with professional and lay membership to discuss problem cases and advise on hospital policy (Fleischman and Murray 1983). They can be seen as providing a form of arbitration between the parents and doctors on the one hand and state interference on the other, but their creation is voluntary and they are not part of State legislation. Whether they will lead to 'better' decisions for infants remains to be seen. With or without the influence of these committees and in spite of the more flexible modifications that, under pressure from doctors, were made to the original legislation, it is inevitable that American paediatricians and parents continue to feel extremely vulnerable to legal action (Moskop and Saldanha 1986). It is not surprising to learn that many more infants are now subjected to excessive treatment and the cruel and pointless prolongation of suffering.

It is noteworthy that parents who, more than any other individual or group, must bear the consequences of these decisions were almost completely ignored by the drafters of the Baby Doe Rules (Angell 1983). One can readily understand why their sense of injustice is particularly acute in a society whose government, at the same time as introducing this legislation, was also threatening to reduce the funds available for the care of handicapped persons in the community.

In the United Kingdom, there is no similar legislation, although 'right-to-life' groups have lobbied for its introduction since the 1981 trial and subsequent acquittal of Dr Leonard Arthur, a paediatrician accused of the murder (later, attempted murder) of an infant with Down's Syndrome. Indeed, as a reaction to this trial, a Limitation of Treatment Bill was proposed which, with appropriate safeguards, would allow the withdrawal of life-sustaining treatment up to 28 days after birth (Brahams and Brahams 1983). While this Bill would provide some legal protection to paediatricians and might remove some of the absurdities of present distinctions between the legal killing of fetuses and the illegal 'killing' of newborn infants of the same 'age', most of us would still be reluctant to see State involvement either to enforce life or dictate death. There is merit in doctors and parents continuing to trust each other in seeking the least detrimental solution for an infant even if it causes much anguish and uncertainty. Legalizing infanticide might erode much of this trust. What parents and doctors need from society and from government are not new laws but more understanding of what congenital abnormality can mean, more compassion for the afflicted infants, more appreciation of family realities in individual circumstances and considerable latitude to work out the dilemmas in the best interests of the infant and family.

Regulations like the Baby Doe Rules and the activities of 'pro-life' activists could force paediatricians to go too far in keeping babies alive far beyond all reasonable hope of healthy survival. These pressures are bound to increase the suffering of infants and the harm done to families. They might even lead to parents taking legal action against paediatricians somewhat similar to the recent 'wrongful life' suits directed against obstetricians. Persisting with the cruel use of new technologies to keep infants alive for no purpose beyond a personal belief in the sanctity of life or fear of legal sanction is in itself one of the worst forms of child abuse and constitutes a victimizing abandonment of our responsibility to do no harm to patients.

New dilemmas : resuscitation for 'pre-viable' infants and the survivors of late 'therapeutic' abortions

To achieve uniformity and make comparative statistics meaningful, it is desirable that all births over 500g should be recorded. Gestational age may be inaccurate and is too subject to misinterpretation to be reliable as a criterion for registration purposes. Nevertheless, for various reasons including sensitivity to the mother's 'feelings' the recording of extremely low birthweight infants is extremely variable. Maternity units will notify only some still births under 28 weeks and there will be inconsistent recordings of infants born under 28 weeks gestation who are born with signs of life yet perhaps 'not capable of being born alive' as interpreted under the Infant Life Preservation Act of 1929.

With tinier and tinier babies being born alive, the moral and legal considerations in treatment become more troubling and certainly more difficult than the medical and technical ones. Most newborn resuscitation in hospital is carried out by junior doctors who quickly develop the practical skills to resuscitate almost any infant born with signs of life and even some who, by definition, are stillborn. In almost all circumstances their responsibility is clear. They should resuscitate all infants of whatever gestation age, birthweight, or apparent abnormality until a more considered judgement can be made, usually by a senior doctor, on the advisability of continuing life support. For infants under 1000g birthweight there is evidence that early aggressive management, including intubation and assisted ventilation, offers the best chance for survival.

In my view, an exception to the above general 'rule' is when an infant is born with signs of life after an attempted 'therapeutic abortion', an increasing problem in recent years (Rhoden 1984). Possibly because of the increasing threat of exposure by a hospital 'mole', and the resulting medico-legal implications, more and more of these babies are being identified. A paediatrician may be asked to resuscitate and treat a tiny live-born 'abortus' in spite of the fact that a short time earlier a gynaecological colleague made a deliberate attempt to kill it. Like the obligation to render medical aid to the condemned man injured in a botched execution, should doctors be obliged to rescue these infants? At present the law confers protection on every infant born alive and paediatricians have a duty to care for them. However, I do not believe that this care should necessarily include aggressive methods of resuscitation and intensive care. These infants may have been damaged as part of the abortion procedure. It is unlikely that they will be wanted by the mothers who earlier sought their demise. They will be difficult to place for adoption. They should be allowed to die. Pressures to provide aggressive resuscitation and intensive care for these infants should be resisted.

This new dilemma is one of the ironies of an abortion legislation which considers some fetuses expendable, overlapping with the law that grants live-born infants full protection. We need to ensure either that abortion never results in live-born infants, or modify the law to recognize a different status for these infants.

ALLOCATION OF SCARCE RESOURCES

The provision of resources has failed to keep pace with the increased demand for newborn intensive care. At the level of *macro allocation* (decisions about which services to provide to which groups), there are many reports which indicate the inadequate state of neonatal care in the country as a whole (Speidel 1986). At the same time there is anxiety that providing intensive care to a relatively small number of infants is expanding at a rate detrimental to the resources available for other services including those for older children. The need to limit use of resources makes doctors very uncomfortable. On the one hand they are realistic enough to recognize that a 'blank cheque' is impossible, yet they insist that they must have freedom to do and spend whatever is necessary for their patients. They consider the 'common good' as secondary to the individual patient, a view that brings them into conflict with health economists whose primary concern is to make maximum use of resources for the health of the community as a whole (Mooney 1984).

Paediatricians will argue that, if difficult decisions about rationing resources have to be made, it makes economic sense to give priority to prevention rather than to the treatment of end stage disease, and that prevention is one of the key elements in child health and paediatrics. Skimping on the care of vulnerable newborn infants is false economy. Preventing avoidable handicap by high quality perinatal care is not only a blessing for individual families but within limits is cost-effective (Sinclair 1987).

At the level of *micro allocation* within a neonatal nursery (choices about which individuals should benefit from the resources available), deciding to be selective in the use of skills and technology on the basis of what seems best for the infant has already been discussed. To me, this seems morally at least as defensible as a decision to refuse admission because the unit is full, short of nurses, or lacking in medical staff; deciding not to use IPPV (intermittent positive pressure ventilation) because there are no more respirators. Yet these decisions will become necessary everywhere on purely economic grounds if we shrink from developing criteria based on what seems best for infants and families, including an assessment of expected quality of life, a concept apparently abhorrent to some philosophers and the US Government. Providing intensive care for all infants whatever their weight, gestation age, or condition, apart from the potential for harm to them and their families, may seriously affect the ability of an overloaded and understaffed unit to provide adequate care for other infants. This may have serious consequences for some who might otherwise have had every expectation of survival and a healthy future.

REFERENCES

Angell, M. (1983). Handicapped children: Baby Doe and Uncle Sam. *New England Journal of Medicine*, 309, 659–61.

Annas, G. J. (1984). The Baby Doe regulations: governmental intervention in neonatal rescue medicine. *American Journal of Public Health*, 74, 618–20.

Brahams, D. and Brahams, M. (1983). The Arthur case: a proposal for legislation. *Journal of Medical Ethics*, **9**, 12–15.

British Medical Journal (1981). Withholding treatment in infancy. *British Medical Journal*, **1**, 925–6.

Budin, P. (1907). *The nursling: The feeding and hygiene of premature and full-term infants*. Caxton Publishing Co., London.

Campbell, A. G. M. (1982). Which infants should not receive intensive care? *Archives of Disease in Childhood*, **57**, 569–71.

Campbell, A. G. M. (1984). Children in a persistent vegetative state. *British Medical Journal*, **289**, 1022–3.

Duff, R. S. and Campbell, A. G. M. (1973). Moral and ethical dilemmas in the special-care nursery. *New England Journal of Medicine*, **289**, 890–4.

Duff, R. S. and Campbell, A. G. M. (1976). On deciding the care of severely handicapped or dying persons: with particular reference to infants. *Pediatrics*, **57**, 487–93.

Duff, R. S. and Campbell, A. G. M. (1980). Moral and ethical dilemmas: seven years into the debate about human ambiguity. *Annals, American Academy of Political and Social Science*, **447**, 19–28.

Ferngren, G. B. (1987). The status of defective newborns from late antiquity to the reformation. In *Euthanasia and the newborn: conflicts regarding saving lives*. (ed. R. C. McMillan, H. T. Engelhardt Jr. and S. F. Spicker), pp. 47–64. D. Reidel Publishing Co., Dordrecht.

Fleischman, A. R. and Murray, T. H. (1983). Ethics committees for infant Doe? *Hastings Center Report*, **13**, (6) 5–9.

Fost, N. (1981). Ethical issues in the treatment of critically ill newborns. *Pediatric Annals*, **10**, 383–9.

Ingelfinger, F. J. (1973). Bedside ethics for the hopeless case. *New England Journal of Medicine*, **289**, 914–15.

Kelly, G. (1950). The duty of using artificial means of preserving life. *Theological Studies*, **11**, 203–20.

Kohl, M. (1987). Moral arguments for and against maximally treating the defective newborn. In *Euthanasia and the newborn : conflicts regarding saving lives*. (ed. R. C. McMillan, H. T. Engelhardt Jr, and S. F. Spicker), pp. 233–52. D. Reidel Publishing Co., Dordrecht.

Ladd, J. (1980). Medical ethics: who knows best? *Lancet*, **2**, 1127–9.

Mooney, G. (1984). Medical ethics: an excuse for inefficiency? *Journal of Medical Ethics*, **10**, 183–5.

Moskop, J. C. and Saldanha R. L. (1986). The Baby Doe rule: still a threat. *Hastings Center Report*, **16** (2), 8–14.

Rachels, J. (1975). Active and passive euthanasia. *The New England Journal of Medicine*, **292**, 78–80.

Rachels, J. (1986). *The end of life: euthanasia and morality*, Oxford University Press.

Rhoden, N. K. (1984). The new neonatal dilemma: live births from late abortions. *The Georgetown Law Journal*, **72**, (5), 1451–1509.

Rhoden, N. K. (1986). Treating Baby Doe: the ethics of uncertainty. *Hastings Center Report*, **16**, (4), 34–42.

Robertson, J. A. and Fost, N. (1976). Passive euthanasia of defective newborn infants: legal considerations. *Journal of Pediatrics*, **88**, 883–9.

Sell, E. (1986). Outcome of very very low birth weight infants. *Clinics in Perinatology*, **13**, 451–9.

Shepperdson, B. (1983). Abortion and euthanasia of Down's syndrome children—the parents' view. *Journal of Medical Ethics*, **9**, 152–7.

Silverman, W. A. (1981). Mismatched attitudes about neonatal death. *Hastings Center Report*, **11**, (6), 12–16.

Sinclair, J. C. (1987). High technology, high costs, and the very low birth-weight newborn. In *Euthanasia and the newborn: conflicts regarding saving lives*. (ed. R. C. McMillan, H. T. Engelhardt Jr, and S. F. Spicker), pp. 169–89. D. Reidel Publishing Co., Dordrecht.

Speidel, B. D. (1986). Skimping on the care of the newborn is false economy. *British Medical Journal*, **293**, 575.

Stinson, R. and Stinson, P. (1981). On the death of a baby. *Journal of Medical Ethics*, **7**, 5–18.

Young, E. W. D. (1984). Societal provision for the long-term needs of the disabled in Britain and Sweden relative to decision-making in newborn intensive care units. *World Rehabilitation Fund Inc.*, New York.

7

Management of the child with a heart defect: ethical dilemmas

ELLIOT A. SHINEBOURNE

Almost all congenital heart abnormalities can be palliated if not corrected. Some infants, however, will be palliated only for a short time. In theory, the majority of uncorrectable defects could be treated by heart or heart/lung transplantation. A shortage of donor organs precludes this. There remain some complex heart anomalies which result in a short life expectancy even with palliation. The family and paediatric cardiologist then face the question 'should this life be prolonged?' rather than 'can it be prolonged by surgery?'

Are there circumstances when a heart operation is possible, but it is preferable or justifiable not to operate? The paediatric cardiologist has to treat (or not) the child, not only the cardiac abnormality. The child does not exist in isolation. Neither the child's heart nor the child can be considered independently of other persons concerned with the care of the child. For the newborn this is first the mother, and/or the father. Additional factors affecting management include associated abnormalities, the range of possibilities indicated by the family's social circumstances, the availability of expertise within a given hospital, and the extent to which a society elects or can afford to allocate scarce resources to a particular child.

Should coexistent abnormalities in the child influence treatment? If a child has two medical conditions it may be wrong to treat one without taking account of the other. An example is a child with severe mid-cavity obstruction in the right ventricle (double chambered right ventricle). The child has no symptoms related to the heart but is at risk of sudden death because of the severity of the obstruction. This same child has spinal muscular atrophy, a condition where there is progressive weakness of all muscles including those concerned with breathing. The concern is that if an operation requiring an anaesthetic were carried out, it might not be possible to extubate the child post-operatively. The operation may lengthen life, but because of weak respiratory muscles the child may remain dependent on a ventilator. The child's life expectancy is short but his quality of life within the family, though limited, brings fulfilment, and heart surgery may interfere with this. Here it would be correct not to operate.

Now, if the child did not have weak muscles but rather a chromosomal abnormality such as Down's syndrome, should this child have an operation? Again the answer is clear cut. Surgery should be carried out because the risk is low and the child's life expectancy will be increased. Though intellectually impaired, a child with Down's syndrome can form warm relationships with his family and others. Should then all children with Down's syndrome and a congenital heart abnormality be treated like children chromosomally normal? I would argue that there are circumstances where coexistent Down's syndrome does influence the decision (Bull *et al.* 1985).

Although rare in normal children, the commonest heart abnormality found with Down's syndrome is a complete atrioventricular septal (or canal) defect. Instead of two valves separating the atria from the ventricles, there is a common valve with large holes above (atrial septal defect) and below (ventricular septal defect) the common valve. Reviews of published literature indicate a hospital mortality for surgical correction of around 20 per cent with additional late deaths (Abbruzzese *et al*; Chin *et al.* 1982; Mavroudis *et al.* 1982). An optimistic estimate of 10-year survival would be 70 per cent. While some patients will have a technically perfect result others will not.

What if a child with Down's syndrome and an atrioventricular septal defect does not have surgery but is treated medically? In a group of such children followed up at our hospital, there was an 80 per cent 15-year actuarial survival (Bull *et al.* 1985). Many of these children presented at an age when surgery was in any case contraindicated because of secondary damage to the lungs. None the less, the actuarial survival in the non-operated patients is comparable with, or better than, in those treated surgically in the previous decade. Should, therefore, children with Down's syndrome be treated in the same way as otherwise normal children, and what advice should we give the family? There is evidence that medium-term survival is better with medical treatment, but death from progressive lung damage is inevitable in the third or fourth decade. Surgery carries a higher risk of early mortality but a prospect, albeit small, of adult life without cardiac disability. Life expectancy in Down's syndrome, even with a normal heart, is less than in a normal population. Furthermore, over the age of 35 years an increasing proportion of patients with Down's syndrome developed presenile dementia, particularly Alzheimer's disease. I would suggest that the frequent association of Alzheimer's disease in adults with Down's syndrome may be a reason for considering the early decades of life to be more important than a possibly longer life after surgery.

Acknowledging that the way in which information is presented may influence the decisions made, our experience has been that many parents of children with Down's syndrome and an atrioventricular septal defect elect for medical, not surgical, treatment. Conversely, the majority of parents with chromosomally normal children and the same defect choose surgery. An interpretation of Federal Law in the USA may consider it unlawful not to operate in these circumstances. In our opinion, however, the decision not to operate because of coexistent Down's syndrome may at times be equitable and not unethical. If the parents wish for surgery, especially if the child presents in the first three months of life, then operation should not be refused.

In otherwise normal children, should the nature of the cardiac anomaly itself sometimes be a contraindication to surgery? A diagram is shown of a complex anomaly with a common valve in the middle of the heart which leaks backwards and where there is only one main pumping chamber or ventricle. There is no direct blood supply to the lungs. Pulmonary blood flow is derived from the aorta via a tube or arterial duct present in the fetus. This duct will close spontaneously in the few days after birth, and death will follow if nothing else is done. The heart condition can never be cured surgically but could be palliated for a while. The affected child will be blue and breathless. The question is whether or not to palliate the child, as even with palliation quality of life will be poor.

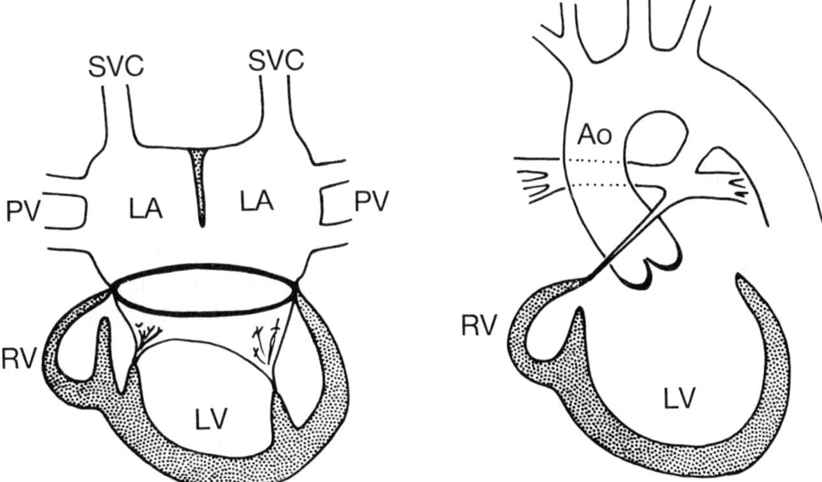

Fig. 1 Diagram of a complex congenital heart abnormality for which surgical treatment is unlikely to alleviate symptoms.
Two symmetrical left atria (LA) enter a left ventricle (LV). Each of the atria receive both blue blood (from superior vena cava, SVC) and red blood from pulmonary veins (PV). The right ventricle (RV) is rudimentary. A single great artery, the aorta (Ao), takes blood from the heart, blood reaching the lungs only via an arterial duct which is likely to close spontaneously resulting in the infant's death.

If the mother were aged 40 years, having her first child and wanting everything possible to be done, she might wish for palliation even if afterwards the child's life were miserable. It would be difficult or wrong not to operate if that were her expressed wish. What if, on the other hand, the parents are young married students, but the pregnancy is unplanned? Both wish to pursue their careers and do not want their baby to suffer. They may choose not to take on the burden of care. If they did not wish for palliative surgery to be undertaken, I would accept that view. Finally, consider the case of the unmarried mother of 14 years, who wants the child to have surgery, but whose mother, the baby's grandmother, does not; neither do the rest of the family. Although debatable, I think the decision of the mother of the newborn child, even though she is young, should be supported and prevail.

The previous paragraph may imply that parents decide whether or not surgery should be undertaken. If after full explanation parents definitely want surgery, their wishes should be respected. But if they do not want palliative surgery, should they make the final decision? The formal responsibility for not operating rests with the physician (paediatric cardiologist). The doctor has a duty to give as accurate as possible a prognosis on the future of the child with or without surgery, but his own views will influence the way in which the information is given to the family. Furthermore, the baby's progress may well be uncertain. Because of the uncertainty of outcome, it may be cruel to ask the parents if they want their baby to have an operation or to die. It is also dishonest, for in most cases the parents are coerced, consciously or unconsciously, by the doctor's opinion.

Even in the developed world there are not unlimited resources for health care. If the view is taken that all children with congenital heart disease should be operated on, this assumes all available resources should be used for all children. One of the few abnormalities for which conventional surgery remains unsatisfactory is the hypoplastic left heart syndrome. This is an anomaly where the left ventricle, the main pumping chamber of the heart, is grossly underdeveloped and the ascending aorta is tiny. In the few centres in the world where palliation is attempted, the mortality is still very high. An alternative approach would be infant heart transplantation (to be discussed later). Even if this were a possibility, donor human hearts will always be in short supply. If transplantation becomes acceptable, choices will still have to be made as to which children should be treated. Coexistent abnormalities will then influence the choice of which child to treat and a chromosomal abnormality such as Down's syndrome will be a contraindication.

Continuing the question of allocation of resources, surgery to correct congenital heart disease is expensive. Not only does it require the time of skilled nurses, doctors, and physiotherapists, but also the heart–lung machine, sterile fluids, cannulae, and tubing are expensive. In poor countries surgery for congenital heart disease poses an excessive demand on resources. The incidence of congenital heart disease is 8 per thousand live births, and 2.5 per thousand will die in the first year of life if untreated. In Britain, the United States, or Scandinavia, the infant mortality rate is less than 10 per thousand live births. In poorer countries, such as the Sudan or Nigeria, the infant mortality rate is greater than 100 per thousand live births. In these countries many hundreds of infants who may die from diarrhoea or malnutrition could be treated for the same cost as that of one open heart operation. Children dying from congenital heart disease represent about 20 per cent of all infants dying in the first year of life in developed countries, but only 2 per cent of those dying in poor countries. It is difficult to justify the cost of open heart surgery in the latter.

To return to the original question, should surgery be offered to all infants with congenital heart disease who can be operated upon? The answer sometimes has to be 'no'. The above factors will and should influence the decision.

What then is the ethical framework within which the paediatric cardiologist working in Britain can make such a decision? McCormick (1981) wrote that 'life is not a value to be preserved in and for itself . . . it is a value to be preserved precisely as a condition for other values . . . in so far as these remain attainable'. This value more than any other, is the potential for human relationships. When this potential is adjudged absent or likely to be so because of the poor physical condition of the child, then it may be appropriate not to intervene. In addition, the ability of those who care for the child has also to be considered. This person will usually be the mother or father. Whether they and the baby will be able to form a mutual relationship is a matter of judgement. If the family appears not to want intervention, they should be supported by a social worker, religious adviser, or friend. Society, ethics committees, and religious views provide guidelines and some substantive standards, but these cannot be inviolable rules. The final burden of decision falls on the doctor in whose care the child has been placed.

FETAL ECHOCARDIOGRAPHY: SCANNING THE FETUS FOR A CONGENITAL HEART ABNORMALITY

At present, accurate ultrasound imaging of the fetal heart is not possible in the first trimester of pregnancy. The heart can be accurately imaged only from 16 weeks gestation onwards (Allan *et al.* 1981). Abortion in the second trimester offers a greater risk to the woman than in the first trimester, morbidity of abortion increasing with gestational age (Grimes and Cates 1982). Once the diagnosis of a congenital heart abnormality is made, termination of pregnancy may be considered. This possibility should be considered before the fetal echo is performed. The implications of making a diagnosis of (major) congenital heart disease in the fetus are such that both the echocardiographer and the pregnant woman should be aware of what is involved both in a termination and in having a child with a 'heart problem'.

Termination of pregnancy for congenital heart disease poses an ethical dilemma. For the woman, termination may be carried out to protect her and perhaps, the family, from a perceived burden of care; but abortion may do her harm physically and/or emotionally. As for the fetus, abortion denies the fetus the possibility of life and that life may not be demonstrably awful. That a fetal heart abnormality is present may be relevant to a decision to terminate but this may still be an inadequate reason. Relevant risks are not necessarily sufficient to support a moral judgement. For instance, the reason for a woman to decide to have an abortion for congenital heart disease may be that she believes that all children with holes in the heart will be invalids. Here the reason for the action is relevant but neither adequate nor factually correct, as many holes in the heart close spontaneously and the child may in any case be asymptomatic.

When a cardiac anomaly is detected by fetal echocardiography, who should decide if termination should be carried out? Ultimately this decision should be made by the pregnant woman. In some societies or countries, however, abortion is only allowed in a very small proportion of cases, such as when the woman's life is threatened by continuation of pregnancy. Even if an inoperable cardiac anomaly were identifed in the fetus, the woman would not be allowed legally to obtain an abortion. It could be that she may then seek an illegal abortion with far greater attendant risks to herself. If the law of the country does not allow termination, screening the fetus for structural heart disease may not be ethically justifiable. One argument in its favour may be to alert the medical team to the need for rapid treatment of the newborn child. This reason is insufficient as by careful examination of the newborn the majority of cardiac abnormalities will be detected in any case. Furthermore, if abortion for fetal abnormality is illegal, it would be more sensible to undertake echocardiographic screening of newborn children than of fetuses. The woman's decision about termination, however, will be heavily based on information given to her by her doctors and by the way in which the information is presented. The obstetrician will explain the methods and risk of second trimester abortion while the echocardiographer or paediatric cardiologist will indicate the cardiac prognosis of the fetus with or without later surgical treatment.

Second trimester termination of pregnancy whether carried out by dilation and evacuation (D and E) of the uterus or by instillation of hypertonic urea and a prostaglandin carries a risk. Both techniques are unpleasant for the patient. Dilation and evacuation spares the woman from a long labour and seeing the fetus (Grimes and Schulz 1985), but is traumatic as the fetus is removed piecemeal from the uterus. In instillation abortion, the urea kills the fetus and the prostaglandin initiates labour. Grimes has described instillation abortion as 'A maxi-labour followed by a mini-delivery'.

If a cardiac anomaly is diagnosed in the fetus, which anomalies are sufficiently severe to warrant termination? One way of assessing this is to look at the actuarial survival of patients following correction of the cardiac defect. We do indeed regard such information as crucial when counselling parents before surgery as to the risk of operation. None the less, whether survival curves from one hospital are pertinent to operations performed elsewhere is debatable. Most fetal echocardiographers would regard termination of pregnancy for the hypoplastic left heart syndrome as acceptable (see later discussion on innovative therapy) and termination for a simple ventricular septal defect (the commonest form of hole in the heart) as unacceptable. Transposition of the great arteries is an abnormality where the aorta is connected to the right instead of the left ventricle, and the pulmonary artery taking blood to the lungs is connected to the left ventricle. As a result, blood with a low oxygen concentration recirculates round the body and the child is very blue. Twenty years ago virtually all babies with this condition died. Now that more than 80 per cent would be expected to survive 10 years (or much longer), termination of pregnancy is not usually considered. When there is only a single ventricle, termination may be offered even if under some circumstances the operation carries a similar 80 per cent success rate; quality of life however may be less good. Even for the echocardiographer it is not always easy to know what is the best advice.

It could be argued that the pregnant woman, with or without the father's agreement, should have the right to choose termination if she wishes. But should this right be overriding? Should the ethical principle of respect for autonomy take precedence over other principles, such as those of beneficence, non-maleficence, or justice? While not condoning unfettered medical paternalism, I would argue that the doctor does have a duty of beneficence. That is to say the doctor has a duty to care for and act in the best interests of the patient. If the doctor believes that the patient (here the pregnant woman) ought to be protected from the risk of making a choice which she might subsequently regret, perhaps he should exercise this duty in her interests (e.g. by refusing termination for a moderate-sized ventricular septal defect). There is little doubt that some harm is done to a woman by a termination and harm is certainly done to the fetus. By supporting the request for termination or by providing termination, the doctor may not be fulfilling a duty of non-maleficence. What about the fetus? The argument is easily sustained that the fetus' best interests are not promoted by its death.

The woman's conflict is whether to continue to allow her body to be used for the development of a fetus with an abnormal heart against her duty to protect the life of the fetus. Presuming that her own personal or religious views do not preclude abortion, her decision will be based on her perceptions of the amount of extra care the baby will require and the extent to which the baby's life expectancy and quality of life will be adversely affected by the heart condition.

In advising her, the paediatric cardiologist's own views on abortion and his attitude to duties owed to the fetus will also play a part in the manner in which he helps the woman come to a decision. His first duty is to discuss with the woman, before scanning her fetus, what might be found and what the implications might be, especially when fetal hearts are scanned as part of a routine screening programme. The cardiologist should also provide a fair guide to actuarial survival and the quality of life expected for the fetus and indicate the risks to the woman of second trimester abortion. It is inevitable that the information will be prejudiced by the particular values and ethical stance of the paediatric cardiologist which perhaps should also be made explicit. It is also important to realize that caring for a child with a congenital heart disease who dies young may bring joy to the family as well as sorrow.

EXPERIMENTAL OPERATIONS

Many simple congenital heart abnormalities such as defects in the ventricular or atrial septum can be corrected with a low mortality. To achieve better results generally requires elimination of error and proper application of what is already known. There remain, however, complex defects such as transposition of the great arteries or univentricular hearts, where the existing operations still have a significant mortality and sometimes an imperfect functional result. To improve management requires introduction of new operations. This experimental surgery should be part of a 'research' programme.

'Research' has been defined as either the act of searching (closely and carefully) for or after a specific thing or person (*Shorter Oxford English*

Dictionary), or as 'a systematic investigation to increase the sum of knowledge' (*Chambers Everyday Dictionary*). The British Paediatric Association defined 'therapeutic research' as research in which a procedure is of potential benefit to the subject. However, it is the procedure that is therapeutic, not research as such. Introducing a new operation on the heart should constitute 'therapeutic research', that is to say, it should be part of a carefully planned development (Shinebourne 1984). Certainly the surgeon will have admirable reasons for wishing to try something new and better to help his patients. But as Ramsay (1970) has commented, 'In this age of research medicine it is not only that medical benefits are obtained by research but also that a man rises to the top in medicine by the success and significance of his research'. This applies particularly to operations such as inserting a totally artificial heart or neonatal heart transplantation, where media coverage may have professional advantage whatever the outcome. None the less, new operations have to be attempted to advance medical treatment. Unnecessary suffering or death, however, may result from uncontrolled repetition. Thus the performance of a new operation as part of a planned research programme may be ethically justifiable but haphazard experimentation by many different surgical teams, possibly resulting in unnecessary mortality, may be deemed unethical.

Informed consent

In that informed consent is one means whereby autonomy is safeguarded, we should note the inherent problems in providing unbiased information to permit consent to a new operation or invasive procedure.

Informed consent should include an adequate explanation of alternative treatments available and also as clear as possible an analysis of the ratio of risk to benefit. Recommendation 4 of the United States National Commission Protecting Human Subjects of Biomedical Research (on children) states that, for a new treatment 'The relation of anticipated benefit to risk should be at least as favourable to the subjects as that presented by available alternative approaches'. This is particularly so with innovative cardiac surgery. The notion of a learning curve for a new operation is widely recognized. The first time a new operation is performed there may be technical difficulties not previously met; with practice or as a result of improvements in technique the probability of success becomes higher. This applies equally to new 'medical' procedures such as balloon dilatation of narrowed coronary arteries, pulmonary, or aortic valves. The first patient in whom a new procedure is performed is at greater risk than those to follow; yet no patient (in particular a child) should be operated on more for the benefit of future patients than for himself. Resolution of this ethical dilemma is difficult, but the patient (or person entrusted to give proxy consent on his or her behalf) must be fully informed of the risks and of the other procedures available.

Neonatal heart transplantation

Although most congenital heart abnormalities can be corrected or palliated, a few newborn infants have such a severe anomaly that replacement of the heart offers the only alternative to letting the child die. Opposition to neonatal heart transplantation may be because, while technically possible, rejection during childhood may be thought inevitable and the child's quality of life will be poor. Objection may be because of the difficulties of obtaining donor hearts and the belief that removing the heart of an anencephalic or irreparably brain-damaged baby is wrong. It may be felt that it would be bad for society because of the possible abuse of such a system in that donor hearts might be taken from brain-damaged babies while they still had some capacity, however small, for forming relationships. Objection may be on the grounds of cost and inappropriate use of scarce resources. Finally, we should ask if we wish to live in a society where a good intention, saving one baby by heart transplantation, has the secondary effect of more rapidly disposing of another baby with no brain. Perhaps this devalues the worth of the imperfect. I think the primary concern for the physician, however, is whether there is any realistic chance that a particular baby who has a heart transplant will live to form human relationships with others.

As with all research interventions in children, because of the problems of obtaining informed consent, and because of the need to protect children from exploitation and harm, new procedures should, where possible, always first be carried out on adults. Older children are more able to indicate their views than younger children, while neonates are potentially the most vulnerable group of all. At major centres the five year survival for adult heart transplantation is of the order of 60–70 per cent; death usually results from infection or rejection. Similar results are probably now possible in children although development of malignant disease may be an additional complication.

With this background it is perhaps useful to consider the treatment options for the hypoplastic left heart syndrome. In this defect the left ventricle is extremely small and unable to perform its normal function of pumping blood round the body. In addition the aortic valve is atretic and the ascending aorta often only two or three millimetres in diameter rather than the normal one centimetre. The anomaly occurs in about one in every 12 000 live births and causes one quarter of cardiac deaths in newborns. Hitherto the majority of these babies have been allowed to die. A complex two-stage surgical approach has been developed by Norwood *et al.* (1983) in Philadelphia. Some success has been achieved with this but mortality remains high and the long-term outlook questionable. Transplantation with a human heart has been tried once, unsuccessfully, in England where there has been a moratorium on further neonatal transplants while the ethical, legal, and resource implications are reviewed. In view of the increasing success with heart and heart/lung transplantation in children, it is inevitable that human heart transplantation will be used to treat this anomaly. As the procedure will have a chance of success in the particular baby so treated, it will become no longer unethical. Transplantation with a heart from another species, however, still remains unethical because as yet there is no realistic hope of a reasonable survival time. The ethics may change if problems of interspecies rejection can be effectively countered: questions of ethics can never be separated from questions of good or ill effect.

REFERENCES

Abbruzzese, P. A., Livermore, J., and Sunderland, C. O. (1983). Mitral repair in complete atrioventricular canal. *Journal of Thoracic and Cardiovascular Surgery*, **85**, 388–95.

Allan, L. D., Tynan, M. J., Campbell, S., and Anderson, R. H. (1981). Identification of congenital cardiac malformations by echo-cardiography in mid trimester fetus. *British Heart Journal*, **46**, 358–62.

Bull, C., Rigby, M. L., and Shinebourne, E. A. (1985). Should management of complete atrioventricular canal defect be influenced by coexistent Down's Syndrome? *Lancet*, **1**, 1147–9.

Chin, A. J., Keane, J. F., Norwood, W. I., and Castenada, A. R. (1982). Repair of complete common atrioventricular canal in infancy. *Journal of Thoracic and Cardiovascular Surgery*, **84**, 437–45.

Grimes, D. A. and Cates, W. Jr. (1979). The comparative efficacy and safety of intra-amniotic Prostaglandin F2alpha and hypertonic saline for second-trimester abortion: a review and critique. *Journal of Reproductive Medicine*, **22**, 248–54.

Grimes D. A. and Cates, W. Jr. (1982). Instrumental abortion in the second-trimester: an overview. In *Second-trimester pregnancy termination*, (ed. M. J. N. C. Keirse *et al.*), pp. 65–79. University of Leiden Press, The Hague.

Grimes, D. A. and Schulz, K. F. (1985). The comparative safety of second-trimester abortion methods. In *Ciba Foundation Symposium 115*, pp. 83–96. Pitman, London.

Mavroudis, C., Weinstein, G., Turley, K., and Ebert, P. A. (1982). Surgical management of complete atrioventricular septal (canal) defects. *Journal of Thoracic and Cardiovascular Surgery*, **83**, 670–9.

McCormack, R. A. (1981). *How brave a new world?* SCM Press Ltd., London.
Norwood, W. I., Lang, P., and Hanson, D. D. (1983). Physiological repair of the aortic atresia—hypoplastic left heart syndrome. *New England Journal of Medicine*, **308**, 23–6.
Ramsey, P. (1970). Consent as a canon of loyalty with special reference to children in medical investigations. In *The patient as person*, pp. 1–58. Yale University Press, New Haven.
Shinebourne, E. A. (1984). Ethics of innovative cardiac surgery. *British Heart Journal*, **52**, 597–601.

8

The care of the sexually active adolescent girl

JOHN HARE

Of the several rights bestowed on the citizen of the United Kingdom on his or her sixteenth birthday none invites more interest or controversy than the right to participate in heterosexual intercourse. Before that date sexual relationships are illegal, and any adult member of the opposite sex involved in such relationships with a minor is committing an offence in law. For girls especially, the 'age of consent' has been built up in our society as a major milestone in life, attracting cultural and commercial, as well as legal, interests. After she reaches this age a girl is her own mistress; free to form sexual relationships, use contraception, become pregnant, and, if she wishes, marry, although for this last parental consent is needed for the next two years. Before then she is supposedly untouchable and almost sacred; the forbidden fruit in the garden.

But forbidden fruit is usually all the more desired, and the issue of sexuality in the adolescent girl has always fascinated older men and women. From classical stories such as Daphnis and Chloë, through the crude and rumbustious attitudes of the Middle Ages and the sordid dealings of the Victorian underworld we find our own age no less interested. In recent years the success of the novel *Lolita*, the film *Mona Lisa*, and the advertising campaigns for a brand of jeans that depended for its appeal on whether or not the 15-year-old model was wearing anything under them are typical of the response to this topic. On 21 September 1987 the *Guardian* newspaper, in an editorial comment on the sensational content of some of its tabloid competitors, declared that 'ours is a society that is relentlessly forcing back the boundaries of teenage sexuality', despite a strong but superficial attitude favouring a return to conservative moral values. For teenage sexuality is big business; it sells newspapers and much else, and 'in any contest between the market and morality, the market will win every time'.

Fiction and fantasy are the acceptable face of unpalatable reality; underage girls *do* indulge in sexual activity and directly flout the law, and how I as a physician and gynaecologist should respond to them is the subject of this chapter. I shall not discuss the question of sex and health education, although doctors will usefully become involved in the planning and delivery of such programmes. Nor shall I concern myself with assault, or rape. I shall assume the girl is sexually active of her own volition, and concentrate on three main clinical situations when she might seek help: sexually transmitted infection, the request for contraceptive advice and supplies, and pregnancy.

Before the clinical discussion, however, it would seem important to review the legal, medical, and sociological aspects of the age of consent. Certainly there is no natural or universal law concerning this and Barron (1986) notes the worldwide variation to be from 12 years in India to 18 years in the Republic of China. Kinsey *et al.* (1953) reported that the age of consent varied in the several states of the USA from 14 years to 21 years, with 18 years being the commonest age set. Answers from enquiries made to the London embassies of the countries of the European Community reveal that within this tightly-linked group differences remain. In the United Kingdom, Luxembourg, the Netherlands, and West Germany the age of consent is 16 years, although in Germany the girl who cannot be proven to be 'chaste' would appear to lose some of her rights in law. In Italy the age is 18 years, in the Irish Republic 17 years, and in Greece and Denmark 15 years. In Spain there is no law directly governing this matter, but by the extrapolation of related statutes it would appear that permission may be assumed by a girl and her partner at an age which may vary between 12 and 18 years. No replies were forthcoming from the embassies of France, Belgium, or Portugal.

The medical hazards of pregnancy in teenagers are well reported, and it is generally accepted that the younger the girl, the greater the risk involved. However these results are invariably biased by the legal strictures involved; below the age of consent the pregnant girl is a shameful object, either hiding herself or hidden by her relatives. Pregnancy is often discovered late, and antenatal care lacking. Many problems are created by neglect rather than by nature, and certainly for 14- and 15-year-olds the dangers have been overstressed.

It would seem, therefore, that there is no international or natural standard by which an age of consent can be set down; the only general agreement being that prepubertal coitus is wrong and that above the age of 18 years girls should be entitled to make up their own minds about when to enter a liaison, assuming, that is, that they are of sound mind and that no physical, mental, or economic duress is applied to them. What happens in practice also needs to be known.

In their monumental work on female sexuality Kinsey *et al.* (1953) recorded that 3 per cent of the American women they questioned had had intercourse before the age of 16 years. Underage coitus was more common in lower social class groups, those of lower educational attainment, and those who married early. There was a slight rise in the proportion of sexually experienced girls in successive decades, from 2 per cent in those born before 1900 to 4 per cent in those born between 1920 and 1929. In Kinsey's survey Catholic girls were far more likely to have had underage coitus than Protestant or Jewish girls, and the devout adherent to any religion less likely than the lukewarm.

The incidence of underage coitus in Britain was fully explored by Michael Schofield in *The sexual behaviour of young people* published in 1965. He reported that very few girls (0.1 per cent) had had intercourse before the age of 14, and the figures for before 15 and 16 were 1 per cent and 3 per cent respectively. Underage girls were almost always introduced to intercourse by an older boy; only 3 per cent claimed initiation with a partner of their own age or younger. Almost always first intercourse was unplanned. Early starters at intercourse (whom Schofield defines as those who started at 16 years or under) tended to come from working-class rather than middle-class homes, to come from less religious homes, and to have left full-time education at the minimum statutory age. Although their attitude to sex was often romantic, it was less so than those who experienced their first coitus at a later age. Only a few girls claimed to have enjoyed their first coitus, but unexpectedly early starters said they did so more often than the later starters. Despite the apparent lack of enjoyment most repeated the experience fairly soon—of teenage girls 63 per cent had intercourse again within a month, 34 per cent within a week and 2 per cent within 24 hours.

Schofield concluded from his study that young sexually experienced girls, far more than boys, were rejecting family influences. Relationships between parents and daughters were commonly strained and these girls were less likely than others to seek or receive advice on sexual matters from their parents. In the same way religious influence meant less to the experienced than the unexperienced teenage girl, although they were just as likely to come from church-going families. If they did seek advice on sexual matters it was more usually from friends of their own age than from adults.

Just over a decade later, in 1978, Christine Farrell in *My mother said . . .* produced statistics that can be used for comparison. In her sample she found that 12 per cent of the girls and 26 per cent of the boys claimed to have had full sexual intercourse before their sixteenth birthdays. Although boys from higher social groups were less likely to be sexually experienced than those from lower groups, this factor appeared irrelevant for the girls; for girls religion was a marker of activity in that those who stated they were members of a Protestant non-conformist church were less likely to be sexually experienced than those who belonged to other churches or no church at all.

To my knowledge no later study has been undertaken on this subject in such depth, and therefore for the purpose of this chapter I will assume that roughly one in eight girls is sexually active for some time before her sixteenth birthday. For most the period of sexual activity will have been less than a year; for some it will have been longer and for a small minority much longer.

SEXUALLY TRANSMITTED DISEASE

Of the three medical encounters I have to discuss, the consultation for sexually transmitted disease is perhaps the easiest and least controversial. This is a typical 'medical' situation; a patient who suspects that she might be ill or diseased, seeking the advice of a physician who she hopes will have the skill to recognize and heal her. Having identified that she is underage the doctor should at this point ask her if her mother (or another close relative) is aware of the situation and urge that she is asked to attend to chaperone the examination and witness at least part of the consultation. If this proves impossible or the girl is adamantly opposed to it, it is ethically acceptable and correct that the consultation should continue. Especial care must be taken over genital examination, for which, strictly speaking, an underage girl is unable to give consent; this must be conducted by a senior doctor who is both skilled and sympathetic. The examination must never be repeated for teaching purposes, and the rules of chaperonage must be strictly applied.

The level of sexually transmitted disease in underage girls is far from insignificant. The incidence of gonorrhoea recorded in 1982 from clinic returns was 6.4 per cent per 100 000 of population for girls under 16 years, around three times the recorded level for boys of the same age. This rate had remained constant for five years, despite a slight fall in the reported incidence of gonorrhoea amongst the total female population. Apart from syphilis, where the figures are too low to be of significance, detailed analyses of age groups are not available for the prevalence of other sexually transmitted conditions, but one can assume that the figures are comparable.

If the girl is found to be infected with a sexually transmitted disease and requires treatment, such treatment can be given and follow-up arranged using the general principles already outlined. As with adults, contact tracing should be carried out where appropriate and the girl asked to identify her sexual partners under the usual arrangements for confidentiality. Additionally the girl identified as underage should be interviewed by a social worker or trained counsellor who can gently make a full exploration of her sexual relationships. Inevitably in some, problems such as child abuse will be uncovered, or other situations from which the girl recognizes she needs help to escape. If such recognition occurs, all necessary help can be arranged by appropriate professionals.

There remains, however, the situation where such help is not sought or is positively refused. The girl may see herself as a normal member of a substantial minority who follow natural instincts which lead to a law being broken in the United Kingdom by what would be perfectly legal behaviour elsewhere. She may consider her sex life her own affair which she herself can manage, and the risks that she takes over sexually transmitted disease acceptable. Moreover she may justifiably claim that it was by her frankness to the doctor that she put herself in her present position. Most women who attend sexually transmitted disease clinics refer themselves, and their general practitioners are either left unaware of the attendance or informed later. Most underage girls who attend are aged 14 or 15, and will be fully aware that by giving a date of birth indicating that they are just 16 they will circumvent many problems. During one such consultation I became suspicious that my patient was misrepresenting her age. Leaning my hand, as if by accident, on the portion of the notes marked with the registration data I casually enquired 'What was your date of birth?' to be met with the firm answer 'What it says in the notes'.

The problem has arisen, therefore, because the girl has been open and honest about her age and has truthfully revealed information which is of no direct importance in the medical management of her case. Had she not done this her primary medical management would not have been any less effective. Given these factors the ethical position seems clear; medical trust and confidentiality must remain paramount. Advice and counselling should be available and the law must be explained: and if parental help and support is not available other help, including contraception, may need to be offered; but the trust with which she has approached her doctor must be honoured.

Thankfully most of these girls will be in the 14- and 15-year age group and can be recognized as the tail of a normal distribution curve which happens to be cut off by the line on the graph at 16 years which represents the law. Doctors may feel as individuals that what these girls do is morally or biologically wrong; they may strive as citizens to create a moral climate where premarital and underage sexual activity become less common; but they cannot call such activity medically abnormal or aberrant.

Although the law has been flouted, police authorities will normally take no action in such cases, provided the girl has passed her fourteenth birthday and the boy or man was no more than ten years her senior. A much more serious problem arises if the girl is under 14 years. Then the offence committed is in law more serious, and the chances that exploitation or abuse has occurred are much more likely. Nevertheless the same principles will apply, and painstaking counselling and discussion will always need to be carried out. Almost always a way will be found to be of help, even if this is initially only an arrangement to keep in touch and have further discussions. Only if all else fails and the doctor is convinced that his patient is being exploited or abused should an unauthorized break of confidence be considered. This would be through the local Social Services Department, never directly to the police authorities.

CONTRACEPTION

The question of contraceptive counselling presents different problems. Here we have a girl presenting as a well person for advice and help on how to run her life. If she presents to her general practitioner, her age and history are known; if she refers herself to a separate family planning clinic, she may choose to falsify or conceal some of these details. However if her details are known it is obvious that she intends to be party to the law being broken, and to encourage another person to do the same. For many doctors the stumbling block is that they feel they too are being drawn into the criminal circle by facilitating this act.

Farrell found that very few young people use a medically prescribed contraceptive at the first incident of coitus. Reporting on 16–19-year-olds, but stating that these figures are true for the younger group who have intercourse before the age of 16, she states that only 8 per cent of girls were taking oral contraceptives at the age of first intercourse. At the time of that experience 43 per cent claimed no contraceptive usage, 36 per cent that their partner used a sheath, 10 per cent that he practised withdrawal, and 1 per cent that they were using the safe period, chemicals, or other unspecified methods. For subsequent episodes younger girls tended to rely on withdrawal or the sheath, with eventually 36 per cent of sexually active 16-year olds taking the oral contraceptive pill. Eleven per cent of sexually active 16-year-olds claimed never to have taken any birth control precautions.

It would seem from these figures and from those quoted earlier on patterns of sexual behaviour that the question the underage girl is asking her doctor is not 'Should I start or continue to have sexual intercourse?' but 'How can I best guard against pregnancy resulting from continuing to have sexual intercourse?' Of course the doctor has a full counselling role to play, and this will include the potential dangers of underage sexual activity, but his attitude must be positive rather than negative. Abstinence may be the ideal solution for most if not all, but it will be acceptable to few. Above all he must show sympathy and understanding and give the impression that he has time and interest. According to Farrell under half of the teenage group felt that their doctor was easy to talk to and only half felt that he had the time to discuss contraception with them. Unfortunately young girls seemed to experience such problems in communication most commonly. Having discussed the matter, the doctor may feel free to suggest, prescribe, or fit the method of contraception he thinks most appropriate for that girl, which will almost always be the diaphragm, sheath, or hormonal method.

The greatest fear that prevents young girls from attending for birth control advice is the fear that their sexual activity will be revealed. In Farrell's series this reluctance decreased with increasing age and becoming engaged (and of course married). Less than half of the 16-year olds were happy that their confidence would be kept, and such worries increased if the doctor appeared to have little time or was difficult to communicate with. Such fear also accounted for a great deal of reluctance to attend special family planning clinics, not because the integrity of the staff was questioned but because of the risk of being seen entering or waiting in a clinic which obviously dealt with this single problem.

The question of confidentiality in contraceptive advice to underage girls has recently had a full and thorough legal airing, and it would seem worthwhile to detail the discussion here. Mrs Victoria Gillick, a mother of five daughters then under the age of 16 years, sought to challenge the DHSS ruling on the availability of contraceptive advice and supplies to underage girls by requesting an assurance from her local Health Authority that none of her daughters would be given abortions or contraceptive treatment while they were under the age of 16 years, and that should any of them seek advice in a family planning clinic she would automatically be contacted and informed. Not receiving such an undertaking Mrs Gillick sued both the local Health Authority and the DHSS on this matter. She had no success in the High Court, and so took the matter to the Court of Appeal.

The Court of Appeal found in her favour (*British Medical Journal* 1985). Lord Justice Parker ruled that:

> ' a girl under 16 could neither by her consent deprive any assault of its criminal nature, nor validly prohibit a doctor from seeking parental consent. Moreover, any doctor who advised a girl under 16 as to contraceptive steps to be taken or afforded contraceptive advice or abortion treatment to such a girl without the knowledge and consent of her parents, save in emergency, infringed the legal rights of her parent or guardian. Except in cases of emergency the proper course was to seek the parents' consent or apply to the court.'

The question of what constituted an emergency was left undefined.

The case then went to the House of Lords, where this ruling was overturned by the Law Lords by a majority of three to two (Dyer 1985). Lord Fraser, the senior Law Lord, stated that there was:

'no statutory provision which compels me to hold that a girl under the age of 16 years lacks the legal capacity to consent to contraceptive advice, examination and treatment provided she has sufficient understanding and intelligence to know what they involve'.

The crux of his judgment was:

'The only practicable course is, in my opinion, to entrust the doctor with a discretion to act in accordance with his view of what is best in the interest of the girl who is his patient. He should, of course, always seek to persuade her to tell her parents that she is seeking contraceptive advice and the nature of the advice she receives. At least he should seek to persuade her to agree to the doctor's informing the parents. But there may well be cases and I think there will be some cases where the girl refuses either to tell the parents herself or to permit the doctor to do so, and in some cases the doctor will, in my opinion, be justified in proceeding without the parents' consent or even knowledge provided he is satisfied on the following matters:

1. that the girl, although under 16 years of age, will understand his advice;
2. that he cannot persuade her to inform her parents or allow him to inform her parents that she is seeking contraceptive advice;
3. that she is very likely to begin or to continue to have sexual intercourse with or without contraceptive advice;
4. that unless she receives contraceptive advice or treatment her physical or mental health or both are likely to suffer;
5. that her best interests require him to give her contraceptive advice, treatment or both without parental consent.'

He warned, however, that doctors ought not to regard this as a licence to disregard the wishes of the parents whenever they feel it convenient.

Another Law Lord, Lord Scarman added that:

'The principle of the law was that parental rights were derived from parental duties and existed only so long as they were needed for the protection of the person and the property of the child. Parental right yielded to the child's right to make his decisions when he reached a sufficient understanding and intelligence to be capable of making up his own mind.'

Despite this judgment, opposing views are still heard. The General Medical Council (GMC), while recognizing the Law Lords' ruling, stresses that:

'If the doctor is not satisfied of the child's (under 16 years old) ability to understand, he may decide to disclose the information learned from the consultation, but if he does so he should inform the patient accordingly, and his judgment concerning disclosure or advice must always reflect both the patient's best medical interests and the trust which the patient places in the doctor'. (GMC 1986)

The question here is of emphasis. Anybody can invent a case where confidentiality would have to be broken, for example a seven-year-old child with sexually transmitted herpes virus infection in my own practice. However, the GMC ruling by its layout and its emphasis suggests that the girl's immaturity will often be the deciding factor, rather than an extreme exception to the rule. This impression is dangerous.

The ethical problem crystalizes in the Scarman judgments. Sexual maturity is one of the signs of the passage of childhood into adulthood, and sexual responsibility is one of the burdens that needs to be taken up as adulthood approaches. If of her own free will a girl has assumed this burden she has taken over the responsibility for it from her parents, and we must assist her to bear it. This assistance must be caring, honest, and positive, and the younger she is the more assistance she will need. Usually such assistance will also come from others, especially parents, but she has the right not to ask for this, or to reject it if it is given. Above all this right entails the liberty to make mistakes; the best advice should be given to try to prevent this, but she has the liberty to be wrong.

PREGNANCY

There remains the most difficult issue of all to discuss, the question of pregnancy in the underage girl. That such pregnancies occur is obvious to all, but the extent of the problem may surprise many. In 1985 in England and Wales there were 9600 reported pregnancies in girls under 16 years, excluding spontaneous miscarriages before 28 weeks' gestation, for which there are no ways of collecting statistics (OPCS 1987). Fifty-six per cent of these (5376) ended in pregnancy termination, and 44 per cent (4224) of these girls had babies. A significant and worrying feature of the underage girls seeking abortion is how late they do so. Thus girls under 15 years make up 0.4 per cent of those having termination before 9 weeks of pregnancy, 0.8 per cent of these between 9 weeks and 12 weeks (which represents the upper limit for optimum safety), 1.3 per cent of these between 13 and 19 weeks, and 2.2 per cent of those having the physically and mentally traumatic experiences of pregnancy termination at 20 weeks or over. The corresponding figures for 15-year olds having abortions are 1.5 per cent of those before 9 weeks, 2.2 per cent of those between 9 and 12 weeks, 3.7 per cent of those from 13 to 19 weeks, and 4.8 per cent of the total over 20 weeks. The lack of someone to confide in and fear of betrayal of confidence contribute very largely to the upward trend in these figures, especially in the 20 weeks and over group, which should be less representative from the younger girls as it contains a high number of woman undergoing termination because of fetal abnormality detected by amniocentesis.

Even if we accept that guaranteed confidentiality will lead to sooner consultations and a safer outcome whatever the management, three situations may create further dilemmas. These are:

1. When a pregnant underage girl wishes to continue with her pregnancy, and her parents or guardians wish her to undergo pregnancy termination.

2. When a pregnant underage girl wishes pregnancy termination and her parents or guardians wish her to continue with the pregnancy.

3. When a pregnant underage girl seeks pregnancy termination, and her parents or guardians know neither that she is pregnant nor that she is seeking termination.

Before discussing these situations we must look at the working of the abortion law in this country. Most terminations are carried out under clause 2 of the Abortion Act 1967, which allows an abortion to be carried out if, in the opinion of two doctors, 'continuation of the pregnancy would be a threat to the physical or mental health of the pregnant woman greater than if the pregnancy were terminated'. The ethics of pregnancy termination is a large and much debated subject, and no room can be found in this chapter to explore it in detail. Suffice it to state that, by general consensus, social, cultural, and economic factors are taken into account in the decision and for those cases where the decision rests largely on these factors, this clause is invoked.

In general it is always better that parents are aware of their daughter's pregnancy, and support her in the decision she has made concerning it. However, if there is disagreement it could almost never be right for the daughter to be forced to have a termination performed against her will, certainly not on social, economic, or cultural grounds; however adverse the circumstances, the girl must have the last word. In severe mental handicap when the girl is truly unable to grasp what has happened to her, a case could be made for the parental duty to make a decision, but apart from this, very few medical conditions demand such intervention.

The girl's attitude in such cases is often acquired from her parents, and any inconsistency is theirs. In one case I sat bewildered between mother and daughter when, in response to her mother's demand to know who gave her the 'nonsense' idea to go on with the pregnancy, the girl retorted forcefully 'you did'. The evils of abortion and the profligate and unworthy nature of those who sought it had been the main thread of the mother's teaching on sexual matters, and now, faced with the situation herself, she realized too late that this was not what she had meant to say.

At the other extreme, no one should compel an underage girl to have a child she does not want. If she asks for the pregnancy to be terminated, is mentally capable of making up her own mind, has been fully counselled, and is under no duress or misapprehension, then her decision should be final. One can have immense sympathy with parents who for religious, moral, or ethical reasons reject termination and wish their daughter to have her baby, but the decision is not finally theirs. Her view is paramount, although a court action on her behalf by a social worker might be necessary. I must stress that I have never known of such a case.

Less understandable and equally unacceptable is the decision not to terminate a pregnancy for other reasons, in particular in order to 'teach her a lesson'. This situation arises much more commonly with the older girl, but especially if her behaviour is reckless and antisocial, perhaps having led to a pregnancy previously. Parents, doctors, and nurses may all feel antagonism towards her and decide that she needs to be taught a lesson. However undesirable the girl's behaviour may appear this attitude is never acceptable; no one should be made to bear a child as punishment for antisocial behaviour.

Cases do occur in the third group; cases where the underage girl presents pregnant, requesting a termination with her parents or legal guardians being kept unaware of the situation. Almost always this is a panic reaction, and befriending by a counsellor who can help the girl break the news to her family is what is most needed. Rarely, this request will hide an incestuous relationship or one with a close family friend, and again counselling and skilled help is required. But sometimes, albeit uncommonly, what the girl is making is a considered request with the best interests of the family in mind.

Two cases come to my mind to illustrate this. The first involved the daughter of an immigrant family from southern Italy, where the father and mother both felt strongly about their strict traditional code of honour. I have often idly speculated as to whether the common phrase 'my dad'll kill me if he finds out' fulfils strictly the first clause of the Abortion Act (the continuation of the pregnancy represents a threat to the life of the pregnant woman) but in this case the general practitioner agreed with the girl; violence against her or her boyfriend was highly likely if either parent found out. Despite her age, I terminated the pregnancy without parental consent. The other case was different; a loving family, close-knit but already badly shaken and traumatized by circumstances beyond their control. The eldest daughter, depressed by these events, unthinkingly laid herself open to rape, from which she became pregnant. In her view severe damage would have been done to the family had her plight been revealed, and she did not feel this was justified. To me her judgement seemed mature although the risk to her was considerable, but after counselling I went ahead and terminated the pregnancy.

The age of consent is arbitrary; even in similar civilized societies there is no general agreement. For most it is a useful guideline to acceptable behaviour, and the fact that one in eight girls flout it does not mean that it automatically needs adjusting downwards. However, as with any legal restraint on moral or personal behaviour, sympathetic help must be available for those who find themselves outside the law. Confidentiality and trust are paramount. In most cases parental support, and reconciliation, sometimes after initial trauma, is most of what is required. In a minority of circumstances, however, for various reasons this may not be possible. Then the doctor must accept that he is dealing with a young adult who is trying to pull together what remains of her life, and he must afford her the courtesy, confidentiality, and rights of adulthood. However unhappy it may make us all, these include the liberty to make a mistake.

REFERENCES

Barron, S. L. (1986). Sexual activity in girls under 16 years of age. *British Journal of Obstetrics and Gynaecology*, **93**, 787–93.

British Medical Journal (1985). Teenage confidence and consent. *British Medical Journal*, **290**, 144–5.

Dyer, C. (1985). Contraceptives and the under 16s: House of Lords ruling. *British Medical Journal*, **291**, 1208–9.

Farrel, C. (1978). *My mother said . . . .* Routledge and Kegan Paul, London.

GMC (General Medical Council) (1986). GMC's revised guidance. *British Medical Journal*, **292**, 570.

Kinsey, A. C., Pomeroy, W. B., Martin, C. E., and Gebhard, P. (1953). *Sexual behaviour in the human female*. W. B. Saunders, Philadelphia.

OPCS (1987). *Abortion statistics for the year 1985*. Office of Population, Censuses and Surveys, London.

Schofield, M. (1965). *The sexual behaviour of young people*. Longmans, London.

9
The care of patients with sexually transmitted diseases

A. MINDEL

INTRODUCTION AND HISTORICAL PERSPECTIVE

Historically, sex and the management of patients with sexually transmitted diseases have always involved a host of moral and ethical dilemmas, and the medical profession's conduct has generally been dominated by fears, misconceptions, and prejudices existing in society at the time. If one looks back to the late nineteenth and early twentieth centuries 'Victorian morals' then forced the government to introduce legislation in an attempt to control the venereal infections which were widespread in the community at that time. The Contagious Diseases Acts of 1864, 1866, and 1869, and the Royal Commission on the Poor Law of 1909 required or recommended compulsory detention in hospital of infected prostitutes and patients with venereal infection; and the Royal Commission on Divorce of 1912 considered that the passing on of a venereal disease was an act of cruelty and the strongest grounds for divorce. Patients with venereal infection were also liable to lose their livelihood (House of Commons Report 1911).

Sentiments within the medical profession were equally intolerant and short-sighted. Sir Francis Champneys, a renowned physician, wrote in 1917 that 'it is better that venereal diseases should be imperfectly combated than that, in an attempt to prevent them, men should be enticed into mortal sin which they would otherwise avoid.' (Champneys 1917). Some even advocated the refusal of treatment. 'You have had the disease one year, and I hope it may plague you many more to punish you for your sins, and I would not think of treating you' (Royal Commission on Venereal Diseases 1916).

Punitive legislative measures and narrow-minded sexual attitudes did little to control the sexually transmitted diseases (STDs). The problem was reaching crisis point in the early years of this century. An example of this can be found in a serological survey concluded in 1914, which showed that 12 per cent of adult males and 7 per cent of females in London had evidence of syphilis (Adler 1980). With this background the government formed a Royal Commission under the chairmanship of Lord Sydenham of Combe; evidence was first taken in 1913 and the final report was made in 1916 (Royal Commission on Venereal Diseases 1916). The impetus of a Royal Commission and the implementation of its recommendations were undoubtedly boosted by the growing number of cases of gonorrhoea and syphilis among troops fighting in and returning from the First World War (Rout 1922; Parran and Vonderlehr 1941). The Commission recognized the difficulties despite the moral overtones within the community, and recommended the setting up of an open access medical service, funded mainly from central government. The extensive clinic system of today, consisting of over 200 clinics nationwide, reflects the implementation of the Royal Commission's recommendations.

Despite the fact that a national STD service has been available for 60 years, many physicians and members of the public still see the specialty as having a social stigma, and indeed many clinics, even some within prestigious medical schools, are still situated in basements or prefabricated builidings, away from the main hospital complex. The liberalization of attitudes to sex in recent years has led to a better understanding of the sexually transmitted diseases and their control. Unfortunately, much of the demystification of the STDs and improvement in attitudes is in danger of being swept aside with the wave of moral indignation apparent within society since the advent of the AIDS (Acquired Immune Deficiency Syndrome) (*The Sun* 1985; *Daily Telegraph* 1983).

CONFIDENTIALITY

Protection of patients' confidences forms the cornerstone of medical practice in this specialty. Indeed, the National Health Service Act of 1946 forbade the dissemination of information about a patient with a venereal infection to any third party without the patient's consent. Two further measures, the National Health Service (VD) Regulation 1968, No. 1624 and 1974, No. 29, also embody this principle. To quote from the latter act:

> 'Every Regional Health Authority, and every Area Health Authority, shall take all necessary steps to secure that any information capable of identifying an individual obtained by officers of the Authority, with respect to persons examined or treated for any sexually transmitted disease, shall not be disclosed except:
>
> (a) for the purpose of communicating that information to a medical practitioner, or to a person employed under the direction of a medical practitioner in connection with the treatment of a person suffering from such a disease or the prevention of the spread thereof, and;
>
> (b) for the purpose of such treatment or prevention.' (National Health Service (VD) Regulation 1974)

It is apparent that the physician looking after patients with sexually transmitted infections has a dual responsibility. On the one hand, there is the protection of the patient's confidences, on the other is the public health responsibility—prevention of further spread of the infection. The physician will, in most circumstances, encourage patients to inform contacts, stressing the possibilities of asymptomatic infection, complications, and further spread. The use of skilled contact tracers (discussed below) is often of help. Problems arise when the patient is unwilling to inform contacts and when the physician is aware of the identity of the contacts. In these circumstances each case should be dealt with on its merits. That is to say, contacts of patients with minor infections, without serious long-term consequences, can probably be ignored. If the consequences are potentially more serious, some physicians would advocate that an attempt should be made to find and treat the contact irrespective of the patient's wishes. This is not my view, nor indeed, the view of most doctors working in genito-urinary medicine.

In recent years, with greater public awareness and acceptance of sexual matters generally, and with the growing complexity and possible long-term consequences of some of the illnesses dealt with by genito-urinary physicians, general practitioners, doctors in other specialties, and dentists are increasingly requesting more information about their patients. Many patients are unwilling for their doctors to know the details of their history and diagnosis. The GP may be an old family friend and may be unaware of the patient's sexuality and sexual practices. The patient may feel that this information could prejudice his future management, or that details of his sexual activities may inadvertently be divulged to a third party.

The current practice in most genito-urinary medicine clinics is not to divulge any information to another doctor unless the patient was originally referred by him, or the patient requests that the doctor be informed. In the case of a more serious illness it is generally suggested that the patient informs the general practitioner or allows the clinic to do so. If the patient refuses, the refusal is respected. This argument is becoming more difficult to sustain in the light of infection that may have serious consequences for the patient and his partner; for example, the association of chlamydial infection with pelvic inflammatory disease, the possibility of the development of chronic hepatitis in a hepatitis B carrier, or the possible association of human papilloma virus with carcinoma of the cervix. In these circumstances, many physicians would consider that placing more pressure on the patient to inform the GP was acceptable.

There are two other circumstances in which it would be desirable for other health care personnel to be aware of the patient's diagnosis. First, if the patient has an infection that can be transmitted by blood or blood products (e.g. hepatitis B or human immuno virus (HIV)) and secondly, when the infection may be transmitted to a newborn baby (e.g. herpes simplex virus, hepatitis B, gonorrhoea, syphilis, chlamydia, HIV, or the human papilloma virus). In both these situations I believe that the physician responsible for the patient's management should be informed. In the second, this will enable the physician to inform the patient of the risks to the baby, and of any measures that can be taken to reduce the risk.

UNLAWFUL SEXUAL ACTS IN THE CONTEXT OF GENITO-URINARY MEDICINE

The genito-urinary physician will often deal with patients who have been involved in criminal sexual activities, including prostitution, rape, underage sex, incest, and child abuse.

It is beyond the scope of this chapter to deal with all these issues. As an example of some of the problems I will consider the question of prostitution and underage sex. Genito-urinary clinics often deal with prostitutes. When this is so, not only is one dealing with an unlawful activity, and a profession one may or may not approve of, but one is also dealing with an activity in which the individual may have put or may still be putting numerous other people at risk of acquiring a sexually transmitted disease.

Case history

June was 31 and had been 'on the game' for five years. She attended the clinic every month for a check-up. On average she had two or three partners per night and estimated that she had had at least 50 sexual partners since her previous visit. She usually insisted that her clients used a condom; however, she had several 'regulars' who did not. The examination was normal and she was asked to re-attend one week later for the results of cultures and serological tests. She was advised not to have sex until the results of her tests were available. Unfortunately, she said that this was not possible. The serological tests for syphilis came back strongly positive, suggesting a diagnosis of early infectious syphilis.

This case demonstrates some of the difficulties in dealing with cases of this sort. First, the majority of her contacts were anonymous, making contact tracing almost impossible. Secondly, prostitutes are often unwilling to inform regular clients about the infection as this may be damaging to business. Finally, this patient continued to ply her trade pending the results of the test, putting even more people at risk. The best one can hope to do in these circumstances is to win the patient's confidence, suggest that she attends regularly for testing, and also that she always insists on condoms.

Females under the age of 16 who are involved in heterosexual relationships and males under the age of 21 who are having homosexual sex who attend STD clinics pose a number of interesting moral issues. First, the patient may have engaged in an unlawful or criminal act. More importantly the physician may consider that this sexual activity may have caused physical or emotional damage to the patient. The doctor may have a moral dilemma between protecting the patient's confidence and taking action to prevent further harm coming to the patient. Where a female has willingly participated in sexual activity and when, for example, she is 15 years old with a regular boyfriend, perhaps 18 months her senior, I do not believe there is any problem. On the other hand, when an STD is diagnosed in a young child and when the sexual partner is older, the problem is more complex. The parents may not know that the child is sexually active or has been sexually abused and the child may not wish them to know. Divulging information to the parents may be a breach of confidence. The problem is compounded if the child's sexual partner is a member of the family. In these circumstances I believe that the infection should be swiftly treated and the child referred to a suitable alternative agency, for example a paediatrician, or general practitioner, a medical social worker, or other professional counsellor, for futher follow-up and counselling.

BEING UNFAITHFUL

Sexual intercourse with a person outside a stable relationship (including extramarital sex) is often the source of sexually transmitted diseases and many patients with a suspected STD will present to genito-urinary physicians.

Case history

Cathy was a 28-year-old married personnel assistant, who presented to the clinic with a vaginal discharge which she had had for two weeks. She had had a brief affair with a colleague while her husband was abroad on business. The discharge was found to be due to gonorrhoea and chlamydia and successfully treated. She refused to inform her husband. However, two days later he developed a discharge. He went to his GP who referred him to a local STD clinic where the same two infections were diagnosed and treated. He wanted to know what he was being treated for and how he had contracted the infections.

Cases such as these place the physician in a difficult situation, particularly if he or she deals with both partners. The physician cannot apportion blame or allow any feelings or suggestions that one or other party has acted improperly to cloud his judgement. In addition, extreme care to avoid any disclosure about the other partner is paramount. It is always useful to ascertain what the patient already knows, as this may help to delineate the areas to avoid. Breakdown of the relationship can be a consequence and the utmost sensitivity and discretion are needed.

HOMOSEXUALITY AND BISEXUALITY

Homosexual and bisexual males constitute a sizeable minority of patients with sexually transmitted diseases (British Co-operative Clinical Group 1973). Although sexual intercourse between consenting males over the age of 21 was legalized in 1969 (Report of the Committee on Homosexual Offences and Prostitution 1957), intolerance of, and misconception about, homosexuality are still widespread in society. Such prejudice in the medical profession can form a significant barrier to the adequate care of the homosexual patient. To deal adequately with the management of a homosexual man with a suspected STD, the physician will need to be free of prejudice, to be non-judgemental, comfortable with his or her own sexuality, and knowledgeable about sexual practice in homosexual men and with the homosexual lifestyle generally.

Unfortunately, there are still members of the medical profession who display gross intolerance when it comes to homosexuality. This issue has been discussed at a recent Annual Representative Meeting of the British Medical Association (British Medical Association 1987) and has been the subject of a recent leader article in the *British Medical Journal* (1985). This lack of tolerance has been particularly virulent in relation to AIDS, and is discussed in detail below.

Considerable difficulties can arise when one is dealing with the female partner of a bisexual man when she is unaware of his sexual orientation. The following case highlights this problem:

Case history

Jack was a 34-year-old married man. He also had occasional, usually anonymous, homosexual contacts. He presented to the clinic with a widespread rash, which proved to be secondary syphilis, and he was asked to bring his wife to the clinic for tests. He initially refused but subsequently agreed, provided we did not divulge either his diagnosis or more importantly his sexual orientation. His wife attended and although she had no clinical evidence of the disease, the serological tests proved positive.

This problem is not just one of protecting both patients' confidences, but also the thorny issue of whether the wife should know about her husband's homosexual activities, which could put her at risk of contracting many serious infections, including hepatitis B, syphilis, and HIV. One certainly cannot tell her of his diagnosis or sexual orientation, but one can tell her that she has syphilis and that it is sexually transmitted. One could also give her general information about syphilis, possibly indicating that many cases are contracted through homosexual contact and leave her to draw her own conclusions. Extreme caution would be required with this approach to avoid any possible reference to her husband. I suspect many physicians, myself included, would steer away from such an approach, preferring to be relatively non-committal.

CONTACT TRACING

Contact tracing, as its name implies, is the process of identifying people who may have been the sexual partners of patients with an STD and ensuring that they are interviewed, investigated, and treated appropriately. The method of contact tracing favoured in the UK and the USA relies on the patient being encouraged to ensure that contacts are informed. Confidentiality, the effectiveness of treatment, and the need to prevent further spread are stressed.

Difficulties sometimes arise when the patient refuses to inform his or her contacts; particularly in the context of infection which may be asymptomatic (e.g. syphilis, HIV infection, hepatitis B, or human papilloma virus). If simple persuasion fails, the patient can be offered a confidential contact slip using a coded diagnosis to give to his contact or contacts. A contact slip is a piece of paper with the originating clinic's name and address at the top. A patient's clinic number (but no name or other identifying characteristic) is written on the slip. The patient's diagnosis is written in a predetermined code, recognizable to all genito-urinary medicine clinics. The code consists of letters followed by one or more numbers. The code for candidosis, for example, is C7. The slip is given to the patient who can then, should he or she so which, pass the slip or slips on to the sexual partner or partners. The use of coded diagnoses, and patient numbers only, ensures the protection of confidence. Alternatively the skills of an expert health advisor can be employed. On occasion the patient may allow the health adviser to visit the contact. Considerable tact, skill, and sensitivity are required for these home visits. Sometimes, in very delicate cases, particularly those involving marital infidelity, contacts are brought into the clinic under the pretext that their partners may have a minor complaint such as a water infection. If no evidence of infection is found, the contact can be reassured without difficulty. On the other hand, if an infection is diagnosed the physician will have to decide whether to tell the contact the diagnosis or to continue the ruse and talk about 'water infections'. Sometimes this telling of untruths or half-truths becomes very complex and tortuous. There are inherent ethical problems in this approach. First, one is lying to the person. Secondly there is the question of withholding information which may be vital to health. I believe that every patient has the right to know his or her diagnosis, and early disclosure often builds up confidence and helps in the management.

On occasion a patient will agree to bring a contact to the clinic, provided that the contact is not told of his or her own diagnosis. I do not believe that the physician should ever give an undertaking to a third party not to discuss the medical details of a case with a patient. This would be an act of collusion and deception. Instead, great stress should be placed on confidentiality and the need for treatment.

INFECTION WITH THE HUMAN IMMUNO VIRUS (HIV)

The recent HIV epidemic has raised a number of important moral and ethical issues. Many are similar to the issues already discussed in relation to the other STDs, namely confidentiality, contact tracing, and homosexuality. However, the severity of the infection and the fact that it is transmitted largely amongst homosexuals pose some new and important problems. An additional factor is the enormous impact the disease has had on society's attitudes to sex, sexually transmitted diseases, and homosexuality. There are many reasons why society is unlikely to return to 'traditional' sexual morality—including effective and safe contraceptives, ability to treat the 'common' sexually transmitted diseases, the changing role of women in society, and the fragmentation of family life. Despite this, the impact of AIDS is likely to lead to a more questioning attitude to the potential attraction and risks of sex.

It is beyond the scope of this chapter to deal with all the ethical issues raised by AIDS; it will cover only two of the more contentious, the role of the doctor, and the ethics of HIV testing.

The doctor and AIDS

Doctors and other health care personnel have always been at risk of contracting diseases (some potentially fatal) from their patients. Examples of this include Lassa fever, hepatitis B, and tuberculosis. This risk had to be balanced against the doctor's traditional role as a healer and has always been regarded as part of the moral duty of the medical profession (Volberding and Abrams 1985). The risk of infection with AIDS deserves some closer inspection. When the epidemic first started there was a certain amount of understandable fear about the possible risk of transmission to health care personnel. It soon became obvious that the risk, except in the case of major accidents involving blood, was negligible (Miller *et al.* 1986; Volberding and Abrams 1985). Despite these reassurances, problems have persisted and have led to suboptimal care being given to many patients. Some of the difficulties we have encountered include general practitioners unwilling to have AIDS patients on their lists, trouble finding in-patient hospital beds, and inability to obtain investigations including certain blood tests and endoscopy. It has become increasingly obvious that factors other than the doctor's perceived risk have determined and continue to determine the conduct of doctors when treating patients with AIDS or HIV related problems (Guy 1987). These include overt, or more commonly hidden, homophobia, and the idea that because the patient has put himself at risk this somehow negates the duty of the doctor to care for the patient. The latter concept is particularly illogical and prejudiced, as many people have so-called 'self-inflicted' illnesses and are accepted for treatment. We have found that the best way to deal with these issues is by education and negotiation. It is vital that doctors remember that they have a duty not only to treat patients but also to help the community to put the disease in its proper perspective.

HIV antibody testing

There has been considerable debate about the value of taking blood for human immuno virus antibody testing (British Medical Association 1987; Adler and Jeffries 1987). In order to have a framework for assessing the benefit of HIV antibody tests, one first needs to understand the meaning of the test itself. The presence of HIV antibodies in a patient's blood means that he or she has been exposed to the virus and may develop AIDS at some future date. It does not indicate how long the infection has been present, nor does it indicate if the patient is currently infectious.

A positive result may have other consequences for the patient. These include possible difficulty in obtaining medical and dental care, ostracism at or even dismissal from work, and difficulty in obtaining life assurance. (Miller *et al.* 1986)

There are now three circumstances in which, in my view, the test is justified. The first is when the patient requests it and understands its meaning and possible consequences. The second is when it may be helpful in dealing with a clinical problem. The third is in the context of the blood transfusion service, where prevention of spread to a third party is the objective. In both the second and third cases informed consent should be obtained. Some clinicians feel that in the context of a clinical problem it is perfectly reasonable to take the test without informing the patient of its purpose. They argue that we do not inform or seek consent for other tests, so why should HIV be different? This argument is flawed on two counts. Firstly, the consequences of a positive test are different from those of any other test. Secondly, the medical profession should be moving towards more information for patients rather than less (Adler and Jeffries 1987).

Spread from mother to baby is an important source of infection in the neonate (CDC 1984) and routine antenatal screening is now being considered. The implications of a positive test in these circumstances are even more complex. There is the risk of spread to the baby who may go on to develop AIDS. There is also the possibility that the mother may develop AIDS in the early months or years of the baby's life. Finally there is the issue of termination of pregnancy. Screening may be suitable in high risk populations, for example where the hospital sees a large number of intravenous drug users; but is of questionable benefit in the routine antenatal population. I believe that this particular debate still has a long way to run, particularly as the actual risk of the neonate acquiring the infection is still unclear, and the natural history and outcome of infection in both mother and baby are still being studied.

What about mandatory screening in high risk populations in an attempt to prevent spread? Universal screening violates personal liberty (Gillon 1987), and is unlikely to prevent spread of the infection. Indeed there is now considerable evidence to support the view that education and voluntary screening have helped to decrease the transmission of HIV amongst homosexual men in New York, San Francisco, and London (Weller *et al.* 1984; McCusick *et al.* 1985; MMWR 1985; Stevens *et al.* 1986; Weber *et al.* 1986; Carne *et al.* 1987). Whether similar success can be achieved in other high risk groups remains to be seen. I do not believe that there is any justification for mandatory screening at the present time.

REFERENCES

Adler, M. W. (1980). The terrible peril: a historical perspective on the venereal disease. *British Medical Journal*, **281**, 206–11.

Adler, M. W. and Jeffries, D. J. (1987). AIDS, a faltering step. *British Medical Journal*, **295**, 73–4.

British Co-operative Clinical Group (1973). Homosexuality and venereal diseases in the United Kingdom. *British Journal of Venereal Diseases*, **49**, 329–34.

British Medical Association (1987). Agenda of the British Medical Association's Annual Representative Meeting Motions, 359–74 (Insertion in issue 6 June) *British Medical Journal*, **294**, 12–13.

British Medical Journal (1985). Intolerance 1980s style. **291**, 1745–6.

Carne, C. A. *et al.* (1987). Prevalence of antibodies to human immunodeficiency virus, gonorrhoea rates, and changed sexual behaviour in homosexual men in London. *Lancet*, (**i**), 656–8.

CDC Update 1984. Acquired immunodeficiency syndrome (AIDS). United States. *MMWR*, **33**, 661–4.

Champneys, F. (1917). The fight against venereal infection. A reply to Sir Bryan Dontin. *Nineteenth Century*, **82**, 1052–4.

Daily Telegraph (3 May 1983). 'Wages of Sin', a deadly toll.

Gillon, R. (1987). Testing for HIV without permission. *British Medical Journal*, **294**, 821–3.

Guy, P. J. (1987). AIDS: a doctor's duty. *British Medical Journal*, **294**, 445.

Leads from the MMWR (1985). Declining rates of rectal and pharyngeal gonorrhoea among men. New York City. *MMWR*, **252**, 327–31.

McCusick, L., *et al.* (1985). Reported changes in the sexual behaviour of men at risk for AIDS, San Francisco 1982–4. *Public Health Reports*, **100**, 623–9.

Miller, D., Jeffries, D. J., Green, J., Harris, W. J. R., and Pinching, A. J. (1986). HTLV-III—should testing ever be routine? *British Medical Journal*, **292**, 941–3.

MMWR (1985). Centers for Disease Control: Self reported behavioural change among gay and bisexual men, San Francisco. **34**, 613–15.

National Health Service (Veneral Diseases) Regulation (1968). S.I. No. 1624. HMSO, London.

National Health Service (Venereal Diseases) Regulations (1974). S.I. No. 29. HMSO, London.

House of Commons Report (1911). *National Insurance Bill to provide insurance against loss of health and for the prevention and cure of sickness and for insurance against unemployment and for the purposes incidental thereto*. 4, No. 198, HMSO, London.

Parran, T. and Vonderlehr, R. A. (1941). *Plain words about venereal disease*. Reynal and Hitchcock, New York.

Report of the Committee on Homosexual Offences and Prostitution. (Wolfenden Report) (1957). Cmnd; 247, HMSO, London.

Rout, E. A. (1922). England and venereal disease. *British Medical Journal*, **I**, 975.

Royal Commission on Venereal Diseases (1916). Final Report of the Commissioners. (Cmnd 8189), HMSO, London.

Stevens, C. E., *et al.* (1986). HTLV-III infection in a cohort of homosexual men in New York City. *Journal of the American Medical Association*, **255**, 2167–72.

The Sun (7 February 1985). AIDS is the wrath of God, says vicar.

Volberding, P. and Abrams, D. (1985). Clinical care and research in AIDS. *Hastings Center Report*, **15**, 16–18.

Weber, J. N., et al. (1986). Three-year prospective study of HTLV-III/LAV infection in homosexual men. *Lancet*, **i**, 1179–82.

Weller, I. V. D., Hindley, D. J., Adler, M. W., and Meldrum, J. T. (1984). Gonorrhoea in homosexual men and media coverage of AIDS in London 1982–3. *British Medical Journal*, **289**, 1041.

10
Ethics in a college health service

RAANAN GILLON

Most college health services—sometimes known as student or university health services—are combinations of straightforward general practices skewed, but by no means confined, to a late adolescent/early adult age-group of patients, and occupational health services for the institutions of which they form a part. Thus the ethical issues faced by practitioners in college health services comprise all those faced by general practitioners, plus all those faced by occupational health physicians, plus the additional ones of trying to reconcile the two roles. Because it would be worthless to try to address the enormous range of ethical problems that arise in both general practice and in occupational health in a short chapter, I shall instead sketch one commonplace case history that may arise in our own practice, and indeed in any other general practice, and pursue some of its ethical implications.

A FICTITIOUS CASE HISTORY BASED ON ACTUAL EXPERIENCES

An 18-year-old girl comes to my open clinic and says that she and her boyfriend had an accident last night—the sheath they were using had burst. Could I do anything to help her? I ask her what she would do if she became pregnant. 'I couldn't have a baby now—I'd definitely want an abortion'. We have a fairly brief discussion (about 15 minutes). What she has come for is post-coital contraception and she also wants to start the pill. She has no moral worries about these courses of action. I prescribe her the post-coital pills and ask her to make an appointment to discuss contraception and have a proper medical examination. She is reluctant to wait—'couldn't you do it now, doctor?' I point out that there are 15 other patients waiting in the open clinic and she agrees, somewhat reluctantly, to make an appointment. A week or so later I see her again to discuss contraception. I point out some of the harms and benefits of alternative courses of action (including the advantages in terms of protection from viral diseases that condoms provide, and the fact that there is a remote but definite risk of nasty things happening as a result of taking the pill, even of dying, although I emphasize that these are very low probability risks, somewhat comparable at her age with the risks of travelling in motor cars). She is definite that she wants the pill, and after a full history to exclude additional risk factors, and medically examining her, I prescribe the pill.

Two or three weeks later I am telephoned by an anxious sounding woman from Scotland, who says she understands I have been seeing her daughter, who won't tell her why. What is going on? Has her daughter been put on the pill? Fortunately I have a terrible memory and I explain that I cannot remember anything about whether or not I have seen her daughter but that in any case I would not be able to discuss her without my patient's explicit permission. We have a somewhat prolonged discussion and *I think* we part on reasonably friendly terms, although I do not think she accepts my attempt to explain my position by asking her what she thinks I should tell her daughter supposing that the positions were reversed, with the mother as my patient and the daughter wanting to know if her mother were on the pill.

There is nothing very remarkable about this vignette, which is in fact a fictitious compilation and condensation of several real events, but which could perfectly well have been a single case history. Yet it illustrates several of the ethical issues that arise recurrently in my work and, I am sure, in the work of most general practitioners.

CONTRACEPTION, POST-COITAL CONTRACEPTION, AND ABORTION

My patient's request for post-coital contraception raises for her and for me the moral issues of abortion, for post-coital contraception works by preventing implantation of the fertilized ovum which is of course a human embryo. It seems to me clear that the standard Roman Catholic line on this is accurate—namely that a genetically new human individual starts when a sperm fertilizes an ovum. Nor is this fact undermined, as is sometimes claimed, by the facts that occasionally this early embryo may divide into identical twins, that it may turn into an hydatidiform mole, that it does not implant into the lining of the uterus for several days, and that it takes time for the new genetic mix to be finalized (Dawson 1957). The ethical debate turns not on this somewhat mundane description of the biological facts, but on what it is morally permissible to do to this new human individual and why. For my own part, a newly fertilized ovum is at the beginning of a spectrum of development of a human being, at one end of which is a human *person* with the full moral status that people have, and at the other end of which is a human being with only the *potential* to be a person, and with no more moral status than this potential affords. That, I would (but here do not) argue, is a matter of decision, and depends primarily on the value the pregnant woman places on that embryo and to some extent on the value society places upon it. Thus, so far as I am concerned, the newly fertilized ovum does not fall within the *scope* of our normal moral obligations to other people and, (to skip a lot of controversial argument), it is, I believe, morally justifiable to kill this early human being if to do so is desired by the pregnant woman, produces net benefit over harm, and is sanctioned by society. (The same does not apply to actual people even if their mothers would like to kill them, even if to do so would produce a net benefit over harm, and even if to do so were socially sanctioned.) So much (in brief summary) for my moral views about the matter. What relevance have my views so far as the patient is concerned? That question seems to point to a second type of moral question in general practice, namely the moral relationship between doctor and patient.

THE DOCTOR–PATIENT RELATIONSHIP

The doctor–patient relationship is paradigmatically or typically a relationship based on agreement between two people. One offers to use his special skills to try to benefit the other medically in a way that respects the other's views and with as little concomitant harm as possible, within the limits of his professional and personal skills and norms. The other asks, explicitly or implicitly, for such assistance and, having been told what can be done, has the option to accept or reject the doctor's proposed course of action. (The question of payment is not, as I see it, central to the relationship, though it is obviously true that *one* of the motives—at any rate for most doctors—for being a doctor will be remuneration, usually above average remuneration.) Thus the relationship is based fundamentally on *agreement* between two people that one should exercise his special skills in order to benefit the other in an agreed way and with as little concomitant harm as possible.

So the moral views of the doctor obviously have relevance to the doctor–patient relationship, both as they have in *any* relationship between people—ordinary relationships require mutual respect and this usually requires people not to do anything to someone else without the other's approval—and conversely not to require of others actions that the other believes to be unjustified. In addition the doctor, as one who is committed to exercising his skills to benefit his patient with minimal harm, should surely only do, in the context of respecting his patient, what he considers would be beneficial and minimally harmful to that patient. Now, that might sound like a recipe for rampant medical paternalism, but it certainly is not. For if the doctor takes seriously the requirement of respect for the person who is his patient, he will give very great weight indeed to what his patient considers would be harmful and beneficial when coming to his decision about how to act.

How does all that relate to the fictitious history cited above? First, if the doctor believes that to kill a human embryo is morally indefensible then it seems clear to me that he should not participate in such a killing or prescribe post-coital contraception (and the same would apply to abortion, of course). But he should make it clear to his patient that this decision is the result of his own moral perspective. It should then be open to the patient to seek a doctor who shares her moral perspective. (It should also in my view be open to society in co-operation with the medical profession to decide how many doctors with anti-abortion moral views which they wish to allow to influence their treatment of their patients it is prepared to accept, and in what sort of specialty and geographical distribution.)

What about the matter of contraception? Again, there are some doctors who believe that contraception is morally unacceptable and once more I see no reason to impose prescribing of contraception on such doctors. Once again, however, they should make it clear that they are refusing on moral grounds; it should remain open to the patient to seek a doctor who shares her moral perspective. The same remarks apply to a societal involvement here as in the case of abortion.

I, however, have no moral qualms about contraception, but the basic medical obligation to act to benefit the patient with minimal harm still remains, as in every doctor–patient relationship. As I indicated in the story, I explained to my patient that my own view these days is that the safest form of contraception is the sheath (with post-coital contraception and/or abortion if this fails). This greatly reduces the risk of wart virus transmission with its low probability but apparently definite risk of cancer of the cervix, and of *herpes genitalis* virus transmission with its recurrent and currently ineradicable episodes of painful sores, and of transmission of the more traditional venereal diseases. In addition, the sheath seems to afford a high degree of protection against transmission of the probably fatal AIDS virus, and although heterosexuals are, in Britain at least, still relatively unscathed by this organism, the risk is steadily increasing. Moreover the sheath does not carry the small but definite risk of causing death that the pill carries.

However my patient said that although she understood all that, none the less she and her boyfriend had tried the sheath and he 'couldn't get on with it: it ruined our sex life'. She was prepared to take the risks and wanted the pill. I acceded to this on the grounds that making such risk assessments about one's life is ultimately one's own business and that it is not the task of the doctor to try to impose his own risk assessments on his patients. As I see it, it is his business to *advise* his patients on the relevant medical facts, not to act if he really believes that his action would be morally unacceptable, and to try to benefit his patient with minimal harm. But (in the normal case) it is only his business to try to benefit his patients at all in so far as they want or at least are prepared to be benefited by the means he proposes. If a patient is not prepared to use the sheath (or any medical treatment the doctor advises) then so be it: the doctor, prima facie at least, should offer other available options until his patient finds one she accepts as optimally beneficial and least harmful.

In my view, one of the greatest harms for many people is having their own assessment of how they intend to run their lives and of what risks they are prepared to incur in order to do so overridden by someone else. It may sometimes be justifiable to do so despite that, but the harm of thus overriding people's autonomous decisions about their goals and the risks they are prepared to take in pursuit of those goals should not be underestimated. Indeed for Charles Fried one's risk budget, as he calls it, is part of what makes one the unique person one is (Fried 1970). Clearly sufficient harm to others may justify overriding people's personal risk budgets, as may sufficient mental impairment; and, as indicated, a doctor does not have an obligation to act if he believes that to do so would be morally unacceptable. But in the normal case such factors do not apply and I believe that respect for the person who is one's patient requires his or her assessment of what one proposes to be decisive. On rare occasions such decisions may both conflict with medical advice and be fatally mistaken: a poignant example is given by Sir Richard Bayliss of a Christian Scientist who rejected medical assistance and died of her easily remediable thyrotoxicosis (Bayliss 1982).

INFORMED CONSENT

It is that principle, of respect for one's patient and his autonomy, or self-determination as Justice Kirby calls it (Kirby 1983), that seems to me to be at the heart of the requirement for informed consent, a phrase which simply describes the proper process of agreement between a doctor and a patient about what the doctor shall do for the patient. Thus when a doctor offers to try to benefit his patient medically, there seems at least a prima-facie moral obligation for him to specify the benefits he expects and also the risks he sees as possible, so as to enable the patient to decide whether or not to accept those risks in pursuit of those benefits. I write 'prima facie' because several factors may modify this prima-facie obligation. One such factor is that many patients wish to hand over the decision-making processes, including the assessment of risks and benefits, to the doctor. In those circumstances it seems perfectly justifiable on exactly the same grounds—respect for the patient's autonomy—to respond to that wish. But the starting assumption should surely be that people want to make their own decisions on the basis of the best available relevant information. Again, people vary considerably about what they consider to be relevant; for example about how *much* they want to know about the risks and benefits and available alternatives and about how great a probability of danger has to exist for it to be relevant to their decision. Many people want to know only about major or substantial risks, but a few are interested in low probability risks. Again the moral objective should surely be to try to match the information offered to the information desired.

WHEN OBLIGATIONS TO OTHERS CONFLICT WITH WHAT THE PATIENT WANTS

Some people, however, would like to spend hours talking about their particular problems and their possible solutions and the risks and benefits of each alternative. Here a further moral factor may justifiably override the prima-facie obligation to respect that patient's autonomous desires—notably one's obligations to others, including but not only, one's other patients. When a patient wants to know in such great detail about all the available alternatives (incidentally a perfectly reasonable, indeed admirable, desire, so it seems to me) that it threatens one's obligations to others, then it may be necessary to explain that one simply has not got the time to pursue the matter in greater depth and instead to point the patient in the direction of an appropriate medical library. This is an unusual but by no means unprecedented outcome in my own practice and when it happens the patient may well come back very pleased to have done some profitable research on his own problem, and often as a result may be considerably better informed about it than I am. In my experience people are perfectly ready to understand that one may not be able to spend as long as they would like dealing with their problems, because of one's concomitant obligations to others. If one has taken a reasonable degree of trouble to answer their questions and discuss their problems, they are usually quite ready to accept it when one calls a halt. Precisely the same sort of reasoning applied when my patient in the story who came to the open clinic and wanted me then and there to go through the fairly lengthy process of discussing contraception and examining her prior to starting the contraceptive pill. When I explained that there were 15 other patients behind her in that morning's queue who also wanted to consult me, she understood and made a later half-hour appointment. In both sorts of case, considerations of justice seem to me justifiably to override my prima-facie obligation to respect my patient's autonomy.

CONFIDENTIALITY

Finally, my case story concerns the medical obligation of confidentiality. Here my views have changed. When I started to practise medicine I think I believed that I had an absolute duty of confidentiality to my patients—something akin to the absolute duty or confidentiality which I understand Roman Catholic and other Christian priests consider themselves to have to those who confess. In more recent years and with an increasing interest in medical ethics I have shifted away from this absolutist position (as indeed from all absolutist moral positions) and now adopt a view that makes medical confidentiality a very strong, but not absolute, obligation. The obligation is strong enough for doctors and nurses not to tell enquirers—including parents and academics, sometimes as indicated to their surprise—even whether or not a patient has consulted us, let alone disclose why, or what our findings were; unless of course we have the patient's permission to do so. It is strong enough for us to have added a condition to the non-medical and non-nursing employees' contracts of employment requiring them to undertake strict standards of confidentiality about any information they acquire concerning patients (including the need to avoid gossiping about patients—something that we are all, alas, tempted to do. Setting ourselves a moral standard is one thing, living up to it is quite a different thing!) We do not write these requirements into the terms and conditions of service of the doctors and nurses, although each of us has a copy, simply because we believe that strict standards of confidentiality are already part of the existing professional obligations of doctors and nurses.

All that said, I am now fairly clear that confidentiality is not an absolute obligation (*pace* Kottow 1986), and have argued more thorougly for this elsewhere (Gillon 1986). In brief, neither a principle of respect for autonomy nor a utilitarian concern to maximize welfare, the two strongest justifications for upholding medical confidentiality, can justify doing so *whatever the consequences*. At some level of harm to others confidentiality has to be overridden, from either perspective. If, for example, it would be very likely that I could save someone from being murdered by breaking a patient's confidence (and the probability as well as the degree of harm must be very great) then I suspect that I would decide that I ought to break that confidence. This produces a problem about how we can and ought to explain to patients both that we believe confidentiality to be a very strict obligation and that, none the less, we do not consider it to be an absolute obligation. The solution—by no means, I recognize, satisfactory—that we have come up with in our practice is to describe our confidentiality as in 'medical confidence', and that is the heading on our medical questionnaire that we ask all new patients to complete as a sort of medical data base concerning their health. So far no one has asked me what exactly 'medical confidentiality' means, but when the time comes I shall explain, as the GMC (General Medical Council 1987) and the BMA (British Medical Association 1984) explain, that there are rare cases in which doctors may feel obliged to override their strong duty of confidentiality. Although, as indicated above, I believe this non-absolutism to be morally justified, most doctors, including I must confess myself, are in practice reluctant to be explicit in advance about our readiness to break confidentiality in certain sorts of cases (for example, when ordered to do so by a judge, or where it seems necessary to avert very great harm to others). Usually this reluctance stems from a belief that it would frighten patients and prevent them from being honest with us and thus prevent us from doing our medical best for them. It seems to be an area that needs far more professional and public discussion.

CONCLUSION

In conclusion, my case history points up some common moral problems that arise in general practice. As may be apparent, the sort of reasoning that I have tried to apply to them is based on four prima-facie moral principles, and consideration of their scope (what they apply to). These principles are discussed by Beauchamp and Childress in their admirable textbook on medical ethics (Beauchamp and Childress 1983), and are defensible from a wide variety of moral perspectives, religious and secular, utilitarian and deontological, virtue based or principle based, which is why they seem so attractive for medical ethics with its pluralistic requirements. The four principles are: (1) the principle of respect for autonomy, fundamental to most moral interactions between equals but perhaps not as widely recognized in the past in medical ethics as is now beginning to be the case; (2) the principle of beneficence (benefiting others); (3) the principle of non-maleficence (avoiding harming others), (2) and (3) forming the linchpins of traditional medical ethics; (4) and the principle of justice or fairness.

Thus in my case story the moral questions about post-coital contraception and abortion concerned primarily the scope of our moral obligations to each other (and especially of course our obligations not to kill each other); do these obligations include embryos and fetuses in the same way as they include other people? (And if so, why: if not, why not?) The various questions about assessing harms and benefits to patients are questions about the principles of beneficence and non-maleficence; and the questions about respect for one's patients, about keeping their secrets, and about obtaining their informed consent to what one proposes to do for them, are largely about the principle of respect for autonomy. Finally the questions about distributing one's time and resources between different people, especially between different patients, are largely questions about justice. I have discovered no nice formula (and do not expect to) whereby these different prima-facie moral obligations can be ranked or otherwise manipulated into some form of standard decision process. But I do find that the principles themselves and the question of their scope are of some help in trying to think more clearly about the medico-moral problems I encounter in my practice. My thanks to Beauchamp and Childress who first made me think systematically about these principles in the context of medical ethics.

REFERENCES

Bayliss, R. (1982). A health hazard. *British Medical Journal*, **285**, 1824–5.

Beauchamp, T. and Childress, J. (1983). *Principles of biomedical ethics* (2nd ed). Oxford University Press.

British Medical Association (1984). *Handbook of medical ethics*, BMA, London.

Dawson, K. (1987). Fertilization and moral status: a scientific perspective. *Journal of Medical Ethics*, **13**, 173–8.

Fried, C. (1970). *An anatomy of values*. Harvard University Press, Cambridge, Mass.

General Medical Council (1987). *Professional conduct and discipline: fitness to practise*. GMC, London.

Gillon, R. (1986). *Philosophical medical ethics*, Wiley, Chichester.

Kirby, M. (1983). Informed consent: what does it mean? *Journal of Medical Ethics*, **9**, 69–75.

Kottow, M. (1986). Medical confidentiality: an intransigent and absolute obligation. *Journal of Medical Ethics*, **12**, 117–22.

11
Ethics in general practice

MICHAEL LINNETT

In this book, ethical problems in many branches of medicine are considered. Because of the often intimate nature of his relationship with an individual and with his family, all these problems may involve the general practitioner, since the situation which generates them may be declared first to him; and if specialist opinion is needed, he may well again be consulted to help make the right decision.

But in family medicine, what is ethically a 'right' decision, and how do we reach it? In this chapter an attempt will be made to discuss some of the ethical difficulties confronting a family doctor in his daily work. It would be a rash man who felt he could utter generalities on standards of conduct and moral judgements: the difficulties arise in the contrast between the perceived and often changing standards and moral judgements of society on the one hand, and the problems of the individual patient and doctor on the other. It is significant that the discussion of ethical problems has now become a major subject. Were we more certain, if less scrupulous, in the past? Are our motives and habits of thought less trustworthy now, that we have to be guided? How much of ethics is special pleading to support us against the accusations and even litigation that have lately darkened the trust that existed between the community and the professions?

Trust should be the linchpin of the relationship between the patient and his own doctor, yet the fundamental ethical problem in general practice is found here. Is my doctor telling me the truth? The question is implicit in the patient's anxious question 'are you sure the pills are safe, doctor?' or, more serious, 'are you sure it is not cancer?' To what extent does the profession tell the 'truth'; for truth, and the way it is presented, are central to the existence of trust? And yet, just as in the study of historical events the exact truth is so difficult to define, so the safety of a medicine is difficult to describe, and the extent of the truth a patient can comprehend is variable. If it is the doctor's duty to acquire sufficient knowledge to be able to compare and contrast risk and benefit, it is also his duty to present his conclusions simply and understandably to the patient; and from one point of view it would be unethical for him to dismiss the patient's anxieties with lightweight routine reassurance, for the patient needs convincing facts which he can believe.

The issue of how much a patient should be told about his illness, especially a long-term or eventually fatal illness, has always occupied both patients and their doctors. In the past 30 years there has been a trend towards fuller discussion with the patient of the nature and prognosis of his illness, and many doctors nowadays find a situation much easier to manage when the patient, through understanding, is better able to co-operate in treatment. Yet, although external pressures urge the fullest of revelation to patients, they often fail to realize that for many patients this may place an intolerable burden on them. Patients sometimes protest, 'don't tell me any more doctor, it confuses me and I don't want to know'. More likely, they fear their ability to handle bad news, for who among us, even when we demand to know the whole truth, can be sure of our ability to absorb it and its complications with dignity and courage? And conversely, how often is a doctor humbled by the simple brave acceptance of a patient confronted with disaster?

Until recently a doctor's training and the dictates of compassion, more often than not, led to the shrouding of a serious diagnosis and to withholding the truth. Nowadays, because of the greater medical knowledge of the public, few intelligent patients are in doubt about the general nature of their illness. Some do fear that they are not being told the truth. This is in part because the media both urge the public to find out more about disease and also, on occasion, raise issues of the duplicity and inadequacy of the medical profession. Today doctors feel increasingly bound to be more specific to their patients in order to retain their confidence, and to be able to show what is being done to help them. While it might be good to find that all patients can accept the burden of knowledge, it is unrealistic to expect that all can. Doctors have years of training in objectivity, although they often cannot maintain it. Patients are untrained in medicine, and their reactions will be largely subjective.

Communication, or the lack of it, is at the bottom of most misunderstandings between doctors and patients. In a conversation with a patient there are at least three levels of interpretation of the words the doctor uses. There are the words that are said, for example: 'we think some of the cells are not quite normal'. There are the words actually meant: 'we think the cells may be malignant'. Finally there are the words implied: 'we think you have got cancer'. Patients are mostly quite aware of these subtleties, and some will be relieved not to be faced with a dogmatic statement of disaster while others will resent what they perceive to be an obfuscation of the plain truth. But the doctor must also be aware of the layers of meaning behind a patient's remark. 'You don't *really* want me to come so often for check-ups, do you, doctor?' may mean 'you think the cancer is spreading, don't you?' All doctors have patients who understate (or overstate) their problem. The writer remembers a pleasant, balanced man who cancelled an appointment about his backache with an apologetic request for a visit—on the way home would do. He turned out to have polio, but his main anxiety was for his golf. Happily the attack was mild, and he was playing again in seven weeks. Words, and the meanings behind them, are crucial to the ethics of the transaction between patient and doctor.

The doctor is therefore left with an ethical dilemma: how much does this patient need to know without destroying hope, and with what words is he to be told it? It requires an experienced doctor who knows his patient to be able to find the correct answer to that question and this is why, so often, it needs the combined knowledge and skills of the specialist and the general practitioner to ensure that their patient is correctly but compassionately informed of a serious diagnosis without being left in irrecoverable despair. For a doctor, the breaking of the news of potentially fatal illness to a patient is often a painful and difficult task: dismay at the diagnosis may provoke an urge to minimize the manner in which it is imparted to the patient. Such a desire to spare the patient can hardly be called unethical, and yet according to his circumstances, whether he is a man of affairs whose responsibilities depend on his health, a mother whose care and support of her family are her life, or somebody who is clearly unwilling to face the bitter facts, the doctor needs all his experience and all his empathy to choose the right words and convey the right attitude. Like so many ethical choices, this cannot be learnt by reading, only by example, experience, and an innate awareness of the conflicting currents in the personality of the patient, together with a respect for his autonomy.

As has been said above, trust is the linchpin of the dialogue between patient and his doctor. The patient should have confidence in his doctor, and he will give the doctor much information about himself in confidence. What he says forms the basis of the notes the doctor makes, and of some he does not make because of their sensitivity. There are some things he has to trust to his memory even though it be fallible, for nowadays nobody can be sure that notes will not fall into other hands. Until fairly recently it had been taken as axiomatic that the doctor's notes, which were his property, were part of the contract of confidence implicit between him and his patients. It was understood that their contents would not be divulged to other parties except under the seal of confidence, to a specialist for example, when his help was wanted—the seal of professional confidence. Or they might be used with the patient's express permission, usually in writing, as the basis of a report to a body such as an insurance company. If the contents of notes are disclosed in other ways, confidence is quite rightly in danger.

And yet, in 1971 it became lawful for a judge, in certain circumstances, to order the disclosure in whole or in part of a patient's notes to a third party during or prior to a legal action in which the patient's health was of material importance. This has come to mean that solicitors are increasingly prone to demand, under threat of judicial order, access to the patient's notes in their entirety. This, of course, means that much material of no relevance to the case, sometimes extremely sensitive, can be disclosed without the patient's permission to people who for one reason or another are hostile to the patient's interests. The doctor is therefore placed in a difficult ethical dilemma, for if he refuses to obey a judge's order he places himself in contempt of court; equally if he only discloses part of the notes he may be put under considerable and unpleasant pressure until everything is revealed. He cannot unwrite what has been written at other times when there was no threat of impending legal action: indeed, such notes may be essential to record, for example, the complexities of a psychiatric state, or the result of a test for venereal disease. Is he in future to keep truncated notes and trust the vagaries of his fallible memory? The merits of this course are in a sense strengthened by the threat of legislation requiring doctors to give their patients freedom of access to their notes. Under the Data Protection Act, a patient already has right of access to his own computer-stored records. It may be argued that if a patient makes such a demand, confidence may well have irretrievably broken down, but the doctor is still left with an ethical dilemma.

Reports to insurance companies are normally straightforward. The patient has given written consent to disclosure, and the doctor is allowed to disclose, in reply to written questions, information about his patient's past health and habits. But questioning of patients suggests that they do not always realize precisely to what it is they have consented, and the extent of the information that could be released. Many doctors, it seems, do not reveal information which cannot be relevant to matters of insurance, yet if recorded, would remain on the file of an organization which in common justice should not have it—for example the fact that a young woman had previously had an abortion. Even more sensitively, an insurance company may ask, on the medical attendant's report, whether there has been any reason to suspect that the patient's habits might render him open to venereal infections, including AIDS. While one can sympathize with the company's anxiety not to fall unknowingly into an obligation to insure against certain death, are we yet prepared to agree that a person who is, or is suspected of being, homosexual or someone who, being afraid that he might have contacted AIDS, asked for and was granted a test which established his normality, should have these matters revealed with the possible consequence of being debarred for a time, or even for life, from insurance of life or health? Should a person's homosexuality be placed on record in the documents of an insurance company, possibly to be spread further when the company refusing insurance is approached by a second company wanting to know the reason for rejection? With these questions in mind the doctor has a difficult decision to make. If he consistently refuses to answer the question which seeks to establish whether the applicant runs the risk of AIDS, and all that implies, that fact in itself may raise doubts in the insurers' minds. If he just tells an 'at-risk' patient of the questions, the patient, not having realized that such a question would be put to his doctor, may withdraw his consent to the answering of that question, in which case doubt is sown. If the doctor answers 'yes' to the question, he can be in no certainty that the patient knew that it would be asked, and may not act against the doctor on the ground that he should not have replied to a question which the company should not have asked, since the patient was not to know that these matters would be raised.

The appearance of AIDS and its spread has in fact raised so many new ethical problems both general and particular for general practitioners that in many instances we do not yet know whether there is a consensus of opinion about them. Because the need for confidentiality in hospital clinics is so rightly observed, it now seems possible that a family doctor may not, in some circumstances, be informed that his patient has been found to have had a positive AIDS virus test. Although this does not mean that the patient has the actual disease, it does mean that he is liable to get symptoms in future, and that those symptoms must be looked for if he should fall ill. It also means that if blood tests are taken, or an operation is to be performed, special precautions must be taken for protection of the medical and nursing staff. Because of the nature of his disease, and its implications, it seems hardly possible that the knowledge of a positive result should be restricted to the patient and special clinic staff only, for the consequences of inappropriate handling are too serious. AIDS is not like ordinary venereal disease which can generally be cured on recognition by the doctor: AIDS kills.

It is for this reason that when a patient comes to his doctor asking for a test for AIDS, questions must be asked, before advice is given. Many in the medical profession agree that it is unethical to do a test for AIDS virus on any patient without telling him, for the consequences of a positive test will result in a profound emotional strain for him as he realizes that he now stands a very considerable chance of developing an incurable and fatal illness, and that from that time the pattern of his life will have to be changed because he can infect others. He cannot take out any life insurance, he cannot let himself be involved closely with others, he should not marry, and he will not know when or if the symptoms of the disease will appear. As this chapter is being written, the implications of AIDS and the risks of promiscuity are being absorbed by the population of this country, and doctors are being asked by worried young people whether they should have a test done. Very often these fears can be resolved by discussing their reasons for wanting a test, which are often the result of alarm rather than logic; but sometimes there is a justification of remote possibility, and a negative test will allay the fear.

There is no doubt that our views on the ethical management of the AIDS outbreak will be modified as we see how the passage of the disease through the community alters. At present the informed view is that general screening is both unnecessary and undesirable on grounds of logistics and of unreliability of testing in 'at-risk' groups. If the disease shows signs of rapid spread, however, it seems likely that such groups may have to be tested and appropriately counselled, for the ethical view must favour the protection of the community. A new proposal is the screening of all hospital admissions as one way of determining the spread of the virus through the population. Patients would not be told the results, nor that they were to be tested, and all results would be regarded as confidential. But is it ethical for neither patient nor other health workers to be told of the result if it is positive? Surely those who provide medical care for that patient in future *must* be told. And in view of the reported spread of the virus, an ethical decision both on test and reporting cannot be delayed.

A recent attempt to determine ethical decision by legal decision has been the ruling on whether a doctor prescribing the contraceptive pill for an under-16-years-old girl should keep the transaction confidential between himself and his patient, or should reveal it to the girl's parents. This dilemma directly affects the general practitioner, who may be faced with the difficult position of deciding whether his reasons for breaking confidence and informing the parents are ethically and legally defensible. It is questionable how much of the controversy stirred up by this question has sprung from seeking to use a court judgment to impose conformity, rather than from basing thinking on general professional opinion and individual judgement. The current wave of anti-professionalism makes clear thinking more difficult, but it is sure that in this instance as in so many others, there is no substitute for an informed consideration of the ethical principles involved in each case.

Before the advent of the contraceptive pill and the intra-uterine contraceptive device, family doctors were approached far more often for terminations of pregnancies. The Abortion Act of 1967 postulates four general categories under which abortion may be permitted; and a certificate must be signed by two doctors, one of whom is normally the patient's general practitioner, stating the category under which the proposed abortion is considered to be appropriate. Two phenomena have occurred since the Act. First, the number of unwanted pregnancies has greatly diminished because of better methods of contraception, and it may be that diminution of promiscuity under the threat of AIDS will further reduce their number. But secondly, the Act has generated a feeling that abortion is much easier to obtain, that abortion on demand is now possible. Although this is not so, there is a feeling that the soul-searching investigation of the ethics of each case that used to happen is now of less concern. Quite apart from those with strongly-held religious or other beliefs that proscribe abortion in any circumstances, most doctors now feel less threatened when abortion has to be considered because certain ground-rules have been laid down: but they recognize that the rules themselves are slack enough to allow a certain latitude in their interpretation. We still cannot escape ethical consideration of the state of body and mind of the woman, of her relationship with the father, and of the welfare of the rest of her family, if such there be.

The concept of consent is important for the general practitioner, although the House of Lords has ruled that, at the last analysis in English law, there is no such thing as 'informed consent'. For ordinary purposes the patient's consent is assumed when he or she submits to an examination, or agrees to a minor operation or an injection. The procedure will normally have been discussed, and the patient will usually understand what is to follow. Slightly less straightforward is the consent to an operation where, for example, neither patient nor surgeon may be sure how far the operation is to go. When mastectomy was more frequently done, women were often concerned when they were told that if biopsy, the first stage of the operation, so indicated, the surgeon would immediately proceed to full mastectomy, and many women recoiled from such apparent precipitancy. Some, when the situation was explained, would agree to the full procedure; others, who for various reasons wished to take one step at a time, preferred to await the full biopsy report, and their wishes had to be respected. The family doctor is sometimes consulted before an operation as to how far the consent form allows discretion to the surgeon: patients are often reassured when the meaning of 'discretion' in those circumstances is explained to them.

Another form of consent has caused concern to those involved in drug trials and other forms of comparative treatments in general practice. As a general rule, ethical committees postulate that a trial in which the emergence of a valid scientific conclusion seems unlikely is unethical. But to what extent can or should the proposed drug trial be explained to the prospective participant? Clearly any likely side-effects should be mentioned, together with the monitoring processes which will recognize and treat them. It may be difficult for patients to understand the theory of the double-blind trial, the placebo effect, and the reason why they will not know during the trial whether they are taking drug or placebo. Time has to be set aside to explain these matters simply if the confidence of the patient is to be preserved. And such explanations to each individual participant are quite essential if the charge of using patients as 'guinea-pigs' in experiments is to be avoided. In general practice, where for the most part the drugs to be used have been carefully studied in hospital conditions, risks may spring less from the drug substances themselves than from the manner in which they are used. For example, how ethical is it to suspend, temporarily, treatment of hypertension in order to get a baseline? How ethical is it to divide a population into two cohorts, one of which is to receive the active drug, that is, to have the condition treated, for period x, while the other is to receive a placebo for the same period, the whole scheme to be reversed for a second period y? Ethical committees usually hold, rightly, that in general practice drug trials, any such manoeuvre which was at all likely to disadvantage or harm the patient would be inadmissable without an escape clause by which treatment could be given if danger to a patient in a placebo group were perceived. Trials where the urgency of treatment is such that harm would come to a patient if it were delayed should be done under hospital conditions.

Besides these considerations, multi-centre drug trials in general practice, which yield much information that can be gained in no other way, must be scrutinized by an ethical committee to see that payment to participants does not exceed adequate reimbursement for the work involved, and bears some relationship to the time spent on the technicalities of the work. And it need hardly be said that such trials should in no circumstances be approved where they are an ill-concealed cover for product promotion.

Earlier in this chapter, the question was discussed of how much a patient should be told when a disastrous diagnosis has been made. As life moves towards its end, whether or not the patient recognizes it, a series of decisions has to be made by the doctor and those who care for the patient. At what stage is active treatment allowed to become passive? When does the struggle to contain and defeat the disease process give way to acceptance of its presence and inevitable progression? Particularly if the dying person is being nursed at home, it does not require much perspicacity from the relatives to realize that some drugs are being withdrawn, and others, known to all for their relief of pain and gift of soothing oblivion, are being introduced. While nowadays patients increasingly express their wish, sometimes in writing, not to be officiously kept alive, and relatives may reinforce their plea, occasions arise when in their last desperation at the approach of death, relatives may beseech the doctor not to withdraw treatment, but to seek fresh techniques, to bring in new specialists. The anguish of the relatives of those being nursed in hospital is often not helped by the question 'is he to be resuscitated?'. To say 'no', they may feel, is to admit defeat—should they have said 'yes' in order to take every chance?

It is often the family doctor's task to help the family and relatives to accept that, given an apparently hopeless situation—and here their trust in their doctor comes in again—it is ethical, proper, and merciful to treat pain and discomfort only, and to allow life peacefully to ebb away. Here no amount of legislation can substitute for the compassionate and ethical assessment of individual circumstances. Ethics will usually support compassion in the circumstances, for it guides us to proper moral judgement and standards of conduct.

In this chapter it has only been possible to touch on some of the many ethical problems that may concern the general practitioner. No reference has been made to problems of professional relationships, and only fleeting allusions to contrasts between the dictates of ethical considerations against those of legislation. The fascination of general practice is that it presents so much of life in microcosm, and those who practise can never know what problem will next present itself. For this reason general practitioners have a special need to be aware of the ethical problems in all the decisions they will be called upon to take.

12

Clinical oncology: medical and surgical practice

STEPHEN SPIRO

The management of patients suffering from conditions that are almost invariably fatal causes special problems in their treatment and caring. A respiratory physician frequently encounters malignant disease because lung cancer is the commonest malignancy in the Western world with approximately 35 000 new cases per annum in the UK, and 120 000 in the USA. It is becoming increasingly prevalent in the Third World and will become a major problem there over the next decade. Approximately 80 per cent of all cases of lung cancer are directly related to cigarette smoking and it is the relentless marketing of tobacco products that is sustaining the epidemic. Lung cancer is the commonest cause of death from malignant disease in men in the UK and the USA. It was widely forecast that its incidence would rise above that of breast cancer in 1985 to become the commonest malignancy in women. This has not yet happened, although the two diseases are now virtually equal in incidence. Latest surveys show that health education has perhaps made some impact as the number of new cases of lung cancer in men under 50 is falling; but this trend is not yet visible for women. The incidence in the elderly (older than 65 years) continues to rise.

During the last nine years our unit has developed a special interest in the treatment of lung cancer and most of this chapter will summarize our appraisal of the treatment options for these patients and the dilemmas they pose. The role of clinical trials and the associated ethical difficulties we encounter are also discussed.

The diagnosis of lung cancer is usually a straightforward matter once the patient is referred to a chest physician or surgeon. Clinical examination and the chest X-ray provide most of the circumstantial information, but the diagnosis must be established by obtaining definite histological (tissue) confirmation. In good hands cytological examination of sputum for malignancy can be assumed to be diagnostic but most prefer a biopsy of the tumour itself, usually obtained via the fibreoptic bronchoscope. Although the clinical picture of lung cancer often leaves little doubt in the mind of the physician as to what is wrong with his patient, tissue diagnosis is vital when definitive treatment, for example, surgery, radiotherapy, or chemotherapy, is contemplated. Often the options can only be considered if the cell type of the tumour is known (Table 12.1). Even if the patient's condition is too advanced for surgery or other 'local' treatment such as radiotherapy, the management of disseminated disease will involve decisions which are made easier if one is certain of both the diagnosis and of the specific cell type; the responses to palliative therapy vary considerably according to histological classification.

Table 12.1 Lung cancer cell types and growth rates

Type	Incidence (%)	Volume doubling time (days)	Untreated survival time (months)
Squamous cell	50	90	12
Adenocarcinoma	20	180	18
Small cell	20	33	2–3
Large cell	10	80	10

The age of patients with lung cancer presents special problems. The average age at presentation is rising from approximately 64 years a decade ago to a mean of 66 now. Thus one is dealing with an ageing population, of which many may feel they have lived their 'three-score years and ten', and if the facts are clearly stated to them, they may not wish to undergo major treatment which carries only a small chance of cure and associated significant risks of side-effects and even death. The elderly population, particularly elderly smokers, also have high rates of associated heart, kidney, and cerebral vascular disease, often with a previous history of myocardial infarction or cerebrovascular ischaemic episodes. Diabetes is commoner and frailty, together with deteriorating home support, is also frequent. Thus the physician or surgeon is confronted not only with a difficult disease which metastasises rapidly and requires careful assessment, but an ageing population where life goals may be quite different from that of their younger, enthusiastic physician.

THE TREATMENT OPTIONS

Surgery

The growth rate of the four different cell types of lung cancer separate squamous, adeno, and large cell tumours from the much more rapidly growing and aggressive small cell tumours (Table 12.1). The slower growth of the non small cell lung cancers (NSCLC), together with a less obvious propensity to disseminate, make them more amenable to surgical resection. However, since thoracotomy for lung cancer became established in the 1950s, the overall cure rate for the disease has not improved. What has happened is that the pre-operative selection and post-operative care have greatly advanced, making surgery safer with the immediate outcome much more predictable.

As regards the patient, there remain major difficulties in our choice of advice. Many of those diagnosed to have lung cancer and who apparently have technically resectable tumours have coexistent chronic bronchitis and/or emphysema, the other common pulmonary complications of cigarette smoking. Our ability to predict post-operative lung function from pre-operative values is imprecise. Clearly the quantity of lung tissue to be removed—lobectomy or pneumonectomy—will be a major factor in deciding whether the patient can withstand surgery, but in some cases it is not always certain pre-operatively whether the resection will be confined to a single lobe. Thus it may be necessary to remove so much lung tissue that the patient could not survive and the decision not to operate will be made on those grounds. It is harder with those in whom predicted post-operative lung function will be 'borderline' for reasonable quality of life. There seems little achievement in producing a respiratory cripple: as a result of an attempt to cure one disease, merely bringing another problem to the fore. Great care should be taken to explain to patients considering surgery that their life-style and mobility could be markedly affected. They will be reduced to a much slower walking pace by a pneumonectomy although they may be able to walk just as far, and must understand this inevitable limitation.

Deciding whether to operate on the over-70s is a growing problem. Recent data have suggested that tumours in the elderly grow as fast as in the young and will, if untreated, probably cause their death. Mortality data in the elderly show that the risk of peri-operative death remains twice as high as for those under 65; in the region of 6–7 per cent overall. Explaining these risks to patients is difficult as many may not be used to appreciating risks or making major decisions—particularly concerning themselves. A percentage risk to an individual is a statistical fact but to the person concerned it is 100 per cent if dead, not 6–7 per cent dead.

A small study by McNeil *et al.* (1978) suggested that older patients with operable lung cancer may prefer the 'near certainty' of a period of palliation following radiotherapy to the riskier prospect of surgery with a small but definite chance of immediate death, despite the prospect of cure. The study included only 14 patients but took into account each subject's willingness to take or avoid the risk of surgical mortality and the span of life he would, at the mean study age of 67 years, reasonably expect. The majority of patients were averse to the risks of surgery and would have settled for 2–3 more years of life. This is the only study assessing the patient's response to a defined series of gambles.

In applying the same approach to our patients, most found it impossible to make a decision for or against surgery as they were reluctant to become intimately involved in the decision. Most patients when asked to offer an opinion either became agitated or merely made it quite clear that they expected the physician to advise them what he considered best. Some patients then turned down that advice—but most accepted it. It would appear that provided a patient understands that there is some form of major risk to the procedure and that it does not guarantee cure, and that he is allowed to voice his own philosophy for his expectations and length and quality of life, a decision can be reached without distress. What remains important is for the doctor to complete X-ray and other investigations to assess the tumour and his decision on resectability, before the question of surgery is broached with the patient. The overall health of the patient and the quality of his home support must be included in this treatment advisory process before it is put to him.

Radiotherapy

The great majority of patients with NSCLC prove to be inoperable, either because of obvious extrathoracic metastatic disease or because the chest X-ray or more detailed surgical staging shows the mediastinal lymph nodes to be involved by tumour, rendering surgery unhelpful.

Once the disease has metastasized to lymph nodes in the mediastinum it may cause obstructive symptoms affecting venous drainage back to the heart (superior vena caval obstruction), oesophageal obstruction, or the primary tumour itself may block a major airway causing distal pneumonia. All these symptoms, and many due to extrathoracic metastatic disease such as bone pain, brain metastases, and other neurological symptoms are all indications for palliative irradiation. Provided the patient's general condition is acceptable, radiotherapy will relieve these distressing symptoms to a very great extent in most sufferers and there is little controversy about its use, except that those living some distance from a radiotherapy centre may have to be in-patients during treatment, which may be stressful for both patient and family.

The role of radiotherapy in patients whose disease appears to be confined to the thorax is much more controversial and, I believe, is a much too frequently used method of treatment.

In those whose NSCLC tumour appears technically resectable but the patient himself is unsuitable for surgery because of inadequate lung function, or other systemic disease, or simple refusal, there is a small but reasonable chance that radiotherapy could be curative, and there would be little argument against offering this treatment although the 5-year survival data are conflicting. Radiotherapy has the attraction to the patient (and the doctor) that it carries with it no treatment-related mortality, but it has its own toxicity in addition to tying the patient to a hospital department daily for five to six weeks. The role of radiotherapy in patients who are 'just' inoperable and in those who undergo surgery and, despite a lung resection, have residual disease either as obvious tumour visible to the surgeon, usually in lymph nodes, or reported to be present by the histologist in glands the surgeon removed believing them to be clear of disease, is far more controversial.

Some patients initially considered to be operable are found to have too extensive disease within the chest, shown either with computed tomography (CT) scanning or on mediastinoscopy (a surgical exploration and sampling of nodes, draining the involved lung through a small incision made at the root of the neck). These patients may have been told they have cancer and may be able to have it removed if the investigations are satisfactory. The problem comes when it is realized that surgery is no longer a reasonable option. Many of these patients are still enjoying good general health although they may have some respiratory symptoms caused by the primary tumour. There is to date no evidence that radiotherapy given with curative intent (radical treatment) in such patients significantly improves the five-year survival rate, although it may allay intrathoracic symptoms. Most surgeons, faced with failure for their treatment, feel obliged to offer an alternative treatment; radiotherapy is put to the patient as the natural alternative, and very few radiotherapists are able to turn the patient away in these circumstances. This treatment is usually not given with the patient's full, informed consent. He is often told that surgery was technically not feasible and therefore radiotherapy, which is not constrained to the same extent by anatomical boundaries, should be given. The patient is then subjected to up to six weeks of therapy, causing fatigue, some malaise, sometimes painful swallowing, all for no known or proven long-term benefit. Furthermore radiotherapy, a local treatment, often fails for the same reason as surgery—due to the emergence of distant metastases.

Many patients referred to radiotherapists will have been told the reasons for the referral and it then becomes extremely hard to deny an expectant individual any treatment. The alternative of no therapy until symptoms warrant is a devastating blow for many. As many radiotherapists accept that their treatment has a limited role in this type of presentation, studies have been designed to assess carefully the impact of radiotherapy on these otherwise fit patients, but at the same time accepting that the treatment is not being given with intent to cure. These are basically 'quality of life' studies—randomizing patients to immediate radiotherapy or to conservative management and then applying radiotherapy when symptoms referable to the primary tumour develop.

Most ethical committees require verbal informed consent prior to entry to such a study and this requires the patient to be made fully aware of his disease and that it is unknown whether early or late treatment is advisable. Full discussion with our patients entering this type of study caused major anxiety and depression in many of those who agreed to participate but were allocated to the 'wait and see' arm. It is abundantly clear that it is easier to manage a patient who is given therapy as soon as the disease is properly staged than to attempt to inform fully and gain agreement to postpone therapy. This would appear to be acceptable ethically; but in fact the distress caused to the untreated patients resulted in our own group withdrawing from this type of study. It is often much easier outside the clinical study framework to make up one's mind that radiotherapy is not curative and therefore not in the patient's best interest at that time. It is then reasonable to explain to a patient that the condition is often only slowly growing and may not cause symptoms for a considerable time and any treatment should be postponed until whenever that occurs. Since the first symptoms may well be due to distant metastases and nothing to do with treating the primary tumour site this is often the most sensible option. This, I believe, offers the patient the best potential for radiotherapy, that is, palliation when necessary.

Those who believe in the role of 'wait and see' radiotherapy compared with immediate treatment are constrained by the potential risk of anxiety a patient may experience if informed of the study protocol and having to participate in the decision to risk delaying treatment. This type of informed consent is often impossible to provide. An alternative in an attempt to answer important questions such as these would be not to inform the patient that there are treatment options, but to randomize him and proceed. Strictly speaking this is unethical, and it does not give respect to autonomy but, rather, reflects clinical practice; and yet it may structure treatment in such a way that knowledge can be gained which ultimately will be to the advantage of lung cancer sufferers. However it is unlikely to be as satisfactory a way of obtaining clear-cut data compared with a formal clinical trial having definitive criteria for entry. Hence this question has never been satisfactorily answered.

The other difficult area concerning full information is in those patients who undergo a resection, and histology shows the draining lymph nodes from the lung to be involved by tumour. It has been common practice to offer these patients mediastinal irradiation, a practice based on no convincing evidence of long-term efficacy and often very tough for the patient, following within a month of major surgery. Two recent studies have shown that post-operative radiotherapy in squamous cell tumours with or without involved but resected nodes does not improve five-year survival rates (Van Houtte *et al.* (1980); The Lung Cancer Study Group (1986)). Indeed in one of the studies radiotherapy seemed to be associated with a worse survival at five years (Van Houtte *et al.* (1980)). If note is taken of this data and post-operative irradiation is abandoned, should the patient be given the burden of knowing that the involvement of mediastinal lymph nodes—even resected nodes—is associated with a worse prognosis than was considered pre-operatively? In planning his future commitments this may be vital information, but it is seldom volunteered. It is wrong, I think, to burden most patients with the knowledge that they have residual disease which you do not intend to treat. However, the adoption of this approach will inevitably upset some patients who in retrospect may realize that they were not told the whole truth. Once clinical relapse is evident, treatment can be offered for symptom control and it is easier and more appropriate to tell the patient what has happened on that occasion. Informing patients of residual disease and offering them no therapy causes anxieties, sometimes searches for second and third opinions, and it downgrades their quality of life in most cases. It seems to me futile to tell most patients what they probably do not wish to know. The nearest relative should be informed and discussions as to the necessity of telling the patient gone into very fully with careful exploration why it might be kindest to leave him in ignorance.

Chemotherapy

The majority of patients with lung cancer have metastatic disease and chemotherapy might appear a logical systemic treatment.

Chemotherapy in non small cell lung cancer (NSCLC)

The essential purpose of a cytotoxic anti-tumour drug is both to prolong life and if possible to offer the hope of cure. There are several cytotoxic drugs to which, when given to a patient with lung cancer, the tumour shows a 'response' (i.e. at least a 50 per cent reduction in measurable tumour diameter in two perpendicular directions) in some patients. In NSCLC the number of patients showing responses to single agents is small but when between two and four drugs are combined the response rate increases. It would appear logical that a drug or group of drugs that decrease tumour size will delay death due to that disease. Unfortunately in NSCLC this has not yet been established. The literature abounds with several hundred studies looking at either the simple response rates of cycles of drugs given to patients with measurable disease and noting the length of remission; and comparisons of two or more regimens in usually matched patient populations. In some instances when a particular regimen is shown to be more active than another it is assumed to be effective in prolonging survival and then compared with further regimens. However, there are major pitfalls in these comparative studies:

1. The patient groups must be identically matched for age, disease cell type, disease staging, and patient well-being (performance status). This is often not the case, with gross imbalances in patient selection rendering many published studies of little value.

2. NSCLC tumours grow relatively slowly and the starting point of chemotherapy in the natural history of the tumour will be the factor that has the greatest impact on survival. If a large study is planned, it is necessary to recruit for a long time in order to obtain matched groups of adequate size in order to obtain significant differences (necessary in this disease as responses are generally poor). This can be extremely difficult and most studies succumb to the pressure to publish prematurely or to the arrival of new drugs or 'improved' analogues of existing drugs and have insufficient patience (and patients) to complete the study with adequate statistical security.

3. It is possible that chemotherapy—or at least some chemotherapy—actually shortens survival. It is powerfully immunosuppressive, toxic, and associated with neutropaenia (low white blood-cell count), septicaemia and, in some patients, death. These risks together with anorexia, weight loss, and hair loss often increase with each drug added to the regimen and with dose escalation.

4. There have to date been only a handful of studies controlled by a no treatment arm and in these there has been no survival advantage conferred on the chemotherapy groups. However, within some treatment groups there will be a small number of responders to chemotherapy who live considerably longer than the group mean.

In many centres chemotherapy for advanced NSCLC is readily given—despite the lack of evidence that it prolongs survival. Indeed in the UK there are but a handful of documented patients whose tumour responded completely (i.e. X-ray or other evidence of disease returning to normal) and a complete response is a prerequisite for long survival. It would appear unethical to offer chemotherapy to patients with NSCLC because of the lack of such an advantage, and because of the high incidence of toxicity and the risk of treatment-related death.

Very recently the picture has changed a little with the emergence of more active regimens as newer agents—particularly Cisplatinum and Ifsofamide—seem much more active than previously tested drugs. We intend to evaluate these promising reports and are planning to compare radical radiotherapy given to patients with localized NSCLC, to four courses of chemotherapy followed by radical radiotherapy. Clearly this can only be carried out with the patients' consent but a major ethical dilemma is to try to avoid the complexities, hazards, and toxicity of chemotherapy being explained to all potential entrants when only 50 per cent will be allocated to the combined treatment arm. Hence we intend to use the Zelen model of informed consent. Suitable patients will be randomized for entry to the study. Those randomized to radiotherapy alone will be offered this treatment without being told they are part of a clinical study as radical radiotherapy is considered standard treatment by most radiotherapists. Those randomized to chemotherapy and radiotherapy will be asked to consider entry to the study and the full implications of chemotherapy will be outlined in detail. All patients randomized to this arm must be analysed for survival as a single group whether they receive the chemotherapy and radiotherapy as planned, or in fact refuse chemotherapy and as a consequence receive radiotherapy alone.

Within the framework of clinical trials there also remains a place for chemotherapy in patients with widespread disease. It remains important to evaluate new agents both for toxicity and efficacy and this is often carried out on these patients. These 'phase II' studies must be performed only on patients with measurable disease. The studies are not intended to be curative and often are only designed to adminster a precise number of treatments to evaluate response. Informed consent is essential and most patients faced with advancing disease agree to enter, despite the potential toxicity of the drug being made absolutely clear.

Chemotherapy in small cell lung cancer (SCLC)

While many consider it unethical to treat NSCLC with chemotherapy, the converse is true for the small cell type. Its very rapid growth rate means that the tumour is already very bulky when diagnosed and usually disseminated to bone, liver, and/or brain. This cell type is operable only in about 1 per cent of cases. Small cell lung cancer (SCLC) is much more responsive to chemotherapy and the untreated median survival of 2–4 months can be prolonged to 9–18 months by chemotherapy. Those patients with disease apparently confined to one hemithorax (limited disease) have the best median survival of 18 months.

Chemotherapy has become an accepted form of treatment because it relieves symptoms in 75 per cent of sufferers, prolongs survival, and in about 20 per cent of patients with disease limited to one hemithorax offers survival to two years or more with the prospect of cure in a few cases.

Sadly, the majority of patients with SCLC present with extensive disease (spread beyond the hemithorax) and chemotherapy produces hardly any two year survivors and a median survival in the region of 6–9 months. Most physicians, however, diagnosing this type of lung cancer would offer their patient chemotherapy as worthwhile palliation.

Clinical trials in SCLC are still numerous and much active research into chemotherapy, often in combination with radiotherapy, continues. Most studies are comparative—one chemotherapy regimen versus another, or a combined regimen with radiotherapy. Informed verbal consent has to take into account that the patient has a disease almost certain to be fatal. In experienced treatment centres the expected median survival of these patients is well known and no study is likely to contain a treatment option that is markedly inferior; or at least if it were it would rapidly become recognized as such. Most current studies today, in the absence of any major new drug or choice of treatment, are concerned with well-tried and understood medications.

Most patients asked to enter studies will have been told very recently that they have lung cancer. This fact alone is often rejected or received reluctantly, or renders the patient into a shocked or depressed state. To have to understand in addition the types of therapy available is a further load; and then, the broaching of the prospect of entering a clinical trial and discussing further variables in the treatment is often too much for many patients. We and the patients themselves, whether or not they know this, are faced often with only a possible marginal benefit from any one treatment compared with another. Possible long-term advantages or disadvantages, problems that concern the ethics of many other drug trials, are not relevant in SCLC, or at least, relevant to a minority of potential entrants. One is faced with an entirely predictable disease which can be favourably influenced by chemotherapy in 80 per cent of patients for a relatively short time, but in whom some alternative therapy is to be proposed as a potential improvement. Clearly the extent of information offered has to depend on the patient's intelligence, health, family wishes and support, and his own reaction to the news of his disease.

It is our practice always to inform the patient of the possibility of entering a trial. However, any discussion is preceded by informing him of the diagnosis, the probable prognosis, and the potential benefits of chemotherapy. Patients are also told that chemotherapy is palliative, with a full explanation that only a small number can expect to be cured. Most patients appear to accept this information and are sufficiently trusting to agree to enter studies assessing different therapies. In providing information to consent, the potential benefit of chemotherapy is stressed. It is not volunteered, for example, that after chemotherapy has stopped the disease, after an unknown interval, is likely to relapse. However if this question is asked, the facts are made known.

In a recent study where a further randomization at relapse was made to receive either conservative management or further relapse chemotherapy it became clear that:

(1) many patients become totally confused about their treatment;

(2) the prospect of relapsing seemed to make many patients' attitude to their disease less positive;

(3) there was anxiety in some who were unable to receive further chemotherapy at relapse, and

(4) conversely there was anxiety at the prospect of more chemotherapy at relapse in those who found the initial chemotherapy courses difficult to tolerate.

CONCLUSIONS

The real options in treating patients with lung cancer are depressingly few. If fit and apparently technically operable, patients with NSCLC should be offered surgery. The role of radiotherapy is palliative and its limitations should be accepted by doctors treating patients with lung cancer until disproven. The improvement in median survival with chemotherapy in SCLC seen between 1977 and 1982 has reached a plateau but remains an area of much effort and clinical research.

Ten years ago only 2 per cent of patients with lung cancer entered clinical trials. The number is now probably higher. Since most ethics committees will sieve out the more eccentric and unpredictable studies, it appears that most trials today are based on established medication. Thus patients with lung cancer undergoing treatment will need to be as informed as would appear appropriate for whatever is being contemplated. This can only be done with the medical staff and support teams allowing time to counsel patients and their relatives. The full impact of diagnosis and possible treatments can only be delivered piecemeal to allow understanding and the opportunity for asking questions. In our unit clinical nursing specialists in oncology provide a depth of support and fund of knowledge to our patients that is too seldom available nationwide. Close integration of junior and senior medical and nursing staff with the patient allows trust to be built up rapidly. The explanation of details of proposed treatment (and a clinical trial if appropriate) is then more easily discussed and understood. The attempt must be to treat the patient as a whole, and to involve his family, and then to decide the best policy for the individual. The patient wants to know that he will be looked after by caring people, and he will be more ready to accept advice in these circumstances with confidence.

Thus one might summarize by suggesting that if a patient is eligible for entry into a clinical trial, informed verbal consent should be sought, although, as detailed above, the entire truth about the likely (but never certain) final outcome of the disease could be withheld unless specifically demanded.

The vast majority of patients are not entered into studies. In these cases they should be given their diagnosis. However, how much they are told of what lies ahead has to be the decision of their physician. The more fully he probes the patient, and the care he takes in assessing the family, and the more support he has available in terms of skilled nursing and counselling staff, the better he will be at guessing the correct approach for each individual. However, once you have told somebody the worst you cannot withdraw this. There are occasional patients who demand to know exactly what the future holds so that financial affairs, etc., can be dealt with. But for most a careful approach, the truth but with positive ideas and support, and the thought that there will be some treatment available when the need arises, if it is not likely to be beneficial at the time of diagnosis, is the best we can do.

REFERENCES

McNeil, B. J., Weichsselbaum, R., and Pauker, S. G. (1978). Fallacy of the five-year survival in lung cancer. *New England Journal of Medicine*, **299**, 1397.

Van Houtte, P., *et al*, (1980). Postoperative radiation therapy in lung cancer: a controlled trial after resection of curative disease. *International Journal of Radiation Oncology Biology and Physics* **6**, 983.

The Lung Cancer Study Group. (1986). Effects of post operative mediastinal radiation on completely resected Stage II and Stage III epidermoid cancer of the lung. *New England Journal of Medicine*, **315**, 1377.

13

The epistemology of surgery

MICHAEL BAUM

It is important that medical or surgical interventions be determined on the highest quality of evidence lest untested opinions of efficacy result in a death sentence or a sentence to a life of disability and pain. The greater the scale of intervention, the more toxic or mutilating the treatment, the more irreversible the consequences of such invasions, then the greater is the entitlement of the public to expect unequivocal justification in its support. There is a hierarchy in the cogency of evidence that may be adduced in defence of medical interventions (Green and Byar 1984). Of lowest order is the anecdotal case report. Higher than this would rank case series without controls, or series with literature controls. Higher still might be analyses using computer data bases, or case controlled observational studies. Finally, the summit of this pyramid is held by the randomized controlled clinical trial which, ideally, has been replicated more than once. The reasons why a randomized controlled trial is considered the epitome of scientific validity are worth restating.

Randomization avoids conscious or unconscious bias in treatment allocation. Prognostic factors, whether known or unknown, tend to be balanced between treatment groups. Randomization guarantees the validity of statistical tests of significance. As patients are followed up prospectively, using a clearly defined protocol, missing data are less likely and a biased differential loss to follow-up is avoided. To put it another way: 'alternative strategies should be considered not as an easier route to quicker answers but as second choice methodologies when there are compelling reasons precluding the implementation of a randomized clinical trial' (Ellenberg 1981). Alternative strategies are much favoured by the proponents of alternative medicine, who share disinclinations to subject their panaceas to the hazards of refutation. Therefore the only true demarcation between the practice of orthodox scientific medicine and alternative medicine lies in the quality of evidence available in support of the remedy, rather than the nature of the remedy itself. At the same time, it has to be recognized that there are many occasions when genuine and compelling reasons preclude the implementation of a randomized clinical trial. Paradoxically, it is in the area where the interventions are of the greatest scale, with the most irreversible consequences, that the most compelling reasons are paraded against the conduct of randomized clinical trials, namely the evaluation of major surgical procedures.

A recent paper by Rudicel and Esdaile addresses these issues in a forthright and novel way (Rudicel and Esdaile 1985). After rehearsing all the arguments in favour of the randomized controlled trial, they go on to describe some of the unique reasons why orthopaedic surgeons have been inhibited from evaluating their procedures using the classical methodology. First they describe the ethical issues surrounding informed consent and the disclosure of uncertainty that this entails; next they describe the inbuilt bias that favours a technically simpler operation widely in use, against a complex new procedure. 'A new procedure cannot be studied fairly until the technique is established by experience with the procedure in patients. Once this has been done, it is difficult to generate enthusiasm in the developers of the procedure for conducting a randomized controlled trial'. It is further suggested that the long-term follow-up for most surgical randomized controlled trials makes their performance logistically difficult and expensive. The risk of surgery and its irreversibility demand as much certainty as is possible that the operation prescribed is the correct one. Surgeons have reported that their participation in a randomized controlled trial might jeopardize their credibility with patients by making them appear unsure and indecisive. Finally, these authors suggest that uncertainty is antithetical to surgical training and surgeons may feel that the doctor–patient relationship will be impaired if they appear less than confident.

For these reasons it is worth challenging the stated objections to conventional randomized trials for surgical procedures. First, the ethical issues do not go away in the absence of randomized controlled trials. During a period of genuine uncertainty in any aspect of clinical practice there is the same ethical imperative (or lack of it) to inform patients of this uncertainty, whether they are treated within or without a clinical trial. To do otherwise would be to exercise double standards. Next, the irreversibility of surgery, as already stated, demands the highest order of evidence before the new procedure is widely disseminated in standard practice. This very irreversibility demands as much certainty as possible on the part of the surgeon, yet such certainty cannot be achieved without the results of a properly designed study. It is true that the design of randomized trials favours simpler operations which are not so dependent on the technical skills of the surgeon. There may also be difficulties, though not insurmountable (see Berstock *et al.* 1985; Fisher *et al.* 1980; Ribiero 1978) in undertaking long-term follow-up of large numbers of patients; but this is no reason for not undertaking such trials. Finally, to suggest that surgeons are unique in feeling uncomfortable with uncertainty is false. Quacks depend on the credulity of the public and a surgeon with an overriding belief in infallibility should carefully re-examine his attitudes. Surgical procedures of all degrees of complexity have been evaluated by large prospective clinical trials: for example, trials for coronary artery bypass (Jennett *et al.* 1984), carotid artery endarterectomy (Doll, pers. comm.) and highly selective vagotomy. To illustrate the success of the randomized trial and the pitfalls of non-science in surgery, I will trace the history of treatment for primary carcinoma of the breast.

THE HISTORY OF THE TREATMENT OF BREAST CANCER

Breast cancer has been recognized as a clinical entity from before the time of Hippocrates. An ancient Egyptian papyrus clearly described the disease and its demarcation from acute inflammatory mastitis (Breasted 1930). The ancient Egyptian physicians wisely advised a non-interventional approach. In fact, one of the greatest tragedies in the history of this subject has been the persistent error in confusing activity with progress. Mastectomy of a kind was introduced by the surgeons of the Graeco-Roman period. Probably the first clearly defined hypothesis concerning the nature of the disease and its appropriate treatment can be attributed to Galen. He thought that breast cancer was a systemic disorder due to the retention and excess of black bile (melancholia). As inductive support for this hypothesis, he pointed out that the disease was more common in postmenopausal women, who cease their monthly menstrual loss, and that the menstrual periods were a natural mechanism for clearing the body of excess black bile. The therapeutic consequences, therefore, were self-evident, and for the next 1600 years, women were treated by purgation and bleeding to rid the body of the putative excess of black bile (De Moulin 1983). Local therapy consisted predominantly of cautery and noxious topical applications for the management of offensive and bleeding ulcers. It goes without saying that nothing other than anecdotal support for these remedies existed in the literature.

The first conceptual and, hence, therapeutic revolution dates from the time of Virchow in the 1860s. He demonstrated, by anatomical dissections of cadavers of women who had died of untreated advanced breast cancer, that the disease was commonly seen plugging the lymphatic channels and replacing the regional lymph nodes. He deduced, therefore, that the disease was not a systemic disorder but a localized abnormality, with the spread of the disease along the lymph channels. The cancer was then temporarily arrested in the lymph nodes, which were thought to act as filter-traps. With exhaustion of the proximal lymph node barriers, the more distal lymph node barriers became infected and, ultimately, the disease gained access to the vital organs by centrifugal extension of this process. The therapeutic consequences of this anatomical model were taken up by William Halsted in America, Willhelm Meyer in Germany, and Samson Handley in the United Kingdom, all within a few years of each other (Halsted 1898). All three of these great and influential surgeons developed a radical type of mastectomy, which attempted to rid the body of the primary focus and all surgically accessible lymph node deposits, while avoiding cutting across infected lymphatic channels.

There was never any prima-facie evidence that the introduction of this radical approach improved on the more conservative type of surgery or, for that matter, on sytemic therapy prevalent until the 1880s. On the contrary, publications exist demonstrating that throughout the first 30 years of this century the best result achieved by the radical approach was approximately a 10 per cent ten-year survival, which is almost identical to that achieved by Gross in Philadelphia in the 1880s (Gross 1880). In fairness to Halsted it must be recognized that he successfully reduced the operative mortality and improved the local control of the disease, and no other treatment modalities existed at the time.

It has also to be remembered that the majority of the cases treated in that era would be considered locally advanced today, and excluded from trials of primary local therapy. Surgeons became very frustrated with the failure of the Halsted radical mastectomy to cure breast cancer, but instead of questioning the underlying hypothetical model, they sought improvements by extending the concept to its logical conclusion, leading to the surgical barbarity of extended radical mastectomies and even forequarter amputations. Inevitably there was a reaction against such excess, and we should never forget the contributions of the great and distinguished British surgeon, Sir Geoffrey Keynes. In the face of all established surgical dogma, Keynes introduced a conservative mode of treatment for this disease in the early 1930s, eventually publishing a historical paper in the *British Medical Journal* demonstrating that the results of local excision plus radium needle insertion were equal to any published data advocating the use of the radical approach (Keynes 1937). Perhaps as a result of the intervening war years and Sir Geoffrey Keynes's retirement, this conservative approach never achieved popularity. On the contrary, Sir Stanford Cade, summing up a debate on the merits of the treatment of early breast cancer at the Royal Society of Medicine in 1947, sanctioned the radical mastectomy as the appropriate treatment for Stage I of the disease (Cade 1947). Thus, we have the prospect of two great surgical names advocating diametrically opposite therapies. If the big men could not agree, what were the little men to do?

As throughout the history of our subject, the little men followed the dictates of the authority with the highest profile and the greatest charisma. This can hardly be considered science of any description, but more akin to the behaviour of the faithful within a religious cult. The appropriate scientific response to such a clash of convictions is neatly summed up in the words of Sir Karl Popper:

> 'Instead of discussing the probability of the hypothesis, we should try to assess what trials it has withstood and how far it has been able to prove its fitness to survive' (Popper 1959).

RANDOMIZED CONTROLLED TRIALS OF LOCO-REGIONAL THERAPY

The first truly randomized trials for the treatment of early breast cancer can be credited to the Manchester Christie group, headed by Paterson and Russell (see Paterson and Russell 1959). Since then a host of complementary studies have been completed, with mature follow-up data available for between 10 and 30 years. These studies have compared, in a strictly scientific manner, treatments varying from extended radical mastectomy to local excision, with or without radiotherapy, at the most conservative extreme. In retrospect, the trials of this period were really addressing themselves to two different questions. First, would the use of radical radiotherapy provide the same degree of local control and the same cure rate as radical surgery? In other words, was radiotherapy as effective as surgery in ablating cancer from the regional nodes? The second set of trials were asking a more interesting biological question concerning the relevance of the regional lymph nodes in the putative immunosurveillance of cancer. Thus, procedures that preserved the axillary nodes intact were compared with surgical and radiotherapeutic techniques aimed at total destruction of these nodes (Berstock *et al.* 1985). Observed *in toto*, we can now say with the greatest statistical confidence that although the degree of local control varies directly with the magnitude of the treatment field, no important differences in survival have been detected. Biological extrapolations from these data might suggest one of three conclusions:

(1) untreated lymph node metastases do not act as a source of tertiary spread;

(2) the immuno-suppressive effects of radical surgery or regional radiotherapy are of no clinical relevance; or

(3) the metastasizing capacity of involved nodes is balanced by the

> immuno-surveillance mediated in some way by the intact uninvolved lymph nodes.

Whatever the explanation, these accumulated data support the concept of biological predeterminism. Further analyses of subgroups suggest that those patients with lymph nodes invaded by cancer at the time of diagnosis are those most often predetermined to die (Fisher 1970). As a result of this experience, all but a few die-hards among surgeons and radiotherapists experienced a paradigm shift. The lymph node status of the patient is now looked upon as an expression rather than a determinant of the prognosis. It is a wry pastime to study the attitudes of the die-hards among the medical profession and their attempts to rationalize away the failures of the radical approach. It has been argued that if the patients were diagnosed early as a result of screening programmes, then radical mastectomy would cure them all. Secondly, the failure of radical surgery and radical radiotherapy within randomized controlled trials represents the failure of the surgeons and radiotherapists to deliver the treatment correctly. The therapeutic inductivists still point to the uncontrolled data sets from the great radical surgeons and the centres of radiotherpeutic excellence. Finally, those women who have suffered radical mastectomy and are alive and well to tell their tale 30 years later, are once again paraded as a living tribute to the perfection of the treatments they received. To my mind, this type of conceptual rationalization is no different from the logic adduced by proponents of fringe medicine (Baum 1983).

THE QUALITY OF LIFE AFTER THE TREATMENT OF EARLY BREAST CANCER

It is reasonable for patients to ask whether there is life after mastectomy. The pioneering work of Peter Maguire has clearly demonstrated that about one-third of patients treated for breast cancer by some form of mastectomy will suffer serious and debilitating psychosexual morbidity (Maguire 1982). Of course, the other side of the coin must not be overlooked. Seventy per cent of women provided with a modest amount of rehabilitation and prosthetic advice can enjoy a fulfilling and normal life by drawing on their natural reserves to cope with one of life's major crises. It is a reasonable assumption that the loss of the breast contributes the major component to the psychosexual morbidity of the treatment, but like all medical assumptions, this needs challenging. In 1983, the Cancer Research Campaign (CRC) launched a trial to compare mastectomy with breast conservation for women diagnosed as suffering from early breast cancer. The study was conducted with informed consent, and is unique in having a built-in formal assessment of the psychosexual morbidity in both arms of the trial. The results of this study are, to say the least, counter-intuitive, suggesting that the major contribution to the psychosexual morbidity is not so much the treatment as the diagnosis of the disease itself (Fallowfield *et al.* 1986). This should not suggest for a moment a return to the bad old days of radical mastectomy, but should redirect our attention to the development of counselling services, to enable women to come to terms with their diagnosis and the inevitable threat to their life that this poses.

TRIALS OF ADJUVANT SYSTEMIC THERAPY

If the majority of patients with early breast cancer and positive axillary nodes die within a few years, however perfect the loco-regional therapy, then surely they carry occult micro-metastases present at the time of diagnosis. As that must be the case, then cure can only result from the addition of effective systemic therapy. Experience with advanced breast cancer demonstrates an objective response-rate of the order of 60 per cent, with prolonged cyclical combination therapy, which is twice that expected with an endocrine approach. *Ipso facto*, node-positive patients should be cured by adjuvant systemic chemotherapy. So compelling were these arguments and so beautiful the new hypothesis that many medical oncologists felt it unethical to do randomized trials and, like all inductivists, soon found sufficient corroborative evidence to satisfy themselves. To my mind, such individuals are as mistaken as those who uncritically accepted the Halstedian dogma 70 years ago, particularly as some of these chemotherapeutic excesses can be considered as the medical equivalent to a forequarter amputation! A recent review of the results of randomized controlled trials of adjuvant chemotherapy has arrived at the following general conclusions (Goldhirsch *et al.* 1986).

1. Whatever combination regimen is used there is likely to be a significant delay in the time to first relapse.
2. Although many individual trials have yet to show an improvement in crude survival, a statistical overview of all the available data suggests that a 30 per cent reduction in the risk of dying over the first five years may be achieved following the treatment of pre-menopausal women with node-positive diseases. The benefits for post-menopausal women appear to be marginal.

What, therefore, are the biological implications of these results? First, there is little doubt that the natural history of early breast cancer has been perturbed, lending support to the deterministic model. Whether this perturbation will translate itself into a useful therapeutic advantage for groups other than pre-menopausal node-positive patients remains to be seen. Secondly, the intriguing difference between the behaviour of pre- and post-menopausal women deserves some explanation. The chemotherapy lobby is not short of inductivists and much support has been generated for the concept that the effect of adjuvant systemic chemotherapy is dose-related (Bonadonna and Valagusa 1981). Post-menopausal women seem incapable of tolerating the maximum (?optimum) doses prescribed. This suggestion requires further exploration, with trials of high-dose versus low-dose chemotherapy. To accept the suggestion without prospective studies is to be guilty of a tautology; yet at the same time if older women were incapable of tolerating high-dose chemotherapy, this is certainly an inherent defect of the treatment unless one is prepared to push the drugs beyond the tolerance of the patient, surely a dangerous and inhumane policy. An alternative explanation for this differential effect might be that the cytotoxic drugs are mediating their effect by a chemical castration. This hypothesis has already won some support, following studies of ovarian and pituitary function in women receiving adjuvant chemotherapy (Rose and Davis 1977). It follows, therefore, that to test the hypothesis generated by the trials of adjuvant chemotherapy, one should conduct trials of adjuvant endocrine therapy investigating prophylactic castration and the use of adjuvant tamoxifen.

Trials of prophylactic castration following local treatment for cancer are not new but have suffered in the past from inadequate sample size, leaving uncertainty as to its potential benefit. This subject has recently been reviewed, suggesting that such an approach might indeed produce results of the same order achieved by polychemotherapy for pre-menopausal women, but at the great expense of inducing a premature menopause in young women already facing the threat of loss of the breast (Cole 1970). For the purpose of this chapter however, I wish to concentrate on the trial of tamoxifen therapy, which can be judged to have had the most profound effect on our biological thinking about the disease. The Nolvadex Adjuvant Trial Organisation (NATO) launched a study in 1977 to investigate whether the anti-oestrogen tamoxifen (Nolvadex) would have any benefit for women undergoing mastectomy for early breast cancer (NATO 1983). Approximately 1300 patients were recruited over a period of two and a half years. These consisted of pre-menopausal node-positive cases and post-menopausal node-positive and node-negative cases.

Following local therapy women were randomized to the group receiving tamoxifen, 10mg twice daily for two years, or to an untreated control group. A second-order hypothesis suggested that the women most likely to benefit were those whose primary tumour was rich in oestradiol receptor (E2R) content. Therefore, as a parallel study, attempts were made to collect samples of the tumours from all patients entered into the trial. The published data demonstrated a significantly prolonged disease-free interval in the treated group as a whole, which has recently been translated into a 30 per cent reduction in the risk of dying within the first five years following treatment (NATO 1985).

Paradoxically, a Cox's multivariate regression analysis has failed to demonstrate any interaction between treatment and patient subgroups, divided according to menopausal or oestrogen receptor status. The world overview of similar trials has strongly corroborated this implausible outcome, paving the way for a whole new set of randomized trials of alternative endocrine approaches, with the objective of improving both the length and quality of survival.

In this short historical survey, it can be witnessed that within the passage of 30 years the dogmatic certainty of the Halsted radical mastectomy for all patients with breast cancer has been replaced by a healthy and scientifically honest period of uncertainty. This era of uncertainty has led the way to a reduction in the physical morbidity of treatment together with a recognition of the importance of the psychological morbidity of treatment. At the same time, the use of adjuvant systemic therapy has improved the length of survival for many women with early breast cancer, while the quality of survival has been improved by the replacement of toxic polychemotherapy for a large proportion of these women with the non-toxic agent tamoxifen.

THE ETHICS OF RANDOMIZED CONTROLLED TRIALS

Two trends are emerging that may hamper the progress of scientific medicine, that is, medicine where intuition and theory are backed by sound evidence. Those opposed to experiments on animals may make it increasingly difficult to pursue certain types of experiment. Secondly, the issues of clinical experiments have been exposed to ill-informed and hostile criticism. It would be regrettable if ill-judged litigation frightens doctors and patients away from participation in clinical trials.

Society may not intend to draw a line across the balance sheet of clinical medicine with the cry of 'thus far and no further', but may inadvertently do so. If that happened it would not only delay progress towards new forms of therapy, but also perpetuate various inadequately tested and potentially hazardous procedures now in vogue. Ten years ago, a halt to reliable cancer therapy trials would have helped to perpetuate the indiscriminate use of several ineffective types of immunotherapy; today, such a halt might help to perpetuate ineffective and hazardous types of chemotherapy, and would ensure that surgical procedures continue to be determined by fashion rather than facts.

Four years ago, an elderly woman died after the portal infusion of 5-fluoracil as an adjunct to surgical removal of a rectal cancer. As she was taking part in a controlled clinical trial, this was drawn to the attention of the Birmingham coroner. Summing up, he said, 'The whole idea of concealed controlled trials should be brought to the public notice for proper discussion'. I agree. The time is ripe for public discussion of these very difficult issues, but I would hope it could be between people who have taken the trouble to learn a great deal about the haphazard nature of much of what passes for medical knowledge, and how much more awful medical practice would be were it not for trials. Trials can puncture medical pomposity, and the ethics of how to conduct them can best be debated by people who understand clearly the ethics of whether to conduct them, and the grossly unethical consequences of inadequate experimental design.

With operable cancer of the breast, for example, many surgeons believed that it was enough to remove the lump and treat the remainder of the breast with radiotherapy. Others still consider that inadequate, and believe that removal of the entire breast is advisable. Each practises according to his conscience and neither is judged unethical.

Again, one surgeon might carry out mastectomy for early breast cancer for ten years, and then suddenly switch to lumpectomy and radiotherapy for the next ten years, retrospectively comparing the two approaches. This is done in good faith and would be judged entirely ethical. Yet, it represents 'haphazard' allocation of treatment (depending on which doctor happens to be consulted) without the patients' knowledge of the basis for the allocation. If, on the other hand, a surgeon, uncertain as to optimal treatment, randomizes his patients without their knowledge into one or other treatment, this might be judged unethical by some people. It could be argued, however, that to inform the patient of the nature of the trial is at best unnecessary and at worst damaging in that the knowledge may harm both patient and trial. Perhaps the chief problem is the novelty of the idea that the best treatment may only be determined by a lottery.

ACKNOWLEDGEMENTS

I wish to acknowledge the continuing support of the CRC and, in particular, Dr Nigel Kemp. I also freely acknowledge the intellectual stimulus and encouragement provided by Dr Iain Chalmers, Dr Bernard Fisher, Dr Roar Nissen-Meyer, Mr Richard Peto, and Dr William Silverman, who have been the necessary catalysts that were essential for the synthesis of this philosophical amalgam. Finally, I wish to express my unreserved thanks to all the clinicians and pathologists of the NATO and CRC groups whose extra unrewarded efforts and intellectual honesty made all these trials possible.

REFERENCES

Baum, M. (1983). Quack cancer cures or scientific remedies? *Clinical Oncology*, 9, 275–80.

Berstock, D. A., Houghton, J., Haybittle, J., and Baum, M. (1985). The role of radiotherapy following total mastectomy for patients with early breast cancer. *World Journal of Surgery*, **9**, 667–70

Bonadonna, G. and Valagusa, P. (1981). Dose response effect of adjuvant chemotherapy in breast cancer. *Lancet*, **i**, 1174.

Breasted, J. H. (1930). *The Edwin Smith papyrus*, pp. 403–6. University of Chicago Press.

Cade, Sir S. (1948). Discussion: the treatment of cancer of the breast. *Proceedings of the Royal Society of Medicine*, **41**, 129.

Chalmers, I. (1986). Minimising harm and maximising benefit during innovation in health care: controlled or uncontrolled experimentation? *Birth*, **13**, 155–64.

Cole, M. P. (1970). Prophylactic compared with therapeutic X–ray artificial menopause. *2nd Tenovus Workshop on Breast Cancer*, pp. 2–11, Alpha-Omega, Cardiff.

De Moulin, D. (1983). *A short history of cancer*. Martinus Nyhoff Publishers, Amsterdam.

De Vries, B. C., *et al*, (1983). Prospective randomized multi-centre trial of proximal gastric vagotomy or truncal vagotomy and antrectomy for chronic duodenal ulcer: results after 5–7 years. *British Journal of Surgery*, **70**, 701–3.

Ellenberg, S. S. (1981). Studies to compare treatment regimens: The randomized clinical trial and alternative strategies. *Journal of the American Medical Association*, **246**, 2481–2.

Fallowfield, L., Baum, M., and Maguire, G. P. (1986). The effects of breast conservation on the psychological morbidity associated with the diagnosis and treatment of early breast cancer. *British Medical Journal*, **293**, 1331–4.

Fisher, B. (1970). The surgical dilemma in the primary therapy of invasive breast cancer: a critical appraisal. In: *Current problems in surgery*. Year Book Publishers, Chicago.

Fisher, B., *et al.* (1980). Findings from NSABP protocol No. B-04—comparison of radical mastectomy with alternative treatments for primary breast cancer 1. Radiation compliance and its relation to treatment outcome. *Cancer*, **46**, 1–13.

Goldhirsch, A., Gelber, R. D., and Davis, B. W. (1986). Adjuvant chemotherapy trials in breast cancer: an appraisal and lessons for patient care outside the trials. In: *Breast disease* (ed. J. F. Forbes), pp. 123–38.. Churchill Livingstone, Edinburgh.

Green, S. B. and Byar, D. P. (1984). Using data from registries to compare treatments: the fallacy of omnimetrics. *Statistics in Medicine*, **3**, 361–70.

Gross, S. W. (1980). *A practical treatise of tumours of the mammary gland.* Appleton, New York.

Halsted, W. S. (1898). The radical operation for the cure of carcinoma of the breast. *Johns Hopkins Hospital Reports*, **28**, 557.

Jennett, B., Dark B., and Dworkin, G. (1984). Consensus development conference: coronary artery bypass grafting. *British Medical Journal*, **289**, 1527–9.

Keynes, G. (1937). Conservative treatment of cancer of the breast. *British Medical Journal*, **ii**, 643–7.

Maguire, P. (1982). Psychiatric morbidity associated with mastectomy. In: *Clinical trial in early breast cancer 2nd Heidelberg Symposium.* (ed. M. Baum, R. Kay, and H. Scheurlen), 373–80. Birkhauser Verlag, Heidelberg.

Novaldex Adjuvant Trial Organisation (NATO) (1983). Controlled trial of tamoxifen as single adjuvant agent in management of early breast cancer. Interim analysis at 4 years by NATO. *Lancet*, **i**, 257–61.

Novaldex Adjuvant Trial Organisation (NATO) (1985). Controlled trial of tamoxifen as single agent in management of early breast cancer. Analysis at 6 years by NATO. *Lancet*, **i**, 836–40.

Paterson, R. P. and Russell, M. H. (1959). Clinical trials in malignant disease. *Journal of the Faculty of Radiologists*, **10**, 130.

Popper, K. R. (1959). *The logic of scientific discovery.* Hutchison, London.

Ribeiro, G. G. (1978). Thirty years experience with breast cancer clinical trials at the Christie Hospital in Manchester—clinical aspects. In: *Lecture note in medical informatics no. 4. Clinical trials in early breast cancer, Proceedings*, (ed. H. R. Scheurlen, G. Weckesser, and I. Armbuster), pp. 71–2. Springer, Heidelberg.

Rose, D. P. and Davis, T. E. (1977). Ovarian function in patients receiving adjuvant chemotherapy for breast cancer. *Lancet* (**i**), 1174.

Rudicel, S. and Esdaile, J. (1985). The randomized clinical trial in orthopaedics: obligation or option? *The Journal of Bone and Joint Surgery*, Incorporated 1985, **67** (8), 1284–93.

14
Choices in psychiatry

MAURICE LIPSEDGE

Psychiatrists enjoy enormous power over people, both patients and others, throughout their lifespan, from the time of conception to the disposal of a dead person's property. The psychiatrist can recommend a termination of pregnancy on psychiatric grounds. He can advise on the competence of parents to have the care and custody of their children and can even recommend permanent removal of a child from the care of his parents. He can advise an employer on whether a former patient should be considered for a job. His report on a patient's mental stability may adversely affect that individual's prospects for obtaining a life insurance policy or a mortgage. A psychiatrist might advise on a patient's ability to drive. He might be asked to assess whether an accident victim is malingering in a compensation claim or whether a recipient of permanent health insurance is exaggerating the extent of his disability. He might prescribe an opiate to an addict and in the UK he must notify the Home Office of his contact with such a patient. A psychiatrist can recommend compulsory detention and treatment in a mental hospital for up to six months. He might be asked to present evidence about a patient's mental state so that a court can decide if the accused is fit to stand trial on a criminal charge, and his assessment might provide mitigation for a wide variety of criminal offences ranging from murder, through indecent exposure, to shoplifting. Finally the psychiatrist can determine whether a patient is fit to manage his affairs and he can pronounce on a patient's testamentary capacity and his ability to dispose of his property as he wishes.

Given this immense and wide-reaching statutory and professional power, it is important for psychiatrists to refrain from claiming authority in every problem of living. The psychologizing of social action and of individual conduct has become commonplace. Many problems of thought, feeling, and behaviour are neither medical nor psychiatric and in many deviations of behaviour there may not necessarily be any medical contribution. Thus while psychiatrists may pontificate on social problems (such as football hooliganism, riots, or prostitution), their statements should not be regarded as invested with uniquely psychiatric knowledge. In any case, what constitutes the subject matter of psychiatry is determined by arbitrary decisions. Thus homosexuality was regarded as a psychiatric disorder until the 1973 decision reached by the American Psychiatric Association (APA) which eliminated homosexuality *per se* as a diagnostic entity. This decree followed a vote by the Board of Trustees of the APA, 50 per cent of whom declared themselves in favour of the view that homosexuality was to be considered a mental disorder only if it was 'ego-dystonic', that is, subjectively disturbing to the individual (Spitzer 1981).

Most paternalistic decisions in clinical psychiatry arise in situations where the physician feels that coercive intervention is justified on the grounds of the prevention of greater harm. The psychiatrist arrogates decisions to himself in the paternalistic belief that he is acting in the patient's best interests. The anticipated risks of non-intervention range from death of the patient by suicide or self-starvation in a profoundly depressed patient, through inflicting physical injury on others in the case of an individual regarded as dangerous, to severe deterioration in a patient's psychiatric state in the case of a person suffering from schizophrenia who refuses maintenance treatment with a long-term neuroleptic. Many clinical decisions are value-decisions, i.e. the weighing-up of risks and benefits of alternative outcomes. Consider the decision to recommend that a patient should take prophylactic lithium. This drug is used to prevent episodes of severe depression or hypomania. It is effective in perhaps 75 per cent of manic depressives. The benefit is freedom from relapse, while the risks include a degree of renal damage, hypothyroidism in 3 per cent, weight gain in approximately 30 per cent and intellectual impairment and emotional flattening in many cases. The psychiatrist is unable accurately to predict which patients are at risk of further episodes of major affective disorder, so he generally follows the rough and ready rule of thumb guideline, that two episodes within two years plus a familial disposition to manic-depressive disorder in a patient aged over 40 indicate a probability of further episodes unless chemical prophylactic measures are taken. The psychiatrist's view of the patient's welfare is influenced by the fact that his contact with patients generally occurs at moments of crisis—in the case of manic-depressives during periods of melancholia or of uncontrollable elation, disinhibition, and over-activity.

The physician's 'illness orientation' will make him focus on relapse-prevention at any cost. The patient, however, may find the cognitive dulling induced by lithium to be intolerable and may actually prefer the risks of hypomania (social or professional disgrace, bankruptcy, damage to family life) to a life of unmitigated sombreness.

In recommending treatment the psychiatrist is more than a neutral dispenser of information. He could simply offer the patient a list of side-effects, but such an inventory would deter most patients from trying any particular medication and would not really allow the patient to make an informed rational decision. The physician should take a more active role and explain to the patient that on the basis of probabilities, certain side-effects *might* occur and also what the prognosis *might* be if no treatment is instituted. Given the patient's lack of training and of experience of the natural history of other similar cases it would be negligent for a psychiatrist to refrain from making a recommendation on the grounds that he wished to avoid paternalism in the sense that 'father knows best'. However, an overdogmatic recommendation from the psychiatrist is unjustified, given the softness of the prognostic data, the uncertain incidence of side-effects, and especially the possible inapplicability of actuarial data to an individual case. Psychiatry may aspire to scientific status but in reality it operates as well-intentioned pragmatism.

The imposition of treatment against the patient's will is regarded as justified when the clinician believes that the patient's life would be at risk if coercion is not applied and the patient's condition is allowed to deteriorate.

Case history 1

A 50-year-old man was brought to the attention of the local social services department by his landlady. For one week he had not left his bed-sitting-room. He had remained in bed, eating nothing and taking only sips of water. He had a history of a previous episode of profound endogenous depression during which, while in a depressive stupor, he had lain down in a field in the middle of winter and had got frostbite. His legs became gangrenous and he had had both lower limbs amputated. During this second episode he was brought to the hospital as a compulsory patient under section 3 of the Mental Health Act. He explained his refusal to eat on the following grounds: he was a profoundly religious man, who regarded himself as a grave sinner who believed he had to starve himself as a penance for his misdeeds. He could hear divine commands to this effect. After admission he refused to eat or drink. I decided that compulsory ECT was mandatory to prevent this patient dying of malnutrition. This decision, a paternalistic one, was based on the view that the patient's physical survival was of greater importance than his civil liberties. The risks of ECT (a mortality of 3–9 per 100 000 ECT sessions and perhaps a minor degree of temporary memory deficit) seemed to be outweighed by the benefits. The patient did not give his consent to the electrical treatment. In this case the brain, the organ which effectively gives or withholds consent, is both involved in the disease process and is the direct object of treatment. In insisting on compulsory physical treatment for this patient I demonstrated a belief, probably shared by the majority of my colleagues, that a patient's right to refuse treatment on the basis of personal autonomy can be justifiably overridden in situations of extreme life-threatening mental disturbance. By the same token, I would support the use of forced medication with a tranquillizing drug in any emergency situation when a patient's behaviour is likely to cause immediate physical harm to himself or to other people.

On occasion a psychiatrist might collude with the surreptitious administration of antipsychotic medication.

Case history 2

A man of 60 was admitted to the intensive care unit of a general hospital. He was suffering from heart failure and while undergoing routine treatment of digoxin and diuretics it became apparent to the nursing and medical staff that he was mentally ill. He accused the nurses of poisoning his food and his manner became hostile and threatening. The junior doctor discovered that he had been assessed by a psychiatrist during a previous admission but had vehemently rejected his advice to take neuroleptic medication. The patient had also failed to attend the psychiatric out-patient department for follow-up. I was asked to assess him and to recommend treatment, by the cardiac team. The patient was clearly psychotic and expressed a number of paranoid delusions. In view of his lack of insight, and of the risk that he might discharge himself prematurely, thus putting himself at risk of serious deterioration in his physical health, I recommended that he be given a neuroleptic tablet with every dose of diuretic. In this case none of the basic rules of informed consent was observed, that is, there was no transmission of information about treatment in non-technical language to the patient and he was not given the opportunity to refuse the treatment.

The question of enforced treatment in the case of a patient whose mental state might deteriorate in the absence of medication is illustrated by the following case.

Case history 3

A 25-year old woman had been forced to leave university by the insidious development of paranoid schizophrenia. She had become increasingly eccentric and reclusive and eventually had barricaded herself in her student's residence because she believed that she was being observed by the Special Branch who were keeping her under electronic surveillance and penetrating her brain with lasers. She was admitted to hospital as a compulsory patient and lost all her paranoid delusions after treatment with antipsychotic medication. Her personality deteriorated in that her behaviour became childish and impulsive but as long as she continued with medication she remained free of ideas of persecution. However, because the medication caused excessive weight gain and because she had read about tardive dyskinesia (irreversible continuous involuntary rhythmical movements of mouth and tongue) which affects a proportion of people with schizophrenia treated with antipsychotic drugs for over a year, she refused to continue medication. Although it was highly likely that she would deteriorate and become floridly paranoid again, I did not feel that it was justified to intervene until the state of affairs had actually materialized. I think I was inhibited by reluctance to force physically a person who was not overtly 'ill' to take medication which, however beneficial from the short-term psychiatric view, might indeed cause irreversible neurological damage at some time in the future. In this case the decision not to violate the patient's autonomy was apparently taken because the anticipated deterioration had not yet occurred and I did not feel it would be justified to override her own wishes in what I would perceive paternalistically to be her best interests. Although the autonomy of the patient is generally regarded as morally pre-eminent, it has been argued that paternalism is justified when the decision a person makes is non-rational. The given grounds are that non-rational decisions are not autonomous decisions and that the physician's duty in such a case is to restore the patient's capacity for autonomy. I have some sympathy with this view and it probably underlies many of my more coercive or interventionist clinical decisions. While in this young woman's case it could not be disputed that it would be irrational for her to refuse medication on demonstrably delusional grounds, for example that the drugs had been tampered with by the Special Branch in such a way that they transmitted messages, her refusal to take neuroleptic medication because of the risk of tardive dyskinesia is certainly not psychotic. But it is not always easy to decide when a patient's decision is non-rational.

The standard definition of non-rationality would be when a patient expresses a demonstrably false belief which conflicts with the available evidence. An example is the emaciated anorexic who claims that she is fat. However, the psychiatrist must be a cultural relativist; otherwise he would regard as psychopathological an endless catalogue of beliefs in the supernatural ranging from the existence of evil spirits to the Roman Catholic doctrine of transubstantiation (Littlewood and Lipsedge 1989). He must also make an arbitrary judgement about the distinction between eccentricity and irrationality, and there is an ever-present risk of inappropriately labelling those individuals who fail to conform to society's definition of normal behaviour. Some radical critics of psychiatry, such as Scheff (1966), have claimed that it is involved in a conspiracy to control the behaviour of those citizens who deviate from social norms, and that the psychiatrist is really a 'professional licencer' of the socially imposed role of mental patient. (Cohen and Scull 1985; Ingleby 1981; Szasz 1987).

Psychiatrists have a dual duty, to protect patients from themselves and, on occasion, to protect society from patients. The prediction of danger to others presents the clinician with harder decisions, since an error of judgement might put the community at risk. Psychiatrists have modest skills in predicting dangerousness to self and quite limited skills in predicting danger to others. Psychiatrists in general tend to overestimate dangerousness (Tidmarsh 1982).

Case history 4

A 35-year-old man told me he was having sadistic fantasies involving the torturing and killing of children. These fantasies, which made him sexually aroused, were occurring more frequently and he was deliberately stimulating them by watching sadistic video films. He informed me of these preoccupations at an out-patient clinic the day after a summer bank holiday when the newspapers were full of two child murders which had occurred during the weekend. I advised the patient to come into hospital. Fortunately he agreed to voluntary admission. Had he refused there would have been a major legal problem had I wished to implement a compulsory hospital admission, since the presence of sadistic fantasies alone does not really constitute a mental illness. After a couple of weeks in hospital the patient reported that the sadistic fantasies had become less imperative and he was discharged. Since then he has attended regularly as an out-patient and the fantasies have varied in intensity. He has an 'open invitation' to attend the clinic or to be re-admitted on demand. In the past he has tried the antilibidinal agent cyproterone acetate but could not tolerate the side-effect of depression.

There are other times when one ethical obligation is in conflict with another, as in the dilemma of whether to betray a patient's confidence by warning a potential victim that he might be in danger (Roth and Meisel 1977).

Case history 5

I was asked by another psychiatrist to provide a second opinion on a 24-year-old man who had developed a delusional erotic attachment to a well-known 'page three' model. He had learnt from the newspapers that the model was planning to get married and he had written to her expressing his anger and jealousy and declaring his love. He informed his father that if the woman did marry his 'rival' he would have to kill her. He was a rather solitary, schizoid individual whose hobbies included collecting Nazi insignia and concentration camp literature and studying martial arts. He was an avid reader of Mishima. While the diagnosis was unclear, it seemed to me that he seriously intended to carry out his threat. I would have preferred him to be in hospital for observation during the time of the wedding. He refused to come in and neither his father nor the local authority social worker would co-operate with a formal admission, although his family doctor agreed that it would be justified to protect others. I felt it was imperative to warn his potential victim so I broke the patient's confidence by asking the police to inform the model of the danger. Three days later the patient was arrested while loitering near her home. While I do not know of any British legal precedent to justify this breaking of confidence to protect the potential victim, the outcome of the Tarassof case in the United States provides support for this course of action. In this case a young man who had informed his psychotherapist he intended to harm Tatania Tarassof eventually killed her. According to the 1976 decision of the California Supreme Court (Tarassof vs. The Board of Regents) in some circumstances psychiatrists have a legal obligation to identify those patients who pose a serious threat of physical harm to others and to warn the potential victim of the risk.[1]

Sooner or later there is bound to be a situation where the physician encounters an intravenous drug-using patient whose serology is HIV positive. Despite the clinician's advice the patient refuses to inform his wife and continues to have sexual intercourse with her without taking appropriate precautions to prevent transmitting the infection to her. The physician knows that she is trying to become pregnant and feels that he has an overriding ethical duty to warn her of the risks to the fetus (half the babies born to mothers who are infected with HIV would be infected and at least half of those babies will go on to develop AIDS), and indeed of the risk to herself if she became HIV positive and subsequently conceived, for it is known that pregnancy may precipitate the development of AIDS in women who have been infected with the virus. The husband might be indignant that there had been a breach of confidence.

[1] Since the decision in the High Court on 9 December 1988 (W. vs. Egdell; Chancery division, Scott, J.), it has been suggested that whenever a doctor perceives a patient to be a serious danger to his family or to the public at large, his duty of confidentiality to that patient will be reduced. (Brahams, D. (1988). Comment on a psychiatrist's duty of confidentiality. *Lancet*, 24/31 December, pp. 1503–4.)

My own view is that in order to protect others, such a breach is justified. In other words I have a utilitarian duty to override the patient's wishes in the best interests of the wider community. My violation of this patient's right to confidentiality seems justified because of the threat the patient's behaviour represents to others. Venereologists would disagree with this approach, perhaps because their professional *raison d'être* depends on total confidentiality. As I understand it, the venereologist's utilitarian argument is that breaching one patient's confidentiality will in the long run cause greater harm to the community than the infection transmitted by a single patient, because many people who might be suffering from an infectious condition will be deterred from seeking help unless they can be guaranteed absolute and unconditional confidentiality.[2]

Psychiatrists are currently divided on the issue of whether to supply opiates to heroin addicts (Robertson 1987). The protagonists of prescribing argue that the provision of uncontaminated drugs and of clean syringes and needles will reduce the risk of infection and help control the spread of AIDS (50 per cent of intravenous heroin users in Edinburgh are known to be HIV positive). They also argue that decriminalization and a liberal prescribing policy will significantly reduce exploitation of addicts by organized crime. The opponents of more liberal heroin and methadone prescribing, with whom I sympathize, take the paternalistic view that prescribing more or less 'on demand' would simply lead to a proliferation of opiate dependence, since the major factors in its spread are availability, accessibility, fashion, and peer-group pressure. It might be argued that uncontaminated opiates are very much less damaging from the medical point of view, than say alcohol, which is available both legally and commercially. My answer would be that opiates induce a state of egocentric, almost solipsistic, euphoria in which the addict loses his drive, motivation, and his altruism. My experience of addicts who have used euphoriants continuously since puberty is that they are completely devoid of any moral sense, are unable to tolerate frustration and disappointment and are incapable of planning and working towards long-term goals. Increasing the accessibility and availability of euphoriants would create a community of morally retarded individuals. This restrictive view runs counter to the libertarian views on the prescribing of addictive substances such as those of Thomas Szasz and even a recent *Lancet* editorial (9th May 1987) which recommends increasing the availability of opiates to addicts.

[2] The subject is discussed by Dr Mindel in Chapter 9.

Case history 6

A heroin addict, a patient of mine, went to a friend's flat to obtain heroin. He found that his friend had just taken an accidental overdose and was in a coma. If taken to hospital immediately his life might have been saved. My patient however just stayed in the flat long enough to steal the remaining heroin, the syringe and the needle, and his friend's money, and then left without alerting the emergency services.

REFERENCES

Cohen, S. and Scull, A. (ed.) (1985). *Social control and the state.* Basil Blackwell, Oxford.

Ingleby, D. (ed.) (1981) *Critical psychiatry: the politics of mental health.* Penguin, Harmondsworth.

Littlewood, R. and Lipsedge, M. (1989). *Aliens and alienists: ethnic minorities and psychiatry*, (Second revised edition). Unwin Hyman, London.

Robertson, R. (1987). *Heroin, AIDS and society.* Hodder and Stoughton, London.

Roth, L. H. and Meisel, A. (1977). Dangerousness, confidentiality and the duty to warn, *American Journal of Psychiatry*, **134**, 508–511.

Scheff, T. J. (1966). *Being mentally ill.* Aldine, Chicago.

Spitzer, R. (1981). The diagnostic status of homosexuality in DSM III: a reformulation of the issues. *American Journal of Psychiatry*, **138**: 210–15.

Szasz, T. (1987). *Insanity: the idea and its consequences.* John Wiley, New York.

Tidmarsh, D. (1982). Implications from research studies. In *Dangerousness: psychiatric assessment and management*, (ed. J. R. Hamilton and H. Freeman). Gaskell: Royal College of Psychiatrists, London.

NOTE ADDED IN PROOF

Since this chapter was submitted for publication, the General Medical Council has issued a statement entitled *HIV infection and AIDS: The ethical considerations:* Paragraph 19 of the statement reads as follows:

> Questions of conflicting obligations also arise when a doctor is faced with the decision whether the fact that a patient is HIV positive or suffering from AIDS should be disclosed to a third party, other than another health care professional, without the consent of the patient. The Council has reached the view that there are grounds for such a disclosure only where there is a serious and identifiable risk to a specific individual who, if not so informed, would be exposed to infection. Therefore, when a person is found to be infected in this way, the doctor must discuss with the patient the question of informing a spouse or other sexual partner. The Council believes that most such patients will agree to disclosure in these circumstances, but where such consent is withheld the doctor may consider it a duty to seek to ensure that any sexual partner is informed, in order to safeguard such persons from a possibly fatal infection. (GMC, May 1988.)

15
Ethics in psychotherapy

SIDNEY BLOCH and TERENCE LARKIN

The practice of psychotherapy inevitably requires a vast range of decisions, virtually all of which involve an ethical component. As if this were not enough of a demand on its practitioners, these decisions are made all the more taxing because of the inherent nature of the discipline.

Consider the following aspects as illustrative. The definition of psychotherapy is elusive: is it an art, a branch of science, a blend of them both, or merely comparable to a trusting friendship (Bloch 1982)? Psychotherapists do not belong to a unitary profession: they may be, *inter alia*, psychiatrists, clinical psychologists, social workers, chaplains, lay-analysts, psychiatric nurses, or counsellors of all forms; and each of these disciplines practises with a certain set of assumptions and premises. The goals they strive for with their patients are frequently blurred and ill-defined, ranging from the relief of a symptom through alteration of specific personality traits to some vague notion of 'personal growth'.

The multiplicity of objectives is matched by the number of schools of psychotherapy, each with its own theoretical model of what constitutes normal and abnormal mental health and with its corresponding set of clinical methods. Finally, research into the subject yields limited information about what comprises the therapeutic process, the effectiveness of various modes of treatment, and who is likely to be a successful practitioner (Garfield and Bergin 1986).

This diversity and uncertainty leave the therapist with no option but to grapple with how he will choose from the various conceptual models and from a range of therapeutic goals and methods. As part of this process he is unavoidably buffeted by ethical factors. Our purpose in this chapter is to highlight these factors and to offer, at least in part, remedies for the ethical dilemmas encountered. Many topics compete for our attention but considerations of space preclude covering all of them. We have elected to focus on the most fundamental questions only, namely (a) who should be offered psychotherapy, and (b) how should treatment be conducted, given that it is pervaded by values held by both patient and therapist? Important topics such as confidentiality, research, registration, malpractice, ethical codes, and multiple allegiance obviously merit our consideration, and the interested reader is referred to Szasz

(1974*a*), Thompson (1983), Karasu (1981), Van Hoose and Kottler (1985), and London (1986).

Notwithstanding the vagueness of the subject and indeed because of it, we are obliged to clarify what *we* understand by the term psychotherapy. Helpful to our purpose is a definition by the doyen of psychotherapy research in the USA, Hans Strupp (1968, p. 32). His definition is especially illuminating in informing us what psychotherapy does not include under its rubric:

> '. . . psychotherapy is not faith-healing, religious conversion, or brainwashing, nor does it traffic in the sale of friendship—it may share some elements with all of these activities, but that is not its defining characteristic. What sets psychotherapy apart from other forms of "pyschological healing" . . . is the planned and systematic application of psychological principles, concerning whose character and effects we are committed to become explicit.'

WHO SHOULD BE OFFERED PSYCHOTHERAPY?

The reader may find it surprising that the issue of selecting patients for the 'planned and systematic application of psychological principles' should involve an ethical dimension. Could this question not be handled with an exclusively clinical approach, with research findings serving as a buttress to the enquiry? Yes, but in part only, and for reasons which should become immediately obvious.

Although psychotherapeutic practice is more firmly embedded than ever before in the medical arena and in the Health Service (we may note for instance the recent establishment of many departments of psychotherapy in the NHS led by medically trained consultant psychiatrists), it is disputable whether all the recipients of treatment are suffering from a diagnosable psychiatric disorder. On the contrary, it is apparent that a substantial proportion are not ill in terms of the conventional medical model but rather are wrestling with 'problems of living' (Szasz 1974*b*).

This raises the fundamental question: should psychotherapy be restricted to the medical model and therefore be 'prescribed' only for those with clearly identifiable psychiatric disorders? Practitioners espousing such a position would assign the clinical symptoms experienced by the prospective patient (sometimes in association with relevant features in the personality) to an operationally-defined diagnostic entity. A corresponding form of therapy is then selected from the established range of psychological treatments (Bloch 1986), with its outcome assessed according to narrowly defined criteria based on the initial presenting symptoms. Thus, a satisfactory outcome for a person with depressive symptoms is elevation of his mood, for a bulimic patient the cessation of bingeing and vomiting, and for a socially phobic student the ability to dine in the college canteen or participate in social events. In other words the aim of treatment is to eradicate or ameliorate the clinical features for which help has been sought.

This approach to the application of psychotherapy owes much to its historical origins. Freud (1895) initially developed a mode of treatment designed to deal with neurotic symptoms such as hysterical conversion, phobias, obsessions, and anxiety. Psychoanalysts, including Freud himself, soon began to free themselves from those specific moorings and to explore uncharted waters. The result of that exploration has been the development of a position that analysts, and therapists generally, have a remit to help a much expanded and heterogeneous group of patients.

The medical model in this view is unnecessarily constraining and ill-suited to the psychotherapeutic task; first, because the legitimate goals of treatment may encompass many more aspects than mere symptomatic relief and secondly, because pinpointing a diagnosis and plan of treatment is antithetical to the notion of psychotherapy as a journal of personal exploration. It is as much an educational model as it is a medical one. Thus, the opportunity is provided for the acquisition of greater self-knowledge (self-awareness is a commonly used term) or for the accomplishment of greater self-fulfilment (self-actualization and self-realization are common synonyms). This conception of psychotherapy also embraces the feature of personal growth and development: the patient (this is clearly something of a misnomer) is not so much ill as he is motivated to develop and enhance his potential—whether it be in the sphere of the interpersonal, the spiritual, the sexual, and so on. An enterprise based on such an approach is inevitably open-ended. Treatment terminates at a point agreed by the therapist and patient but which is nevertheless arbitrary. This is not regarded as unduly problematic given the underlying ethos of the quest for self-awareness and self-fulfilment as a continuing process throughout the life-cycle.

The matter is not quite so straightforward, since various schools of psychotherapy have tried to elaborate their own views on what constitute the desiderata for successful treatment. Freud (1937, p. 250) for example, remarks in his essay *Analysis terminable and interminable* that although it is 'not easy to foresee a natural end', the aim of psychoanalysis is:

> ' . . . not to rub off every peculiarity of human character for the sake of a schematic "normality", nor yet to demand that the person who has been "thoroughly analysed" shall feel no passions and develop no internal conflicts. The business of the analysis is to secure the best possible psychological conditions for the functions of the ego; with that it has discharged its tasks'.

Thus, the key aim is to free the ego from unconscious influences that impair its ability to exercise its appropriate executive function over conflicting forces within the psyche.

Existential forms of psychoanalysis conceptualize the process differently through an emphasis on self-confrontation and making choices. As Sartre puts it:

'[Existential psychoanalysis] is a method destined to bring to light, in a strictly objective form, the subjective choice by which each living person makes himself a person; that is, makes known to himself what he is'.

Yet another view is encountered in Jung's (1983) concept of 'individuation', which he sets forth as the primary objective in therapy. The term denotes the process whereby the patient becomes a 'separate, indivisible unity or "whole" ' through the union of his conscious and unconscious experience. New attitudes and possibilities are derived from this union which amounts to the 'rounding out of the personality into a whole'. This focus on all facets of inner experience facilitates the liberation of formerly latent creative potential.

It will be evident from these three representative positions that they all embody an assumption that psychotherapy has very little to do with the medical model and its amelioration of symptoms but much to do with promoting the growth and maturity of the personality.

We have portrayed two polarized positions in our discussion concerning who should be offered psychotherapy, but there are several other views along the spectrum. Spelling these out is not essential to our immediate task, which has been to demonstrate that the question of who should be selected for psychotherapeutic treatment is fundamentally an ethical one. Selection in this field of work cannot be limited to the customary enquiry about whether patient *A* with condition *B* is likely to respond to treatment *C*. The fact is that *A*, *B*, and *C* each generate intricate conceptual problems, and combine to present a challenging ethical dilemma for the practitioner. We have no obvious remedy to offer but hope our account at least clarifies the nature of the dilemma.

ETHICAL ISSUES IN THE PRACTICE OF PSYCHOTHERAPY

Whoever is selected for treatment and whatever goals are set, another set of ethical issues arises as therapist and patient embark on the process of therapy. These are best considered in the context of the relationship that evolves between them. It is the intrinsic nature of this relationship that makes the ethical dimension of therapy so salient.

The two protagonists are virtually polarized with respect to their initial positions. The patient is commonly bewildered and distressed. Becoming a patient is tantamount to giving up some of his autonomy. The situation is possibly aggravated by a sense of shame and embarassment. The route taken to reach the therapist is likely to be tortuous and cumbersome: consultation with family or friend, assessment by the general practitioner, a referral to a psychiatric clinic, a further referral to a specialist psychotherapy unit. Potentially confusing information is offered at each point and, throughout the procedure, the patient is reliant on supposed experts steering him in the right direction.

At long last the encounter with *the* expert! The inequality in this particular relationship is striking—the dependent, vulnerable patient and the ostensibly powerful, omniscient therapist. This dependency increases the power and authority already vested in the therapist. The sense of dependency may be reinforced by the not infrequent practice of the therapist opting to divulge little about himself or about the nature of treatment, this on the premise that such disclosure would interfere with the development of transference (that is, irrational feelings and attitudes experienced by the patient towards the therapist), regarded by some as a central aspect of the therapeutic process. Mystification is the likely result of the above sequence of encounters.

We would contend that the therapist has a primary obligation to dispel the air of mystery through the process of *informed consent*. We would echo the claim of Redlich and Mollica (1976) that: 'Informed consent is the basis of all psychiatric intervention and . . . without it no psychiatric intervention can be morally justified'. But we need to go further than this. The omnipresence of values in the practice of psychotherapy requires that informed consent be conceived as a dynamic process and therefore in need of repeated, detailed scrutiny throughout the course of treatment.

An admirable model of this is provided by Carl Goldberg (1977) who calls for the concept of a 'therapeutic partnership' with its cornerstone being a 'mutually agreed upon and explicitly articulated working plan'. This then becomes the subject of regular reviews throughout the course of therapy. Among the elements of the plan are: identifying goals and methods to reach them; monitoring the efficacy of treatment; and permitting either partner to voice dissatisfaction with any facet of the plan. Moreover, the respective roles, tasks, and responsibilities of both therapist and patient are outlined, discussed, and examined as necessary.

The therapeutic partnership does not necessarily imply an equal share of power, rather an agreement about how the power inherent in the relationship will be allocated at various times. Thus, complete autonomy in the patient whereby he enjoys the capacity to reflect, and to decide and to act freely on the basis of his reflections, may not always be a feature of the therapeutic encounter no matter how desirable this may seem. A patient in the throes of a severe, intense crisis, for instance, may lack the wherewithal to reflect clearly about what constitutes his best interests and, in collaboration with the therapist, agree to a redistribution of responsibility; the therapist is then assigned a more paternalistic role. As the crisis wanes so will this aspect of the partnership require renegotiation, probably paving the way for a restoration of the patient's autonomous state. The essential feature of such shifts is their *joint* recognition and determination by the two partners.

Dyer and Bloch (1987), in reviewing the various models which could be applied to informed consent in the context of a therapeutic relationship, have proposed that the fiduciary model is most apt by virtue of its emphases on trust and time. Arguing against the exclusive reliance on either respect for autonomy or traditional paternalism as models for informed consent, Dyer and Bloch then suggest that a relationship built on trust is more relevant. Thus, the therapist works in such a way as to manifest his trustworthiness and this in turn encourages the patient to invest his trust in him. The process occurs over time and is not a function of a one-off negotiation at the outset of treatment.

Moreover, the fiduciary quality of the relationship enhances in the therapist a specific sense of responsibility. He seeks to identify the particular needs of his patient and to respond to them. Although autonomy is viewed as a goal of the therapeutic encounter, it is not in itself the exclusive basis for the therapist's ethical concern for his patient; he may be required to act paternalistically on occasion, a paternalism which is comparable to the concern manifest by responsible parents for their child.

The acceptance of a therapeutic partnership based on the fiduciary model goes a long way to obviate the ethical pitfalls that are intrinsic to the psychotherapeutic enterprise. The partnership is a necessary condition for sound clinical practice but it is *not* a sufficient condition. The permeation of psychotherapy by values of all kinds comprises a further complication which must be acknowledged. Given that the problems for which the patient seeks help are inextricably bound up with the basic question of how he should live his life (arguably this is true of all forms of treatment) it is inevitable that the therapist faces the risk of imposing his values, whether consciously or unwittingly (Strupp 1974).

Some leading therapists have, in the face of this risk, espoused the concept of a value-free therapy. Carl Rogers (1979), for example, in labelling his model of treatment as 'client-centred' argues for a restriction of the therapist's role to 'facilitator' in the pursuit of the therapeutic goals set by the patient. Although Rogers asserts that 'one of the cardinal principles in client-centred therapy is that the individual must be helped to work out his *own* value system . . . ', he then concedes the potential influence of the therapist in this process when he adds ' . . . with a minimal imposition of the value system of the therapist'. The use of 'minimal' to qualify imposition overlooks the fact that in this context imposition is akin to pregnancy; it either happens or it does not.

Another similar view, proposed by Engelhardt (1973), involves a shift in focus—psychotherapy is not about ethics but about *meta-ethics*, that is, it paves the way for the possibility of ethical decision-making on the part of the patient. The aim lies not in the patient adopting a *particular* set of values as a result of treatment; the therapist is therefore careful to avoid offering specific recommendations, whether explicitly or implicitly, about how the patient shall live his life. Instead, the patient is helped to reach a point where he can make his own choices *freely*, that is, unhindered by unconscious influences. The problem with this position, however, is that in advocating autonomy as the foremost objective of treatment, and more particularly an autonomy which allows a free choice about how to live one's life, he is conducting no more than another form of value-laden therapy. By stressing autonomy as central, the therapist is making a fundamental ethical statement.

In affirming as a value the therapist's commitment to help a patient become autonomous and therefore able to work out *his* own value system both Rogers and Engelhardt are necessarily acknowledging an inescapable feature of psychotherapy, that it is value-bound. To think otherwise is, as Strupp (1974) points out, a fallacy.

Freud was also intent on promoting the practice of psychoanalysis in a value-free way. Indeed, he argued that: 'The [therapist] should be opaque to his patients and, like a mirror, should show them nothing but what is shown to him' (Freud 1924, p.118); and he insisted that the task of therapy was limited to the 'freeing of someone from his neurotic symptoms, inhibitions and abnormalities of character' (Freud 1937, p.216), through making the unconscious conscious. Here Freud was stressing the essential character of the therapeutic task as he saw it: for the patient to reach certain goals, uninfluenced by the therapist's personal beliefs and attitudes.

On the other hand, he also pointed out the educative role of the therapist (Freud 1940). As he put it '[the analyst] must possess some kind of superiority, so that in certain analytic situations he can act as a model for his patient and in others as a teacher' (Freud 1937, p.248).

It is difficult to conceive this hybrid role of mirror, model, and teacher as being value-free, even if the ultimate therapeutic goal in a Freudian analysis is to rid the patient of his neurotic features in order that he may act as an autonomous person no longer governed by unconscious and irrational forces.

A reappraisal by leading figures of the analytic tradition in recent years suggests that psychoanalysts, and indeed all psychotherapists, inevitably incorporate certain values into their work with patients. Thus, Strupp (1974, p.200) asserts:

> 'There can be no doubt that the therapist's moral and ethical values are always "in the picture" . . . he cannot really espouse a "value-free" position. . . . the therapist, whether he acknowledges it or not, does influence the patient's moral and ethical values'.

And Crown (1977) reminds us that the therapist's influence concerning values occurs at both verbal and non-verbal levels. While he may be aware of his utterances and attempt to control these, 'his non-verbal communication through gesture, facial expression, nods of approval or disapproval, can be almost unconscious', with the result that the patient is in danger of becoming subject to a process of conditioning.

Erik Erickson (1976, p. 411) not only echoes these views of Strupp and Crown but also goes beyond them by proposing that psychotherapy is essentially an ethical intervention. In a thoughtful and illuminating paper he concludes: 'What the healing professionals advocate . . . is always part of the value struggle of the times and, whether "avowed" or not, will be—therefore had better be—ethical intervention'.

If therapy must, to an important degree, amount to ethical intervention, the obvious question follows: how shall the therapist go about this task? He could pursue the Rogerian position (mentioned earlier) and make every effort to minimize his ethical role. But the chance of success is likely to be slim—his 'unavowed' values will in all likelihood manifest themselves through his non-verbal behaviour. Indeed, it is unimaginable to us that a therapist could possibly maintain an ethically neutral stance without a crippling level of self-consciousness.

A second option is for the therapist to accept that among his roles *is* that of 'ethical interventionist', with all its complex ramifications, but that this is his 'problem' rather than that of the patient. The patient is thus not 'burdened' by a dilemma that does not belong to him in the first place. The therapist by contrast bears the responsibility of remaining aware of his potential role as moral agent and of regarding his value system as a given factor in his therapeutic work (Serota 1976). As part of the process he must be keenly sensitive to his own values in order to monitor his unconsciously motivated impulses to influence the patient, or to accept, unwittingly, the values which his patients project on to him.

Illustrative is the case of a student who had won a prestigious fellowship in order to write a book, but who had failed to write a word after nine months. It soon emerged that her motivation for doing the project was wholly derived from an unconscious wish to please her father, from whom she had always craved affection and recognition. Presenting him with academic achievement was her sole means of fulfilling this need. The therapist, an academically ambitious person himself, had to grapple with his own confused feeling, wanting his patient to succeed with the book—in accordance with a strongly held value that academic achievement was a worthy pursuit—and yet knowing through his clinical judgement that her 'ambitiousness' was ill-conceived and had caused her much misery throughout her life.

Thus, a sort of 'value-testing' needs to occur constantly to ensure that the intrusion of values into the therapeutic relationship is never ignored but is dealt with in whatever way appears appropriate at the time. This approach will tend to preclude the unwitting imposition of values by the therapist onto the patient.

A more radical option available to the therapist is to make the declaration of his own value system a value in itself. The argument runs as follows: psychotherapy is a means of social influence; the therapist is more powerfully placed to influence his patients than the other way round; the therapist therefore acknowledges this state of affairs; and he is entirely 'transparent' regarding the values he espouses.

The American psychoanalyst, Robert Jay Lifton (1976, 1986), is probably the most eloquent spokesman for this position. Particularly in association with his therapeutic work with US veterans of the Vietnam War, he has elaborated a view whereby the professional avoids the 'trap of pseudo-neutrality and covert immortalization of technique'; instead, he combines attitudes of advocacy and detachment. The process entails the voicing of 'moral advocacies' while at the same time 'maintaining sufficient detachment to apply the technical and scientific principles of one's discipline'. In the case of the Vietnam War veterans, Lifton articulated his anti-war position explicitly according to a principle he dubbed 'affinity'. This involved the coming together of those who had undergone the common experience of fighting an allegedly unjust war and who wished to make sense of it; Lifton participated in this affinity by virtue of his avowed political and ethical sympathies and associated inclination to act on behalf of the veterans.

Several other examples of such affinity have evolved in psychotherapy over recent years, all typified by the therapist assuming a position of moral advocacy. Some homosexual therapists have publicly aligned themselves with the 'gay movement' in providing therapy for homosexual patients (see Bancroft 1981); a distinguished psychotherapist and researcher, Alan Bergin (1980), has evolved for patients who hold religious convictions a school of 'theistic realism' in which the therapist avows specific values derived from the Judaeo-Christian tradition including forgiveness, reconciliation, spiritual belief, supremacy of God, marital fidelity, and primacy of love; and some therapists, working in the context of the State of Emergency in South Africa, have declared their rejection of apartheid and have committed themselves to the support of traumatized Blacks, especially those who have been the victims of detention and torture (Steere and Dowdall 1988).

In all these illustrations, particular constituencies are being served—war veterans, homosexuals, those with a religious commitment, Black victims of apartheid. However, a therapist's explicit avowal of his value system can be applicable more generally. Hence, the therapist may adopt an approach with *all* his patients whereby he will be transparent about his ethical attitudes in various clinical circumstances. As Aponte (1985) suggests, the therapist does this on the premise that: 'Values are integral to all social systemic operations and therefore to the heart of the therapeutic process . . . Values are an essential component in defining and assessing a problem, determining goals, and selecting therapeutic strategies'. The corollary is unambiguous: 'Therapists do not have a choice about whether they need to deal with their values in therapy, only how well'.

Marital therapy with a devout Christian couple serves as a useful example. Both partners subscribed to the chapter in Ephesians (5:22–33) in which husbands are enjoined to love their wives 'as their own bodies', and wives are instructed to 'submit to their husbands in everything'. Aware of his motives, the therapist not only helped the couple to clarify how each partner interpreted these verses in order to suit their own needs but also contributed his own view of Christian marriage when pressed to do so by both husband and wife. He felt it would be disingenuous to participate in a discussion about a crucial ethical matter without sharing his own position. The aim was not to impose his values but to ensure that the couple knew consciously about them, thereby forewarning them of the potential influence of these values in the proceedings.

The interested reader is referred to Aponte (1985), in whose paper on '*The negotiation of values in therapy*', a coherent and useful account of how the therapist can optimize his ethical task is provided.

CONCLUSION

Freud (1937, p.248) commented in *Analysis terminable and interminable* that:

> ' . . . we must not forget that the analytic relationship is based on a love of truth—that is, on a recognition of reality—and that it precludes any kind of sham or deceit'.

This may seem hackneyed in the light of its repeated quotation but it nevertheless remains apposite in as much as it establishes the ethical ideal for all psychotherapeutic practice. We have argued in this chapter that the psychotherapist can but continuously strive to approximate to such an ideal. The therapist's shortcomings demand that all his decision-making be informed by consideration of the ethical dimension of his task.

We have seen how even in the selection process the theoretical assumptions on the part of the therapist may amount to epistemological 'deceit'. Moreover, in supporting Strupp's (1974) assertion that value-free therapy is a fallacy, we have contended that no pyschotherapist can dismiss the pervading influence of his personal system of values, either those specific to the nature of pyschotherapy itself or general ones to do with how a person should live his life.

We have stressed too that the unequal distribution of power inherent in the therapeutic relationship requires that the influence of the therapist's values be addressed lest treatment deteriorates into something akin to indoctrination.

Our appraisal of these various topics leads us to conclude that psychotherapy cannot be practised without admitting the salience of values and that the crucial question facing the therapist is how effectively he can deal with this issue. Specifically, the therapist's major task is to avoid imposing his own values or misusing the power and influence which he holds in the therapeutic relationship. This task may be worked upon in several ways, along the lines considered by us in this chapter.

It would of course be presumptuous for any contributor to this complex subject to attempt more than a clarification of the issues involved. We have tentatively presented a number of approaches which, while they may not provide remedies for the ethical dilemmas faced by the therapist, may at least avoid some of the pitfalls. How each therapist deals with the ethical component of his practice is ultimately a question of individual responsibility, but we hope that our attempted clarification will make the responsibility easier to assume.

ACKNOWLEDGMENT

We should like to thank Dr Michael Lockwood, of the Department for External Studies, University of Oxford, for his careful reading of an earlier draft.

REFERENCES

Aponte, H. J. (1985). The negotiation of values in therapy. *Family Process*, **24**, 323–38.

Bancroft, J. (1981). Ethical aspects of sexuality and sex therapy. In *Psychiatric ethics* (ed. S. Bloch and P. Chodoff), pp.160–84. Oxford University Press.

Bergin, A. (1980). Psychotherapy and religious values. *Journal of Consulting and Clinical Psychology*, **48**, 95–105.

Bloch, S. (1982). *What is psychotherapy?* Oxford University Press.

Bloch, S. (1986). *An introduction to the psychotherapies*, (2nd edn). Oxford University Press.

Crown, S. (1977). Psychotherapy. In *Dictionary of medical ethics* (ed. A. S. Duncan, G. R. Dunstan, and R. B. Wellbourn). pp.264–8. Darton, Longman and Todd, London.

Dyer, A. and Bloch, S. (1987). Informed consent and the psychiatric patient. *Journal of Medical Ethics*, **13**, 12–16.

Engelhardt, H. T. (1973). Psychotherapy as meta-ethics. *Psychiatry*, **36**, 440–5.

Erikson, E. (1976). Psychoanalysis and ethics—avowed and unavowed. *International Review of Psychoanalysis*, **3**, 409–15.

Freud, S. (1895). The psychotherapy of hysteria. In *Studies on hysteria* by J. Breuer and S. Freud, Standard Edition, **2**, pp.255–305. Hogarth Press, London.

Freud, S. (1924). *Recommendations to physicians practising psychoanalysis.* Standard Edition, **12**, pp. 111–20. Hogarth Press, London.

Freud, S. (1937). *Analysis terminable and interminable.* Standard edition, **23**, pp. 211–53. Hogarth Press, London.

Freud, S. (1940). *An outline of psychoanalysis.* Standard edition, **23**, pp. 144–20. Hogarth Press, London.

Garfield, S. and Bergin, A. (ed.) (1986). *Handbook of psychotherapy and behavior changes*, (3rd edn). Williams and Wilkins, New York.

Goldberg, C. (1977). *Therapeutic partnership: ethical concerns in psychotherapy*. Springer, New York.

Jung, C. G. (1983). Conscious, unconscious and individuation. In *The essential Jung* (ed. A. Storr), pp. 212–26. Princeton University Press, Princeton.

Karasu, B. (1981). Ethical aspects of psychotherapy. In *Psychiatric ethics* (ed. S. Bloch and P. Chodoff), pp. 89–116. Oxford University Press.

Lifton, R. J. (1976). Advocacy and corruption in the healing professions. *International Review of Psychoanalysis*, **3**, 385–98.

Lifton, R. J. (1986). *The Nazi doctors*. Macmillan, London.

London, P. (1986). *The modes and morals of psychotherapy*, (2nd edn). Hemisphere, Washington.

Redlich, F. and Mollica, R. F. (1976). Overview: ethical issues in contemporary psychiatry. *American Journal of Psychiatry*, **133**, 125–36.

Rogers, C. (1979). *Client-centred therapy*. p. 292. Constable, London.

Sartre, J. P. (no date cited). *Existentialism and human emotions.* p.81. Castle, New York.

Serota, H. (1976). Ethics, moral values and psychological interventions. *International Review of Psychoanalysis*, 3, 373–5.

Steere, J. and Dowdall, T. (1988). On being ethical in unethical places: the dilemma of South African clinical psychologists. *Hastings Center Report*, In press.

Strupp, H. (1974). Some observations on the fallacy of value-free psychotherapy and the empty organism. *Journal of Abnormal Psychology*, 83, 199–201.

Szasz, T. (1974*a*). *The ethics of psychoanalysis*. Basic Books, New York.

Szasz, T. (1974*b*). *The myth of mental illness*. Harper and Row, New York.

Thompson, A. (1983). *Ethical concerns in psychotherapy and their legal ramifications*. University Press of America, Lanham, MD.

Van Hoose, W. and Kottler, J. (1985). *Ethical and legal issues in counselling and psychotherapy*. Jossey-Bass, San Francisco.

16
Medical and ethical decisions in the pharmaceutical industry

BRIAN W. CROMIE and PETER L. FREEDMAN

INTRODUCTION

The pharmaceutical industry exists to discover, develop, and sell medicine for a profit. This combination of profit and health care also pertains to manufacturers of bandages, bed-pans, thermometers, etc., and for the selling of personal medical and nursing services by doctors and nurses. In all of these, there is potential conflict between patient-care and economics.

A recent symposium published in *The Proceedings of the Royal College of Physicians of Edinburgh* (1987) was entitled 'Are ethics and economics compatible in health care?' The conclusion of that symposium, which dealt largely with allocation of resources, was that ethics and economics were compatible, so long as decisions were made for the best interests of the patient. This also applies to ethics and decisions in the pharmaceutical industry. It is no different from medicine and health-care generally.

Doctors working in the pharmaceutical industry are employed as doctors and are expected to act as doctors, with all the ethical implications of that profession. If there were any deviation from the ethical standard that the interest of patients is paramount, a doctor in industry would not only be failing his profession but failing in the role for which he was employed.

Of course, the interest of patients is defined differently for pharmaceutical physicians, as they seldom have personal clinical responsibility for patients and may have to consider overall patient benefit and risk. Such considerations are not dissimilar from the allocation of scarce resources by politicians and managers in the Health Service to give maximum patient benefit overall. The concept of overall patient benefit despite risk to individual patients is relatively straightforward for vaccines and similar items; it is more difficult in treatment areas where a choice of therapies exists; and new drugs, e.g. for hypertension, depression, or arthritis pose more difficult problems.

No potent medicine is without adverse effect on some people, so the development, testing, and marketing of such products will invariably cause some ill-effects in some patients. The medical director in a pharmaceutical company must be aware of this and balance it against the natural history of the diseases and the therapeutic inadequacies of alternative remedies. If there is a positive contribution towards better management of patients, as judged by the medical director, then it is ethically proper for him to support the progress of the drug.

Many outsiders feel that there are conflicts between patient interests and commercial pressures in the pharmaceutical industry which will put doctors in very difficult positions. In our experience, this is not so; pharmaceutical companies thrive when their products are used at the correct dosage for the correct indication to obtain the best therapeutic results. In fact, both patients and pharmaceutical companies benefit from 'good medicine'.

If pharmaceutical companies are sufficiently misguided and unwise to go against good medical advice, their products will not achieve optimum results and will not be used again. In these circumstances, doctors in industry can have problems. Years ago, the Secretary to AMAPI (Association of Medical Advisers in the Pharmaceutical Industry) told all doctors considering an appointment in the industry that it was a good and interesting life but that they must always be prepared to resign if their ethical standards were compromised. That advice remains sound today.

POSITION OF DOCTORS IN INDUSTRY

Doctors usually join the pharmaceutical industry from hospital registrar appointments or, less often, from general practice. Competition for vacancies in the industry tends to vary in line with the degree of discontent in the profession generally; but, once offered a job, the doctor must decide whether or not to join, and that could be his first and most important ethical decision in industry. He must try to determine the policies of the company and establish his degree of freedom on ethical issues. If these do not conform with his idea of professional independence, he should not join. Equally, he should not join unless he has a positive interest in the discovery, development, and promotion of medicines and agrees with the economic basis for the industry. He should also be prepared to work as part of a team with both medical and non-medical colleagues.

Some doctors who join the pharmaceutical industry are temperamentally unsuited to the role and hide behind a screen of apparent professional ethics, when refusing to co-operate with colleagues. One doctor formally refused to sign an advertisement which claimed that the product was useful in migraine as, in his experience, he had not found it beneficial. It appeared to be a decision taken on ethical grounds but the product had been extensively tested in migraine, it was a licensed indication, and was recommended for migraine by consultants with long and extensive clinical usage compared with the limited personal experience of the young company doctor. All the evidence demonstrated that there was overall patient benefit from the judicious use of the product in migraine and the doctor was misusing ethical arguments.

When one of the authors joined the industry, his general practitioner father-in-law said that if he was able to influence a major pharmaceutical company, he would probably benefit more patients in a month than he could in all of his life-time as a GP. He could have added that the industry doctor had an equal power for harm, either by allowing false claims or, in the above case, by depriving patients of effective therapy.

Doctors in industry, who are medical directors or medical advisers, have a relatively clear professional role and their responsibilities are increasingly well-defined. They now have legal responsibility for submitting registration dossiers and for all medical aspects of advertising copy. Within the limits of their responsibilities, decisions should be taken in the best interests of patients after careful consideration of all available evidence. If they do that honestly, they will not go wrong.

However, not all doctors in industry are in the medical department. Of the 600 or so doctors in the pharmaceutical industry, an increasing number are now involved in senior management and many are directors or chairmen of companies.

These particular doctors must make all the commercial decisions and would be expected to delegate the medical decisions. But in a pharmaceutical company all commercial decisions have a medical element and all medical decisions have a commercial impact. In the event, we have not found any clash and decisions taken with a view to achieving good medicine are in the long-term interests of both the company and the customers, the patients.

CLINICAL RESEARCH

Thus, medically qualified people are to be found in pre-clinical research, medical information, medicines surveillance, and in marketing support activities, such as promotion and training. Whatever the position he or she holds in a company, be it clinical research physician or chairman, the doctor is viewed by colleagues in a special light and carries a fundamental responsibility derived from the medical qualifications.

The clinical research physician has in some ways the most obvious role and has specific ethical duties to address.

In the process of development of a new medicine, it is necessary to establish the efficacy and safety of the compound. The pharmaceutical industry and the licensing authorities are essentially in agreement on the basis for such data generation, balancing good sense and pragmatism as perceived at the time. The industry, the licensing authorities, and the medical profession at large must feel satisfied that, in the search for more effective and safer medicines, good clinical research has been applied. Above all, these three parties have a duty to inform and reassure the public that the interests of the patient are paramount while the search for better medicines continues.

A key step in the development of a new medicine is the first introduction of a compound into the human subject. The final decision rests with the individual clinical research physician who must draw on the accumulated pre-clinical data to make the necessary judgement of whether or not to take this step. Data will have been generated over several years from a large body of experts—mostly from research staff within the company but also from academic workers. There will be numerous reports to review, including the chemistry, pharmacy, pharmacology, and toxicology of the compound *in vitro* and *in vivo* in animals and bacteria

Before the first administration in human subjects, certain basic questions must be answered.

1. Is there sufficient evidence to suggest that the compound may have therapeutic activity to warrant investigation in man?
2. Is there sufficient evidence regarding the absorption, distribution, metabolism, and excretion of the compound in certain animal species to enable calculation of the first doses to be administered to man?
3. Does the toxicological evidence suggest no unreasonable risk?

Provided that these questions can be answered positively, then it is acceptable to proceed to test the accuracy of the projected prediction that the compound has therapeutic potential.

The first phase of human testing, known as Phase I, will be in the form of closely monitored studies on healthy adult volunteers in a specially equipped and staffed clinical pharmacology unit which is preferably located within a hospital. Generally, for such a compound, a dose of one hundredth of the predicted therapeutic dose is used in the initial study, limited to a handful of subjects. The effect on the blood constituents and circulatory system receive particular attention and, thereafter, the dose is increased step by step with similar monitoring in other subjects. Provided the compound is well tolerated after single and short-term repeat dose studies, the decision can then be made to begin evaluation in patients, in what is generally known as Phase II. Human subjects with a well-defined disorder and without other diseases to complicate assessment are required. In this and the later phase of development clinical investigators from hospitals will become partners in the evaluation process and, to that extent, may be said to share the ethical decisions.

In the UK, the licensing authorities grant a clinical trial certificate (CTC) or an exemption order (CTX) for all such studies in patients after considering the dossier submitted to them. This includes reports on preclinical and healthy volunteer studies, as outlined above. The responsibility for the declaration of this information lies specifically with the industry clinical research physician, who is required to sign the application. Although impartial ethics committees are expected to grant approval, and notwithstanding the apparent diversity of parties involved in the question, 'Is it right to administer the medicine with this limited amount of knowledge to these patients?', the industry physician should not ethically and must not legally abrogate his unique responsibility.

Phase II, as described above, may involve 50–200 patients during which evidence will either affirm or not that the compound has therapeutic activity, that a dose range is understood, and that no serious adverse effects have occurred.

Phase III is an extended programme of clinical evaluation including often 1000 patients or more, during which extensive studies are undertaken to test the level of efficacy and safety of the new medicine. The industry physician must take all these data into account and decide if the risk of adverse effects with the new compound is justified by the potential benefit of the treatment, bearing in mind that all existing therapies will also have a balance of benefit and risk and that the main *raison d'être* of drug research is to improve that balance with new medicines. If he considers that the balance is improved, for at least some patients, he then submits the information in a product licence application. The granting of a product licence means that this is held to be the case *at the time* by the licensing authority. Post-marketing surveillance in its various forms will be required to assess the veracity of the judgement. This is vital if serious side-effects which occur at a rate of 1 in 5000 subjects or less are to be revealed.

At all stages of development, the industry physician, at whatever level of management, has a duty to ensure the adequacy of collection and evaluation of adverse reaction data. He should have the strength to persuade colleagues, if he feels that there are sufficient grounds to delay further studies, to stop development or, for the marketed product, to withdraw the medicine.

The use of human subjects for experiment is controversial but inescapable. Different cultures and changing times bring new perspectives. At the turn of the century, Reed used volunteers and fellow scientists in his classic experiments to show that yellow fever transmission depended absolutely on the presence of the mosquito as vector; there were deaths in the experimental group but the lives of many people were spared by the application of this knowledge. During World War II, Mellanby found a group of conscientious objectors who allowed themselves to be infested with the scabies mite. These subjects, at least, participated freely. However, in the US, prisoners and inmates of institutions for the mentally handicapped have been used in the past to study, for instance, the transmission of hepatitis (Mellanby 1973).

In the context of this history it is not surprising that what is done to human volunteers, whether patients or healthy subjects, in the name of research, is a matter of close scrutiny by society. Judgements should be based on an understanding of the issues, and confidence that the experimental practice is open.

Certain groups present special ethical problems. It may be easy to take the view that the use of prisoners in experiments, given the prospect of earlier release, involves undue coercion. Some would hold that unacceptable pressure may also apply if medical students are persuaded to participate in studies by the physicians on whom they depend for advancement. Similarly, research scientists in industry laboratories may feel obliged to submit to 'healthy volunteer' trials for the sake of their team project. However, medical students, scientists, and doctors alike must be subjects in these experiments and be seen to be so, in order to demonstrate to the public a conviction in their own judgements. Bearing this in mind, the industry physician must decide whether it is right to use such groups.

Even if certain groups, such as students, are accepted as suitable for healthy volunteer studies as allowed by an ethics committee, the industry physician must decide if each individual is a proper subject for such tests. That decision can be taken only after the subject has been interviewed and given a comprehensible explanation of the studies, passed a full medical examination and been cleared for participation by the volunteer's usual medical practitioner.

Opinions differ as to whether positive clearance is necessary, or if it is sufficient simply to inform the medical practitioner and allow adequate time for him to respond if he is worried. However, as adverse effects have occurred in volunteers who did not admit to known illnesses or medication, there are strong arguments in favour of positive clearance.

The use of children in research lays bare the essential issue of informed consent and, for that reason, probably requires even greater scrutiny. But it should be emphasized that infants and children are not 'little adults' and that to extrapolate dosage, efficacy, and safety data from healthy adults to children can be seriously flawed.

In a similar way, inability to give informed consent may apply to some elderly patients. Nevertheless, if any advance in the increasing problem of dementia is to be made, studies in such subjects must be performed and the pharmaceutical physician has to take the ethical decision as to what is appropriate.

The problems of ethical decisions encountered by the industry physician in controlling the activities of the investigator, so that clinical trials are conducted properly, should not be underestimated. The guidelines of 'good clinical research practice' are complex and many investigators find them inhibiting. Nevertheless, all protocols are agreed with investigators beforehand. One of the authors was obliged to insist that an eminent academic physician be removed from further involvement in a clinical research programme following his repeated deviation from the protocol, which put the subjects at risk. In another instance, it became clear that false data had been supplied by an investigator, who asked for payment for more completed patient records than could have been included in the trial with the medication supplied to him. Again, the industry physician revealed that the work was suspect in the Product Licence Application and sought ways to prevent that investigator from continuing further malpractice.

PROMOTION

Promotion of medicines to the medical profession is a contentious area which has had much publicity, with claims that some companies push their products in an unethical way and counter-claims that most excesses of promotion are in response to the greed of the profession.

We have never had any qualms about the ethics of promotion as such. However superior a new drug may be, no patient will benefit unless his doctor has heard of the drug and knows its indications and how to use it properly. None of that can be achieved without effective promotion.

In the pharmaceutical context, promotion means the dissemination of information in a way which allows it to be noticed and fully understood by the doctor. There have been criticisms of some of the methods of gaining attention and a doctor in industry can challenge some of these methods; but he cannot deny the basic need for promotion as such.

The problem areas arise when marketing men attempt to 'gild the lily' with exaggerated or unbalanced descriptions of the drug's effect in the expectation that doctors will not prescribe simply on the basis of an advertisement.

When a doctor in the pharmaceutical industry is asked to sign such advertising copy by his marketing colleagues, he may be made to feel unnecessarily narrow and rigid if he refuses to sign. People may ask what harm can result, as all advertisements go only to doctors who are able to make considered judgements. However reasonable such arguments may appear to be, the doctor in the company must allow no lowering of standards. In this, the theme of patient benefit is somewhat tenuous but the professional ethical standing of the doctor must prevent him from drifting away from the true interpretation of the licensed indication of a drug.

The doctor in industry must also see the final advertisement with the illustration, size of print, emphasis, etc., so that the whole advertisement corresponds to the licensed indication and there is no implied claim in addition to the written text. In one example, the medical director approved the text of an advertisement for a product licensed for reflux oesophagitis and was later called to account because the illustration, which he had not seen, implied that the medicine was effective in all forms of peptic ulceration. The doctor had acted in good faith but was at fault in not inspecting the whole, final advertisement and the apparent claim which had not been stated in the text. Under this sort of pressure, the company doctor can feel isolated, particularly if he is the only medical adviser in the company.

DRUG WITHDRAWAL

One of the most difficult decisions for a medical director in the pharmaceutical industry relates to withdrawal of drugs when adverse effects have been reported. It refers back to the need for industry doctors to consider the best interests of patients overall as opposed to clinicians looking after the interests of their individual patients.

The usual pattern of events is that adverse reactions are reported to the company or directly to the regulatory authorities. At first, it is almost impossible to know if the reactions are caused by the new medicine, as there is always a high reporting rate of coincident symptoms and also of diseases associated with the indication for the new medicine. For example, any new anti-peptic ulcer therapy will get reports of patients suffering perforation, gastric cancer, and the like while taking the new product, as those diseases produce symptoms which tend to get treated with anti-peptic ulcer products.

Later, however, a pattern is suggested and it becomes clearer that the severe rash or hypotensive episode or anaemia is due to the new drug in a group of patients who react differently from the majority.

Once a causal relationship has been established, every effort is made to determine the true incidence of the adverse effect, its severity, its improvement after withdrawal of therapy, and the type of patients who are affected. The possibility of interaction with other drugs or the use of unlicensed dosage regimens must also be considered. In addition, data will have been accumulated on the percentage of patients who derive special benefit from the new treatment and who cannot be adequately controlled with other medicines.

Having obtained all this information, the medical director must make the decision as to what course will produce greatest patient benefit and recommend continued sale, perhaps with modified promotion, or withdrawal of the drug.

The decision may have to be taken under enormous pressure of media publicity, where any single apparent severe drug reaction is taken as a reason for drug withdrawal, and with powerful influences of legal advisers and the like. The decision will also be taken after consultation with regulatory authorities and with colleagues world-wide. Nevertheless, in the end, the medical director must make his own decision in the light of overall patient benefit.

As all effective medicines have some risk and as new medicines are introduced with the expectation of a better balance of benefit to risk, the overall situation is constantly changing. For example, the anti-rheumatic drug phenylbutazone was introduced many years ago and gave relief to a vast number of patients. But, as newer non-steroidal anti-inflammatory agents were introduced, it was apparent that the balance of benefit to risk was better for most patients with the newer drug than with phenylbutazone; phenylbutazone was therefore withdrawn from general use, although it is still cleared for the management of ankylosing spondylitis in practice.

On the other hand it is well known that aspirin produces gastric irritation with a recognized incidence of gastro-intestinal bleeding. It is also known that paracetamol can cause liver damage at higher doses, and that this must always be a risk with readily available analgesics. Despite the accepted potential hazard of these two minor analgesis, both aspirin and paracetamol remain on sale because of the widespread patient benefit which they give.

These examples show that decisions have to be taken on the basis of the balance of benefit to risk with new medicines under test and with alternative treatments already available. They must also take into account the needs of individual or sub-groups of patients, as a medicine which has a relatively poor balance of benefit to risk overall could still be of unique benefit to certain patients whose needs cannot be ignored.

REFERENCES

Jennett, B. (1987). Are ethics and economics incompatible in health care?
Mellanby, K. (1973). *Human Guinea Pigs*. Merlin Press, London.
Proceedings of the Royal College of Physicians of Edinburgh, 17, no. 3, 190–5.

17
Ethical aspects of intensive care

M. A. BRANTHWAITE

I have been half in love with easeful death,
Called him soft names in many a mused rhyme,
To take into the air my quiet breath;
Now more than ever it seems rich to die,
To cease upon the midnight with no pain.
from *Ode to a Nightingale*, John Keats.

Intensive care medicine has been defined as a service for patients with potentially recoverable disease who can benefit from more detailed observation and treatment than is generally available in standard wards and departments (Stoddart 1981). These are unassuming, modest words, and yet the seeds of ethical conflict are already apparent.

Potential for recovery is sometimes easy to identify, even in patients with immediately life-threatening disease. Diabetic coma or severe acute asthma are both good examples. The prognosis becomes more uncertain as severity and complexity of illness increase, and urgent decisions are often necessary when the outcome is unpredictable. A question of even greater importance is whether 'benefit' will necessarily follow recovery. This must be so for the previously fit adult with, for example, pneumonia of any severity, but questionable at best in an elderly, debilitated patient with an inoperable, malignant oesophageal stricture. It is easy to offer extreme examples but there is a whole spectrum of disease where 'benefit' is a matter of speculation or personal opinion (Bayliss 1982; Baskett 1986), no doubt influenced by individual perceptions of the value of life, whether their own or that of others.

The concept of 'more detailed observation and treatment than is generally available in standard wards and departments' also begs a number of questions. There is no uniformly acceptable definition of the degree of observation and treatment which can be expected in a standard ward or department. Facilities vary according to financial resources, degree of specialization, and whether or not the service is located in a highly developed or underprivileged society. Even within one country expectations change with time and the advent of new methods and equipment. This means that choice is essential, and arises at many levels. On a national level, what proportion of a nation's resources are devoted to health care? Within the health services, what is the desirable balance between prevention and treatment. To what extent should resources be directed to those whose ill health is essentially self-inflicted—drugs, tobacco, alcohol, promiscuity—as distinct from those who are the victims of misfortune? How far should emphasis be placed on new developments rather than on the routine service? The practice of intensive care underlines many of these dilemmas because it has the potential for limitless expense. The concept of triage—treatment of limited availability delivered to those most likely to benefit—is accepted practice in military medicine or after a major civilian disaster. Apart from these circumstances, it is often resisted by clinicians or regarded as a threat to clinical freedom (Hampton 1983), and yet there is a growing need to accept this responsibility as medical innovation (and therapeutic potential) outstrip resources. Constraint on the indiscriminate application of extravagant measures is necessary on both economic and humanitarian grounds, and the best criterion for selection is a realistic but well-informed judgement of likely benefit.

Decisions in practice are often influenced by other pressures, usually in favour of continuing treatment at all costs. Human instinct is to strive for recovery, an endeavour reinforced by a pattern of medical training so emphatic that it has aroused some notable criticism (Illich 1974). This means that it is far easier to escalate treatment than to withdraw it. There is personal satisfaction in responding effectively to challenge, and pride in achievement if an apparently inevitable death is averted. If death occurs in spite of implementing every possible therapeutic measure, the physician feels absolved of guilt, confident that he has discharged his responsibility in full. Another hidden temptation to secure personal peace of mind lies within the decision to advocate intensive care. There is a feeling that the patient has been given every chance. At the same time the level of direct responsibility is often diminished by transfering it, wholly or in part, to a colleague. Thereafter, the often considerable demands of moment to moment management are carried by someone else.

Further pressure to attempt exceptional measures comes from fear: fear of making an error of judgement which could cost a life; of professional criticism or even litigation; and fear of carrying indefinitely a burden of personal guilt for having 'failed the patient', 'not tried hard enough', 'not given him a chance'. Similarly there is pressure to try any available new treatment, even without previous personal experience, and often a reluctance to transfer seriously ill patients to centres with greater experience of the newer or less frequently used procedures. This is not necessarily in the best interests of the patient and may be no more than indulgence of personal pride. Finally, there is what Jennett (1984*a*,*b*) has described as 'the vicious cycle of commitment'. So much has been done already, how can there be any hesitation now? The fact that so many procedures have been attempted, sometimes with at least partial success, can be used either to advocate that there should be no turning back, or that the patient should not be advised to accept yet another form of unpleasant treatment of questionable value.

The pressures against escalating treatment are far fewer. Most important is an awareness of the 'cost' of intensive care, the practicalities such as dehumanization and loss of dignity, isolation from family and friends, and erosion of the potential for serenity and the corporate family emotion which attend 'natural' death (Rawles 1986). These penalties are perceived more readily by those who work regularly in such an environment than by the majority of clinicians who refer patients to the service but then assume a more distant role. Staff morale suffers, standards deteriorate, and the quality of care for those who *can* benefit is diminished as a result of attempting to provide treatment, often at the expense of suffering, for those who are unlikely to survive.

The influence of these hidden pressures is diminished and decisions on whether or not to initiate treatment become far easier when an accurate prognosis can be given at the outset. Until recently, data gathering and statistical analysis were insufficient to provide useful guidelines, but the advent of scoring systems for intensive care (Morgan and Branthwaite 1986) has clarified some of these issues. At present scoring systems cannot be expected to provide detailed guidance for individual management (*Lancet* 1986), but they allow some refinement of judgement and are beginning to modify the behaviour of clinicians (Chang *et al.* 1986; Zimmerman *et al.* 1986).

It is easy to criticize this approach on the grounds that allowing previous results to guide future policy merely defines a self-fulfilling prophecy. The innuendo is of a culpable, passive fatalism, a persuasive plea to go on trying—yet again, and with only the same therapeutic options. A constructive analogy can be drawn between this 'trial and error' approach and the evolution of management of other potentially fatal diseases. Consider lung cancer—at one time, surgical resection was attempted in a high proportion of those presenting with the disease. Careful analysis of results demonstrated that only certain patients would benefit. Today such patients are selected on the basis of well-defined and widely accepted criteria. Are there individual patients whose chances of survival are diminished because they do not fulfil these criteria and who are therefore either not treated, or treated by less effective means? In all probability there are, but the selection process channels appropriate treatment to the vast majority, sparing those who cannot benefit from the morbidity—in its widest sense—of surgical intervention. The disease is still lethal in a high proportion of patients, with or without operation, so there is no room for medical complacency. Rather there is a need for new methods to be developed, evaluated, publicized, and implemented. The same arguments can be applied with advantage to the practice of intensive care. Unfortunately, the consequences of withholding aggressive and potentially unpleasant treatment are more obvious and immediate, and only in the fairly recent past has it been possible to define comparable groups of patients on whom an analysis of outcome can be based.

So far there has been no consideration of the wishes of the patient or his relatives. This essential ingredient is easy to overlook, especially when decisions have to be taken urgently. Whenever time permits, the feelings of the family should be explored as gently and informatively as possible. In no circumstances should relatives be allowed to feel that they are 'deciding' what should be done. The potential for remorse or guilt is far too great, quite apart from the distasteful possibility of decisions being influenced by the thought of personal gain or the desire to shed burdensome responsibility. Conversely, the medical remit is to advise, not to compel. The majority of patients and relatives prefer to leave decisions to their medical advisers, but uncertainty in the mind of the practitioner can sometimes be resolved more easily if he knows the wishes of the family. This invokes a second obligation—to ensure that the issues have been explained and understood clearly and have prompted a considered response, given as objectively as circumstances allow. The wishes expressed by the patient in particular are likely to be coloured by current events and feelings. Depression often accompanies serious illness and patients who request 'no intervention' may still be grateful if subsequent recovery ensues, with or without the specific treatment in question. It is, of course, easier to accept wishes which have been expressed consistently, well before urgent decisions are imminent and when thoughts are clear. The greatest difficulty comes when the views of the family are at variance with those of the practitioner. This is not particularly common—but then, how many of us convey the options dispassionately? More often the information is given in words which polarize opinion towards that already held by the practitioner. Does this merely pay lip-service to the concept of considering the wishes of the family? Perhaps so, yet an attempt is better than no effort at communication at all. The extent to which well-informed opinion among patients and relatives can modulate patterns of treatment is apparent from the changing incidence of mechanical ventilation for pulmonary infection complicating AIDS, reported from San Francisco (Wachter *et al.* 1986). The growing reluctance to accept mechanical ventilation reflects the adverse immediate prognosis, and an awareness that AIDS itself is likely to cause death within a year or so. And yet:

these patients are often young, active research is in progress, and a cure for the disease may be imminent. Decisions on management cannot be rigid but must take account of individual circumstance and wishes, and respond to advances in medical knowledge.

It is inevitable from this analysis that there are often no clear-cut guidelines on whether treatment should be initiated or escalated. 'If in doubt, proceed' is an excellent maxim, but because it is infinitely harder to draw back than to withhold exceptional measures at the outset, the initiation of intensive care leads inevitably to the second major ethical issue. When (and how) should treatment be terminated or withdrawn, once it is clear that no progress can be made?

Analyses of outcome have identified the worsening prognosis associated with a prolonged need for intensive care, especially when there is multiple organ system failure (Knaus *et al.* 1985). The passage of time permits a clearer appreciation of the situation than may have been apparent at the outset and it is at this stage, when death appears inevitable both statistically and individually, that the intensive care clinician is faced with a decision about what to do next (Scarman 1981). It is at this stage too that the pressures of other competing demands are often felt most acutely—the presence of a seriously ill patient who is not expected to recover may preclude treatment for another with a better prognosis. The dilemma can be considered in three stages. Should new measures be introduced if the situation deteriorates any further? Should existing measures be withdrawn and, if so, to what extent? Should active measures be taken to terminate what is by this stage a synthetic existence made possible only by previous technological intervention?

It can be argued that if the situation has been created by medical action, then there is an obligation to dismantle it when the consequences appear untenable. This question arises most often in the context of brain death, now generally referred to as brain-stem death. Mechanical ventilation maintains the delivery of oxygen to the lungs, so that the heart continues to beat. This physiological system ceases to function when the ventilator is disconnected: the termination is abrupt. Such an action is widely acceptable today, provided specific criteria have been fulfilled (Pallis 1983).

Far more difficult, and far less widely discussed or even perceived outside intensive care units, is the question of how to bring an end to other equally synthetic situations where the criteria of irreversibility are less well defined and some semblance of life would remain for a matter of hours, perhaps a day or two, if specific supportive measures were to be withdrawn. Without intervention of this nature, it is often possible to maintain or substitute function in many of the essential systems for prolonged periods—hydration, nutrition, breathing, circulation, excretion, and so on. Intensive care is designed to provide this service and it does so efficiently. Abnormalities which might pass unnoticed with a lower level of observation are recognized immediately, often prompting a therapeutic action, for example, suction to remove secretions from the lungs. This prolongs the process of dying inordinately—to the distress of patient, relatives, and staff. Distress for the patient can often be alleviated by sedatives—although the apparently quiescent patient is not necessarily pain-free or tranquil, merely unable to communicate the emotions of the fatally ill (Cassidy 1986). The distress of relatives is lessened if they can be reassured that the patient is no longer suffering, but the very mechanism of achieving this precludes the contact which provides fulfilment, the completion and relinquishing of a close relationship (Campbell 1986). Distress to staff is created by witnessing that of others, by harsh self-criticism resulting in a sense of inadequacy or failure, and by inflicting painful, undignified treatment, either by decision or by the implementing of that decision. The staff are in a position to influence the immediate outcome. Is the motive for intervention to terminate an unacceptable situation primarily for the relief of their own feelings?

Before any action is taken, frank discussions between all staff involved in the patient's care, and with the family are essential. Giving relatives an honest, albeit adverse, prognosis when necessary is an essential prerequisite for this approach, and is usually appreciated far more than spurious optimism. Conversely, nothing is more disastrous or destructive of confidence than conflicting opinions provided from different members of staff or, even worse, manifest conflicts between staff about what constitutes optimum management. Exceptional families have such an innate reluctance to accept the inevitability of death that they urge the continuation of measures which are regarded as inappropriate by the staff. Detailed and sympathetic explanation, or an invitation for a second opinion from a practitioner of their choice, usually resolves these infrequent differences.

Once mutual confidence has been established and detailed explanations offered and understood, it is usually easy to change the emphasis of management towards comfort and tranquillity. Specific treatments may be withdrawn—for example, dialysis is discontinued so that the chemical derangements of renal failure prove fatal over a matter of days. No immediate change is perceived and subsequent deterioration is gradual and non-specific. A more overt conflict presents if a patient judged to be terminally ill develops a fever—the decision to withhold antibiotics is obvious, as are the implications. To *withdraw* antibiotics is a more positive step—justified if it can be agreed that death is inevitable and is merely delayed by further treatment. Emotional antipathy increases as measures with more specific and immediate consequences are considered. The concentration of oxygen delivered to a ventilator is reduced. The strength or rate of delivery of a drug supporting the heart is decreased. Fluids are prescribed sufficient to ensure that there is no depletion of body water, but the chemical composition of the fluids is not adjusted to match the worsening body chemistry. Are these measures euthanasia in disguise (Dawson 1986), or a necessary obligation on a humane profession to terminate a state of potential suffering created by their own well-intentioned (but perhaps misguided) efforts? Whose suffering is at stake? The patient can be sedated through euphoric disorientation into a state of oblivion. The relatives are subjected to a shorter period of emotional distress, but may still wonder if it really had to end that way? The staff too are likely to have mixed feelings—their instincts and training are transgressed by withholding or withdrawing support, and the dividing line between a 'passive' measure which allows death to occur naturally (withholding antibiotics) and an 'active' measure which promotes earlier death (reducing the concentration of oxygen) is only one of degree when so much of the life at stake is already dependent on synthetic measures. Conversely, staff may be relieved that a decision to accept the inevitable has been taken and that instructions for active management have been withdrawn. Viewpoints are likely to differ according to age, sex, and professional discipline, and are influenced all too easily by changes of mood, themselves a consequence of stress or fatigue. Conflict between intellect and instinct is almost inevitable but is easier to bear if its origins are understood.

For those filled with repugnance by such an approach, the only alternative is to continue indefinitely with all supportive measures, irrespective of cost or competing demand. This assumes that the methods used to relieve pain and distress are effective and that the family accept the principle of striving indefinitely until all the resources of modern technology have been exhausted. Indecision is avoided and reassurance sought by responding with appropriate scientific logic to the individual problems which present. It is a policy which raises the challenge of irresponsibility and inhumanity—accusations which can be avoided by those who choose to do so, merely by declining to consider them. An alternative refuge is to seek forgiveness in religion for controversial judgements and actions (Habgood 1986). Those with a firm belief may find this reassuring; to those of little faith, it is no more than a comforting transfer of responsibility, a soft option for living with a troubled conscience.

This discussion implies that the outcome of intensive care is either recovery or death. The possibility of survival but without worthwhile recovery must also be considered. It is particularly likely after major head injury, and can lead to the preservation of lives which are devoid of independence, lack any perceived fulfilment, and impose a formidable burden on individual families and society in general. Recognizing when such an outcome is inevitable is easier than knowing when it is highly probable (Levy *et al.* 1985). What level of probability is required before efforts to secure survival are diminished or withdrawn? The longer treatment is continued to ensure that the prediction 'survival but with irrecoverable damage' is correct, the more likely it is that the prophecy will be fulfilled. The mere passage of time allows resolution of associated pathology, whereas the presence of several abnormalities at the outset may, without specific intervention, lead to an early death. The more often such patients are treated effectively at the time of presentation, the more we have an obligation to examine results meticulously and thereby refine managment policies. It is inconceivable that an accurate prognosis will ever be possible in every case and, where doubt exists, treatment cannot be withheld. Thus, paradoxically, the success of new methods leads to new patterns of disability.

A new ethical dilemma has been posed by the ever-increasing application of organ transplantation. The emotionally-charged potential for conflict between responsibilities to donor and recipient was illuminated by public debate a few years ago (*Lancet* 1981). The wide acceptance of criteria for defining brain-stem death and their coincidence with the ultimate cessation of a spontaneous heart beat have provided some reassurance, but there are still individuals and societies who resist the concept of organ donation. As with so many other aspects of medical science, the rapidity with which techniques are developed threatens to outstrip the pace at which their consequences are deemed acceptable. Donating the cornea or the kidneys causes little comment today. Feelings escalate when the organ in question is the heart, and the matter becomes macabre when the transplant teams request permission for 'organ harvest'—the removal of heart, lungs, kidneys, liver, and pancreas. Logic dictates that this is no more than a natural development of transplantation technology—the philosophical debate ended when organ removal from a donor whose heart was still beating became acceptable practice. Unfortunately the matter does not rest there because inevitably the management of the potential donor can be and is influenced by the needs of the recipient(s). Decisions are best reached on the basis of respect for the wishes of the bereaved family, after they have been fully and honestly informed. Individuals who have expressed a wish to donate organs if circumstances permit, and relatives who provide consent, are unlikely to reject the practical implications of offering the recipient the best possible opportunity for recovery. The emotionally fastidious and those without experience of this situation are likely to be more troubled, and passionate feeling can be incited all too easily by brash, insensitive publicity.

Transplantation for potentially fatal disorders of childhood is a particularly emotive issue. The procedure may well prove more successful because of the immunological immaturity of the very young, but the supply of donor organs is necessarily limited and can be associated with even more grief than death of an older subject. To what extent should the malformed fetus, incapable of independent existence, be preserved for use as an organ donor (Harrison 1986)? The concept may seem horrific when first considered, but surely this too is no more than technology proceeding faster than social custom can accept? It is comforting to speculate on the possibility of using the organs of other species, perhaps bred specifically for the purpose. After all, 1984 is now behind us (Orwell 1949).

It is clear from the above that it is easier to pose the ethical dilemmas of intensive care than to provide wholly acceptable solutions. Historically, the same has been true for the physical practice of medicine—the first requirement has always been to clarify the nature of disease in as much detail as possible before the effective treatment can be developed or applied. Perhaps we can take comfort from this for the practice of intensive care. Technological success has presented us with new conflicts. They too need to be identified and explored with wisdom, compassion, and objectivity, before we can hope to achieve their resolution.

REFERENCES

Baskett, P. J. F. (1986). The ethics of resuscitation. *British Medical Journal*, **293**, 189–90.

Bayliss, R. I. S. (1982). Thou shalt not strive officiously. *British Medical Journal*, **285**, 1373–5.

Campbell, L. (1986). History of the hospice movement. *Cancer Nursing*, **9**, 333–38.

Cassidy, S. (1986). Emotional distress in terminal cancer: discussion paper. *Journal of the Royal Society of Medicine*, **79**, 717–20.

Chang, R. S. W., Jacobs, S., and Lee, B. (1986). Use of Apache II severity of disease classification to identify intensive care unit patients who would not benefit from total parenteral nutrition. *Lancet*, **i**, 1483–6.

Dawson, J. (1986). Easeful death. *British Medical Journal*, **293**, 1187–8.

Habgood, J. (1986). Searching for our moral roots. *British Medical Journal*, **293**, 1600–1.

Hampton, J. R. (1983). The end of clinical freedom. *British Medical Journal*, **287**, 1237–8.

Harrison, M. R. (1986). Organ procurement for children: the anencephalic fetus as donor. *Lancet*, **ii**, 1383–5.

Illich, I. (1974). *Medical nemesis*. Caldar and Boyars, London.

Jennett, B. (1984*a*). *High technology medicine: benefits and burdens*. The Rock Carling Fellowship, **1093**. Nuffield Provincial Hospitals Trust, London.

Jennet, B. (1984*b*). Inappropriate use of intensive care. *British Medical Journal*, **289**, 1709–11.

Knaus, W. A., Draper, E. A., Wagner, D. P., and Zimmerman, J. E. (1985). Prognosis in acute organ-system failure. *Annals of Surgery*, **202**, 685–93.

Lancet (1981). Brain death. *Lancet*, **i**, 363–5.

Lancet (1986). TPN and Apache. *Lancet*, **i**, 1478.

Levy, D. E., Caronna, J. J., Singer, B. H., Lapinski, R. H., Frydman, H., and Plum, F. (1985). Predicting outcome from hypoxic-ischemic coma. *Journal of the American Medical Association*, **253**, 1420–6.

Morgan, C. J. and Branthwaite, M. A. (1986). Severity scoring in intensive care. *British Medical Journal*, **292**, 1546.

Orwell, G. (1949). *Nineteen eighty-four*. Secker and Warburg, London.

Pallis, C. (1983). The prognostic significance of a dead brain stem. *British Medical Journal*, **286**, 123–4.

Rawles, J. (1986). Personal view. *British Medical Journal*, **293**, 1432.

Scarman, The Right Honourable the Lord (1981). Legal liability and medicine. *Journal of the Royal Society of Medicine*, **74**, 11–15.

Stoddart, J. C. (1981). Design, staffing and equipment requirements for an intensive care unit. *International Anesthesiology Clinics*, **19**, 77–95.

Wachter, R. M., Luce, J. M., Turner, J., Volberding, P., and Hopewell, P. C. (1986). Intensive care of patients with the acquired immunodeficiency syndrome: outcome and changing patterns of utilization. *American Review of Respiratory Disease*, **133**, A183.

Zimmerman, J. E., Knaus, W. A., Sharpe, S. M., Anderson, A. S., Draper, E. A., and Wagner, D. P. (1986). The use and implications of 'do not resuscitate' orders in intensive care units. *Journal of the American Medical Association*, **255**, 351–6.

18

First, know thy patient: resolving multiple problems in old age

E. J. DUNSTAN

One of the attractions of geriatrics is its difficulty, which often extends to the ethical problems involved. The multiple, medical, mental, and social problems that occur with increasing frequency in those of advancing age make universal rules hard to apply, and demand solutions which may vary almost infinitely according to the different circumstances of each patient. The fundamental need is therefore for a comprehensive and accurate assessment of each patient's problems before ethical decisions can properly be made. This assessment will often require functional and social information as well as good clinical diagnosis and prognosis. Disability, mental impairment, and a shortish life expectancy may alter priorities, but it is important to recognize the range of people whom the geriatrician may treat, from fit 65-year-olds to disabled centenarians, and vice versa, as well as states in between. It does 'the elderly' no service to regard them as a homogeneous mass.

HOW FAR TO GO?

This is perhaps the commonest decision with an ethical aspect which the geriatrician has to make. His fundamental duty is to diagnose and treat the causes of frailty and loss of function, if he can, to supervise rehabilitation to the maximum potential, and sometimes to provide future care where there is insufficient for a degree of independence. The duty to diagnose and treat may be restricted by other considerations, especially of how far this will actually improve the patient's life. This itself requires some diagnostic certainty. In particular, with advancing age and frailty, restoring function and ensuring comfort become more important than extending an inevitably limited life expectancy: although these will usually coincide, they may not. Important factors include the previous level of function (in that long-standing disability inevitably limits the prospects of good recovery), the prognosis of the presenting condition and of the others which are likely to be present, and to some extent the patient's family and social circumstances. Where diagnosis and hence prognosis are unclear, management should be active while there is a reasonable possibility of a good outcome.

The most important reason for investigation, espcecially in disabled old people, is to look for disease that can be treated with benefit. It is really a matter of clinical skill rather than ethical judgement to decide how to do this with the most accuracy and the least discomfort and risk. Unselective investigation is potentially unpleasant and hazardous to frail old people, with their multiple conditions. Conversely, invasive studies may be indicated if they can reveal disease treatable to good effect, for example endoscopic retrograde cholangio-pancreatography for stones in the common bile duct (Cobden *et al.* 1984). A number of modern techniques such as computerized tomography and ultrasound scanning are much less troublesome to the patient than their predecessors, and have made investigation appropriate when previously it might have been wrong.

Providing a prognosis is an important function of medicine. Patients and especially their relatives often want to know what is going on and what is going to happen, and feel better for knowing. Sometimes the prognosis may be important in planning future care, but it is only a relative indication for investigation, and should not be an excuse for indulging medical curiosity. Well-tolerated tests, such as brain scanning, may be justified, while more invasive procedures such as angiography or cerebral biopsy when carried out only to determine prognosis are almost certainly not. Diagnosis for its own sake is intellectually worthy. It is important in maintaining medical standards, for the patient's best defence is the sharpness of his doctor's brain. But this is not a justification for putting patients to discomfort and risk, especially when an autopsy may soon provide more complete information, so long as the relatives can be humanely persuaded to agree to it.

There is no apparent biological, medical, or moral logic in absolute age-bars to particular kinds of treatment, though it may be found empirically that certain kinds, e.g. bone-marrow transplants (Bortin *et al.* 1981; O'Reilly 1983) do not yield useful results above particular ages. Fortunately, such bars do seem to be becoming less common, with dialysis for acute (Oliveira and Winearls 1984) and chronic (Taube *et al.* 1983) renal failure giving good results in some elderly people, albeit the 'young' ones in the latter case. Cardio-pulmonary resuscitation has also been shown to be worthwhile in acute geriatric units (Gulati *et al.* 1983; Bayer *et al.* 1985) and is an acceptable idea to many elderly patients (Gunasekera *et al.* 1986). It has widely been alleged that the restrictions on chronic dialysis in Britain are really to cover for inadequate resources, but if facilities are limited it does seem justified to use them for those with most in quality and duration of life to gain. Economically, retired people remain net contributors, over their lifetime, until well after the age of 65, and to restrict treatment to current economic contributors would deny human worth except in an economic sense.

Although age alone should not be a bar to treatment, it does not follow that therapy should be offered indiscriminately, especially in view of the increased risks of both medical and surgical treatment in old age. Other medical conditions and the functional and mental state of the patient will give some guidance on whether attempts will be worthwhile or not. It is widely accepted by patients, their relatives, and those looking after them professionally that prolonging life is not an absolute obligation in old age, and that exposing frail old people to the hazards of some kinds of treatment is often not worth the uncertain benefits. The circumstance in which decisions on treatment are most often ethically difficult is a life-threatening crisis in a patient with severe, irremediable, disabling disease. Although it it an awesome presumption to say that someone would be 'better off' dead, most people, professional and lay, recognize times when it would be wrong to prevent death. This is well expressed in the negative obligation that 'we are not here to perpetuate misery': treatment with that effect would be an abuse of medical power.

The usual cause of chronic disability where this question arises is disease of the central nervous system, usually dementia or stroke. Philosophically and practically mental function must be the most important human attribute, determining the capacities for practical ability, awareness, and relationships. The doctor, whose contacts are usually brief and episodic, may not be in the best position to judge these: it is easy to forget the human behind the dementia, of whom others, such as relatives and nurses, may be more aware, and it is imperative to listen to their experience in deciding the line of treatment. It is hard to guess the subjective feelings of someone with dementia, but harder still to guess those of someone with dysphasia, when emotional expression, as well as language and comprehension, may be disturbed.

The appropriate policy depends on the nature of the crisis and the specific treatment for it, the costs to the patient of that treatment, the previous quality of life, the prognosis, and to some extent the feelings of relatives. Some intercurrent illnesses, such as fracture of the hip, acute urinary infection, and faecal impaction cause discomfort and loss of function rather than a swift and gentle death, and the quickest way out of the patient's sufferings is active specific treatment. At the other end of the scale, it is hard to see repair of a ruptured aortic aneurysm ever being justified in someone disabled enough to need long-term hospital care on any of the counts listed above. In a more acute condition, the importance of prognosis may be illustrated by the minimal chance of a comatose stroke patient with conjugate deviation of the head and eyes regaining a reasonable quality of life. Here treatment aimed at prolonging life, rather than that aimed at ensuring comfort, is likely to end in a Pyrrhic victory for heroic nursing. The common problem of bronchopneumonia in a patient with very advanced dementia may be seen in a similar light, albeit on a slower time-scale, with recovery from the infection only allowing a further period of deterioration of an already poor quality of life. It is more difficult to decide what is best for someone with a sound mind but severe physical disability and a poor quality of life which cannot be improved in a life-threatening crisis. My presumption would be for active treatment, up to the limit of its tolerability to the patient. Such patients may well have views of their own, which obviously need respect.

The question of euthanasia would, in my experience, seldom be relevant. It has been asked of me twice in a year (556 admissions): in each case the patient had evidence of dementia, and one stopped asking after anti-depressant treatment. Voluntary euthanasia, all that is at present proposed in the UK, would not be applicable to the great majority of severely disabled old people, whose cerebral disease would prevent a legally valid request. Some patients are reluctant to be admitted to a hospital which, when previously a TB and infectious diseases unit, had a reputation of providing a one-way journey, and the possibility of deliberate killing might revive this fear.

Glover (1977, pp. 92–112, 198–9) has denied the difference between active killing and the withholding of potentially life-saving treatment. To the man at the bedside the difference is clearer, even apart from in his own subjective feelings. The former seeks to exclude the possibility of recovery, while the latter allows it. Such recovery can often happen in very frail patients with bronchopneumonia even when antibiotics are not given. In such circumstances both deliberate killing and active treatment may be seen as harmful, and symptom control as the right course. Glover (1977) would also deny the 'principle of double effect' that if 'an action definable as good in terms of its object' can achieve a good effect only at the risk or expense of causing incidental but unavoidable harm, the act is licit' (Dunstan 1981). This denial would seem to assume that the adverse consequence automatically outweighs the good, and that the moral significance of an act arises only from its outcome, and not at all from its intent. As pain may be a physiological antagonist to opiate-induced respiratory depression (Twycross 1984) it may be unnecessary to invoke the principle in the context of analgesia. It may, however, justify the use of opiates in the relief of cough and dyspnoea. The principle does not justify over-treatment, which would discredit it by blurring the distinction between symptom control and reckless or deliberate shortening of life. It is also apparent that symptom control and active treatment are not necessarily mutually exclusive.

PATIENTS' WISHES

In view of the limits on an elderly patient's life expectancy and often his abilities also, I believe that there should be a presumption that the doctor should want for old people what they want for themselves, though this may be restricted by considerations of risk, mental infirmity, and resources. Old people have as much right as anyone else to adequate explanations regarding their medical management, and to refuse measures should they wish. The limited gains and hazards of some interventions, such as cytotoxic therapy for malignant disease, make reluctance to undergo them understandable. The doctor should be under less obligation to press such therapy than he would be with a younger patient with more to gain, so long as he has ensured the patient's understanding. Many old people have exaggerated ideas of the risks and discomforts of any surgery, however, and it is plainly the doctor's duty to dispel these if he believes the surgery to be in the patient's interest. Conversely some acquiesce in their doctors' plans too easily, often without adequate understanding. Older patients however may genuinely want the doctor to decide for them, probably more often than the young, being a more compliant generation, and it is then plainly his duty to do so. 'Autonomy' should not be forced on those who do not want it. Communication is often difficult, and probably more often than not inadequate. Those with some degree of mental impairment may none the less understand enough to decide for themselves, though they may not remember agreeing to some measure. It is then wise to discuss it more than once to ensure that their agreement is consistent.

In geriatric practice medical management tends to cause less difficulty than decisions on future care. The patient may be surrounded by relatives and others who know what's good for him, even if he disagrees, and the doctor may have to reconcile or adjudicate, often taking the patient's part if this is at all compatible with his interests. The most common problem is that of a patient who will consider no alternative to returning home although this will put him at substantial risk. Many, but not all, such patients are mentally impaired, which adds to the difficulty. If persuasion fails, and there is any significant chance of even temporary success, I believe that the doctor should take the risk of complying with the patient's consistent wishes, having set up all the support he can and ensuring the provision of a safety net, such as a bed kept for a few days.

He has the duty to advise, but cannot often (legally) coerce, and should not deceive. It is not uncommon for people to be told, and not just by relatives, that they are going into an old people's home 'for convalescence' or 'a holiday' when permanence is the unequivocal plan. 'A trial' may be acceptable, so long as there is a genuine option of returning home at the end of it. While often understandable, deception is unjustifiable, especially when perpetrated on the demented, who have less chance of protecting themselves from it.

MENTAL INFIRMITY

Dementia has already been mentioned several times, as befits its importance in the problems of old age. The prevalence is about 6 per cent of all over-65s, and 22 per cent of those aged 80 or over (Kay *et al.* 1970), in a high proportion of whom it is unrecognized. The dependency, falls, and incontinence often associated with dementia make it much more common in hospital geriatric practice than in the community.

The capacity to decide, at least on some matters, may be retained some way into the course of dementia, and should be respected if possible. When the patient really is too muddled to consent to treatment, it is common to ask a near relative so to do. The legal force of this is unclear, though it is a sensible move to forestall complaint, as well as being good manners. Relatives may (or may not) be the people most aware of the patient's views and quality of life, and may also feel themselves responsible, even if this is not the case in law. Neither do these factors seem to add up to a compelling moral force. The management of property is another occasion when the capacity to decide is important, and is subject to legal prodecures. The doctor has the professional duty to judge this capacity, and the moral duty to be alert to the danger of exploitation. The slowness of the Court of Protection does not help, creating a temptation to press powers of attorney to the limit or beyond.

Severe mental infirmity may sometimes raise the question of legal compulsion. Even in the demented the presumption should remain in favour of the patient's wishes, if they can be ascertained, which may be difficult in the later stages. It would be absurd for this presumption to be absolute, especially if there is grave risk to the patient or others. In practice, skilful handling can usually secure co-operation, especially in advanced disease, when there may be too little drive left to resist it. There does not appear to be anything in the Mental Health Act 1983 to exclude dementia from the category of 'mental illness' and hence from the possible use of compulsory admission or guardianship, but its provisions are little used. Although homicide and suicide are not common in dementia, the patient may be at risk to himself from self-neglect for instance, or from wandering into dangerous places, and to others from fire or gas explosion. Guardianship orders could quite frequently be useful in ensuring a better quality of life for those liable to self-neglect despite community services, by requiring a specific residence, attendance for treatment (though not the *receiving* of treatment), or access by certain people.

One little oddity is that social workers may be reluctant to arrange transfer of patients to a residential home who are in hospital unwillingly. Although a home may be equally undesired by the patient, it may be more suited to the patient's needs. Compulsory admission under the Mental Health Act is quite frequently used for patients with functional illness (usually depression) in old age as at any other. In such cases the procedure may be literally life-saving, and is fully justified.

The other mechanism for compulsory admission, in practice most often applied to dements, though formally nothing to do with mental illness, is Section 47 of the National Assistance Act 1948. A magistrate must be satisfied that it is in the interest of the patient, suffering from grave chronic disease, or being aged, infirm, or incapacitated, living in insanitary conditions, and unable to devote to himself, and not receiving from others, proper care, to be removed without delay. Dementia can often lead to these conditions being satisfied, but once admitted such patients usually settle down, and it is seldom necessary to renew the order. The condition for which it is usually considered legally impossible to admit under compulsion is the toxic confusional state, which may be due to treatable life-threatening physical illness. Here the combination of medical necessity and reversible loss of mental competence would make compulsion in fact most justifiable.

RELATIVES

Relatives are the backbone of the care of the majority of old people, and this only gives rise to ethical doubt when their motives seem impure—usually guilt, but sometimes greed. They are also often the key source of information needed for management. Conflict often arises between the wishes of the patient and of the family. The doctor's responsibilities are then primarily to the patient's interests (with a presumption in favour of the patient's wishes as well), not to the family. There may be difficulties to be resolved if family co-operation is needed, despite their wishes, or if the patient's wishes have to be compromised to secure that co-operation in his interests, for example when regular relief admissions are needed to enable some time to be spent at home.

The more dependent the patient, the more people will be involved in care, all of whom will need information. It seems often to be assumed that relatives in particular have a right to know all. With increasing disability, mental infirmity, or communication difficulty this is understandable, so that professional secrecy may become hard to observe, especially if discussion is important despite the patient's wishes. As so often in old age, the usual rule may need to be bent a little—though not as much as it often is. Even the sane, alert elderly are often talked *about* and *over*, but not *to*, and their right to medical confidence ignored. That said, our modern rule may be too strict. The Hippocratic Oath reads 'Whatever I see or hear, professionally or in private, *which ought not to be divulged*, I will keep secret and tell no-one' (Lloyd 1978). While staff involved in care may be told what they need to know, the number of disciplines often involved poses a threat to confidences.

Although it is sensible to listen to family views on management, it is important to make clear the fact that decisions are the doctor's. This may also reduce the risk of guilt if there is an adverse outcome. Though the doctor is treating the patient, not the family, their relationships may well affect what he does. The treatment of a severely demented woman living in the bosom of a loving family may, in my view, quite properly differ from that of one who is alone and rejected.

RESOURCES

Most geriatric services, even more than the rest of the National Health Service, have limited resources to deal with increasing need, and a defined population for which they are responsible. The traditional ideal of the doctor doing whatever is best for the patient in front of him is noble and remains unchallengeable when no resources other than the doctor's time and skill are involved. The geriatrician however, has to ensure the availability of care for those, known or unknown, who are in undeniable need, and so may have to offer second best to others in less pressing circumstances: admission might be best, but day hospital care will have to do. Similar pressures may demand swift discharge and transfer to other forms of institutional care. In the latter case, there may be worry that the standard of life may not necessarily be bettered, but so long as it is as good, such moves are legitimate, on the grounds that the unique resources of the hospital are freed for those now in greater need.

In these straightened circumstances the doctor plainly has the duty to seek the improvement of the services. If he has done so and made the best use he can of his resources, the moral responsibility for inadequacies falls on the Health Authorities and the Government.

The question of private care for old people is vexed in the UK at present, especially among social workers. I cannot see a primary moral objection to looking after even disabled and vulnerable old people for profit—indeed, the better side of human nature can make such care very good. It does require both greater degree of business scruple than selling the necessities of life to their less disabled contemporaries, and great care in making arrangements. The doctor is to some extent peripheral to this, except that he is usually the driving force behind discharge, and so could force an inappropriate move upon a patient. He may also have acquired knowledge of individual institutions, which he should put to his patients' service. This seems to me more likely to serve their interests than the 'hands-off' attitude of some social workers (Coid and Crome 1986). The matter in which the demand for beds should not affect decisions is that of active versus palliative treatment, despite the severe pressure and temptation for it so to do.

RESEARCH

This has recently been discussed by Denham (1984). In brief, the number and severity of unsolved problems in old age make an ethical demand for good research. The practical difficulties include the greater risks to frail elderly subjects and the problems of comprehension and consent, especially in mentally impaired patients, whose numbers make study of their condition particularly important. Denham suggests various procedures for dealing with these difficulties, such as testing the understanding of information given, checking mental capacity, and perhaps the participation of non-medical staff in ascertaining consent.

CONCLUSIONS

The complexities of geriatrics require many decisions with ethical aspects. The problems are much more easily described than the inevitably varied solutions, which may unavoidably be imperfect. The keys to ethically sound practice remain a comprehensive view of the patient, expert clinical assessment, and judicious therapeutics.

REFERENCES

Bayer, A. J. Ang, B. C., and Pathy, M. S. J. (1985). Cardiac arrests in a geriatric unit. *Age and Ageing*, **14**, 271–6.

Bortin, M. M., Gale, R. P., and Rimm, A. A. (1981). Allogeneic bone marrow transplantation for 144 patients with severe aplastic anaemia. *Journal of the Americal Medical Association*, **245**, 1132–9.

Cobden, I., Venables, C. W., Lendrum, R., and James, O. F. W. (1984). Gallstones presenting as mental and physical debility in the elderly. *Lancet*, **i**, 1062–3.

Coid, J. and Crome, P. (1986). Bed blocking in Bromley. *British Medical Journal*, **292**, 1253–6.

Denham, M. J. (1984). The ethics of research in the elderly. *Age and Ageing*, **13**, 321–7.

Dunstan, G. R. (1981). Double effect. In *Dictionary of Medical Ethics*, (2nd edn.) (ed. A. S. Duncan, G. R. Dunstan, and R. B. Wellbourn), p. 145. Darton Longman and Todd, London; Crossroad, New York.

Glover, J. (1977). *Causing death and saving lives*. Penguin, Harmondsworth.

Gulati, R. S., Bhan, G. L., and Horan, M. A. (1983). Cardiopulmonary resuscitation of old people. *Lancet*, **ii**, 267–9.

Gunasekera, N. P. R., Tiller, D. J., Clements, L. T. S.–J., and Bhattacharya, B. K. (1986). Elderly patients' views on cardiopulmonary resuscitation. *Age and Ageing*, **15**, 364–8.

Kay, D. W. K., Bergmann, K., Foster, E. M., McKechnie, A. A., and Roth, M. (1970). Mental illness and hospital usage in the elderly: a random sample followed up. *Comprehensive Psychiatry*, **11**, 26–35.

Lloyd, G. E. R. (ed. 1978). *Hippocrates writings*, p. 67, Penguin, Harmondsworth.

Oliveira, D. B. G. and Winearls, C. G. (1984). Acute renal failure in the elderly can have a good prognosis. *Age and ageing*, **13**, 304–8.

O'Reilly, R. J. (1983). Allogeneic bone-marrow transplantation: current status and future prospects. *Blood*, **62**, 941–64.

Taube, D. H. *et al.*. (1983). Successful treatment of middle-aged and elderly patients with end-stage renal disease. *British Medical Journal*, **286**, 2018–20.

Twycross, R. G. (1984). Pain the physiological antagonist to opioid analgesics. *Lancet*, **i**, 1477.

19
Ethics in terminal care

ERIC WILKES

Since all patients die and time is always short, the patterns of ethical behaviour required from the physician will not differ radically from those attitudes shown towards salvageable patients; yet because the pressures are greater, the mind more concentrated, and certain problems recurring, it is justifiable to review ethics in terminal care as if they were to some degree a separate entity.

In the physician's ethical baggage are various bundles with such labels as 'informed consent', 'respect and compassion', and 'the multidisciplinary team'. It is perhaps instructive to see how, under the pressures of the patient's imminent death, these can all be ignored.

It is not likely that a reasonable physician would sterilize a young woman who so desperately wanted a baby that she was knitting baby clothes against the happy day, and furthermore sterilize without any discussion with her or her husband or any attempt to obtain consent. Such behaviour must cause anxiety in the most placid bioethicist; yet I have done this, by agreement with other colleagues, and would have felt uncomfortable with any different approach.

A summary of this case is as follows: A happy couple in their 30s had been married for over five years. At that stage they had not wanted children. Then the wife had fallen ill and had been diagnosed as suffering from an incurable spinal tumour. This gave rise to severe pain so that eventually she was admitted to a hospice. By this time the husband had been given a detailed prognosis but the wife had been told only half the truth about her tumour and had not asked more questions. She coped with a day at a time, as is often the way.

She was not an introspective or imaginative girl but her illness had led her to thoughts of having a child more urgently than during the earlier years of placid and contented drift. The knitting of baby clothes began, and great comfort was obtained through planning for a future that would never be.

Her pain remained difficult to control by medical means so palliative radiotherapy was given—fairly successfully—to the affected area of the spine. This was so near the ovaries that sterilization was an inevitable consequence. In their paternalistic way the doctors considered this irrelevant, for the patient would soon be dead.

Indeed she did die two or three months later without the extra burden of knowing that all her hopes were impossible. How much we were, by our silence, protecting her and how much ourselves will remain uncertain.

THE RIGHT TO KNOW

In theory, patients must have a right to know their own situation, their own diagnosis, and to have time whenever possible to put their affairs in order. One has seen repeatedly over the years sensible and adequate patients denied that right by condescending, evasive, and inaccurate explanations from their doctors. This seems to be especially resented by the younger patients, who often have more emotional and spiritual—as well as financial—preparations to make: but condescension from the doctors—'they talked to us as if we were children'—is never justified. Of course some patients may be confused, and others give definite instructions to the physician that they do not wish to be told, so that the question of telling does not arise. Of course, patients who in theory want to know about grave illness when they are well may be less enthusiastic when strength is eroded by the major disease that will kill them. Others express their knowledge by the vehemence of their denial. But these facts do not explain away satisfactorily that in a recent survey (Wilkes 1984) a third of patients, randomly sampled and excluding sudden deaths, had been given no real idea of their terminal situation.

There is thus strong evidence that the patient's right to know is sometimes still being denied. It is therefore important that opportunity be given for patients to ask. Since situations are continually changing, the rate of information should be controlled by the patient. Often they adjust well but gradually over the months they need to know more. The patient must be in charge of the agenda.

When it comes to prognosis, however, the physician deserves sympathy, because the outlook is usually unpredictable. When a cancer has disseminated or a circulatory disease is apparent, it can be years or even decades between the time of diagnosis and the funeral. If patients or relatives wish to plan for the future, they must learn to live with uncertainty. It is right therefore to forecast realistically yet optimistically, and to bear without fuss the resentment at our not giving details that we cannot possibly know. We can seldom predict with accuracy when a patient will die, or even what will kill him. We can say that of 100 patients in such a state, most will die within three months or two years or whatever, but that some will die perhaps in days, and yet others will outlive us. The fate of the individual patient remains almost as mysterious as it was before the illness had been first diagnosed.

It is necessary to add that in recent years far more patients are being told the truth; that the truth may not be heard or that it is misunderstood, but that too often now it is told insensitively and in stark terms, without further discussion or support, in a way as damaging as the evasiveness of yesterday.

Yet in most cases today, the patients will be told the truth—especially if they ask. It is the responsibility of the doctor to produce such a relationship, so that the patient always feels able to ask. Often, however, the patient knows so much more than the relatives realize, and the importance of non-verbal communication is consistently underrated.

THE RIGHTS OF THE RELATIVES

Despite the determination of doctors to retain and uphold the confidentiality of the doctor–patient consultation, this rule is consistently broken in terminal illness by telling the relatives before the patient. There are many valid reasons for this. The relatives can be expected to know the likely reactions of the patient better than the attending physician. They usually will have to deliver the necessary support and even more of the physical care. Yet initially it seems that relatives are given information not in the company of the patient but behind his back: this can be destructive of mutual trust and of family morale, and can make a difficult situation worse.

There are many relatives who will demand for their patient just this paradoxical combination of care and deception. Often their determination that their partner or parent should not be told stems from their own fears about facing the real situation. They too are in need of time and this request for the over-protection of the patient frequently reflects their need for self-protection.

Most doctors will listen to the relatives' views and yet ignore them if they feel they should. Often simple counselling will, over the days, allow the situation to be resolved. Often the patient's command of the situation will, with or without explicit communication, calm the anxieties of the family. Sometimes however, in an untidy and unpredictable world, the fears of the relatives will be fulfilled, and the demoralization of the patient will be a prelude to the demoralization of the entire family.

If early in terminal illness the relatives are frequently told more than the patient, later this over-involvement of the relatives is too often transformed into exclusion or neglect. While 20 per cent of hospice admissions are social isolates and a quarter of cases are themselves over 70 years of age, family care is not likely to be universally available or of reliably high quality. One is amazed that it is often so good, with unlikely relatives rallying round and surprising even themselves.

The tendency, however, still relies too much on allowing the family to 'get on with it' and to offer help too little and too late. Although early in the illness the relatives may have these excessive responsibilities thrust upon them, we leave the routine burdens of care to them and so neglect the carers themselves until frank breakdown threatens. Then we take the patient away and the relatives feel guilt-ridden failures.

Just as nowadays one helps the mother of the stillborn child to hold and to grieve, so one must try to keep, without inappropriate exclusion or exploitation, the adult relatives involved in care to the end, even if transfer to hospital or hospice has been thought necessary.

It is right to encourage relatives to be present at the last, to be holding hands or to view at the end. Some may even wish to assist in the laying-out. They all need to be praised for their contribution whenever it is reasonable to do this. Discussion and explanation, when the dying has been gradual, may be helpful even at this time, although important questions may only arise later in their grieving. Often reassurance is needed that delays in diagnosis made little difference to the outcome, or that pain-killing drugs did not shorten life. Almost always this is in any case the truth.

THE RIGHT TO TREATMENT

One did not need papal sanction, in the old days, to leave the paralysed, demented, or gangrenous patient to the natural course of events, offering comfort rather than such active interventions as intravenous feeding or amputation. With the depersonalization of our society however, patients and doctors alike have their difficulties, especially when an illness that could formerly have been described as terminal is not necessarily so today.

If a patient collapses or is brought in from home as an emergency, we may know so little of his preceding state that the patient must be given the benefit of the doubt. Age as such has little value as an indicator, for some in their 90s are alert and independent while some in their 70s are more restricted in their abilities.

If a patient is admitted with a severe stroke, alone in the world, and of advanced years, it is unlikely that an attack of pneumonia will be as aggressively treated as with a younger person who has family responsibilities. If a patient who is dependent, confused, and unable to look after himself then falls and fractures the femur, he will usually be operated on if he is fit enough to withstand surgery, for this will facilitate his nursing.

Yet probably the rehabilitation will be unsuccessful and the physiotherapists' efforts limited by the inability to benefit.

What then with the patient who is slowly dying from inoperable malignant disease and who gets, in his frail and vulnerable state, a chest infection that in the last century would have carried him off in a few days and by so doing earned for pneumonia the name of 'the old man's friend'? There are two major indications for intervention, despite the limited outlook for the patient.

Since we are committed to lessen the suffering of our patients, if the infection is causing distress, with breathlessness, spasm, coughing, copious sputum, or other symptoms, then genuine attempts must be made to treat the infection, purely as a measure of symptom control. If by such action we prolong dying rather than living, then so be it. Even if it all takes a little longer, that process should still be more comfortable.

Furthermore, if the patient with pneumonia is likely to die in weeks anyway, we must ask, how valuable is this life to the patient? Many are tired and impatient to be gone, others in their 90s are still as determined to hang on to life as in their teens. A candid discussion with both patient and relatives may be helpful here: but normally if the patient still enjoys the sunshine, the visits of friends, the little, precious delights of the day, active treatment should be given.

It may be that this treatment will fail because the pneumonia is a signal of the natural end. That conclusion has to be acceptable. When there is doubt, discussion with colleagues, especially with the nurses who see more of the patient in the course of their duties at the bedside, is likely to be helpful and permits of a team decision.

My own routine, when there is doubt as to whether the pneumonia is a complication or the beginning of the end, is to review after 24 hours. If it is a complication, the patient's symptoms will be beginning to distress; if it is a natural ending, the patient will be moribund and the question of antibiotics is unlikely to arise. If still in doubt, I treat.

Despite the need for such management to be given by the team and the views of the patient and relatives to be gently sought, the final responsibility should not be that of the relatives, or greater guilt and difficulty may be experienced by them later on. When asked their opinion, often they will feel that the patient already has had enough. When they cannot consider, for example, the taking of their relative off the life-support system, although health-care professionals feel the support to be no longer indicated, one should give the relatives a few more days to adjust and often they will face the inevitable bravely. But basically the doctors' decision should be put in the form of a recommendation to the relatives after discussion with the nursing staff. Difficulties are surprisingly rare.

The aim must be to involve the relatives without abdication from professional responsibilities; and never to short-change the patient in the delivery of appropriate treatment.

THE RIGHT TO DIE

Yet the word 'appropriate' is not enough here. There are patients who cling to life at any cost, who will tolerate all the discomforts of being artificially ventilated when there is yet another exacerbation of their myasthenia gravis and muscle power fails. There will be frail cases of advanced cancer who desperately accept and require the nausea, vomiting, diarrhoea, and hair loss resulting from intensive chemotherapy, even when it has obviously lost all power to cure. Others will seek refuge from modern medicine and ask, calmly and while very obviously in their right minds, that no more active treatment be undertaken. They would rather die than have special methods of palliation or resuscitation which would, if carried out on an unwilling patient who has made his wishes clear, constitute an assault.

This may be unacceptable to the health professional. It may be felt as a distressing or wicked waste, and the power of the Courts sought to override the wishes of the patient, or parent, as sometimes happens in cases where those of certain religious beliefs reject blood transfusion.

What is more subtle and perplexing is when a reasonably objective patient is faced with unpleasant treatment he does not really want, from a doctor trained to exhibit an aggressive therapeutic enthusiasm. Here the medical oncologist may feel that treatment should be continued in a way that is resented by the family doctor, who may be closer to the patient or to the family stresses involved. In such a conflict of views there may be no right answers. What is important, however, is that views should be shared for the patient's sake; so that when a family doctor feels that over-treatment is being persisted with improperly, he should say so to the oncologist and arrange for his review of the patient at an out-patient or domiciliary consultation. This will allow the patient's reactions to be reassessed and the treatment perhaps deferred or postponed, while the patient keeps both doctors as trusted resources for the future programme of care.

If doctors can disagree, how much more can patients and relatives? Most patients have as one of their ambitions the desire not to be a nuisance to their family or their doctor: yet the relative may be campaigning for an unsuitable organ-tranplant or an experimental new treatment to be tried in a desperately inappropriate way. Some patients want to be reassured that they can stop trying and can relax. Others determinedly hang on for the birthday party or the overseas daughter's visit. Some relatives are upset not at the loss of their parent but at the confused, undignified death with a multiplicity of tubes defacing the last hopeless hours. Others will sacrifice anything to give a little pleasure to the dying relative. Still others will squabble over the half-bottle of orange squash left at the bedside of the newly dead.

What guidance can one give when the spectrum of behaviour is so broad? The best advice is to discuss, and to seek counsel from the patient when his physical and intellectual state permits it, to involve the relatives without becoming subordinated to their inexperience and distress, to use the insights of the arts of medicine to do as you would be done by, and to keep making different mistakes rather than the same complacent and predictable mistakes over and over again.

If this were not already difficult enough, we must accept also the restrictions of our society. It is comparatively easy to accept that what may be theoretically available may not always in fact be possible. Expensive treatments are likely to be even more rationed in a few decades than they are now—first, as more will have been invented, and secondly, as their suitability for older patients is more questionable. But there are other, more direct ethical pressures from society that in the real world doctors cannot ignore.

This point is perhaps best summarized in the case history of a rather sad epileptic spinster who devotedly cared for her old mother to the end. By the time of her mother's death the spinster was in her 70s and asked that, if the need arose in the future, she should not be resuscitated. This was some months after the old lady's death, she was not clinically depressed, and she gave these wishes in writing, requesting that all the partners in the practice read the note and that it should be filed permanently in her medical records.

The district nurse usually called to see her for a brief social visit each Thursday morning: but one day a few months later the nurse had to visit a neighbour on a Wednesday so she decided to visit next door while she was in the village. She found the house locked and silent, with no answer to her knocking and ringing. The neighbours gathered round and helped her through a window. She found the door had been barricaded and that the patient was in a deep coma as a result of taking a massive overdose of her anti-convulsant medication. There was even a suicide note addressed to her: but by the chance visit exceptionally early in the week, the patient was still alive.

The nurse summoned the general practitioner who, knowing all the background, while the neighbours watched and waited, sent for the ambulance. She was successfully resuscitated and returned home, annoyed and morose, to die of natural causes some 18 months later.

In a world of lesser evils, while euthanasia or gross neglect are still unpopular with most of the health professionals, who can blame the poor GP? The patient certainly did, and showed her anger unambiguously.

THE RIGHT TO GRIEVE

Anger is certainly a natural reaction and may have an important therapeutic value with patients who have to face the loss of so many hopes. It is therefore important not to resent being the target and scapegoat for the mutilations and disappointments which are attributed to one's ineffectiveness, when they are often inevitable consequences of the disease.

The feeling of impotence and regret must not be allowed to erode one's judgement. Resentment and anger are mainly for patients: but they cannot be exclusively for patients.

Nurses who tend to have closer contact with both patients and relatives need constant support and one has become increasingly conscious of the need for caring for the carers. This used to imply the need for respite care and emotional support for the lonely daughter coping with the endless dependency of elderly parents. Now it should include also the health professionals who, like everyone else, find the recurrent facing of their own mortality neither easy nor pleasurable.

Such support networks—formal and informal—will be tested more than ever, as they are with a dying child, when the young AIDS patients also need terminal care on an ever increasing scale.

CONCLUSION

There are few ethical guidelines to help in the hurlyburly of the day. Yet unfailing respect for one's patient, flexibility in one's approach in the face of widely varying needs, unending support for relatives and colleagues—including when it is least deserved—and the husbanding of one's own strength as part of a team: these comprise a survival kit that permit one to move on to tomorrow's crises and the acceptance, whatever one's religious commitment, that death ends nothing very much and needs, so far as one can, to be cut down to size.

REFERENCES

Wilkes, E. (1984). Dying now. *Lancet*, i, 950–2.

20
Handling life: does God forbid?

HELEN OPPENHEIMER

People with religious faith are not free to manipulate living beings as they may wish. Reverence for God requires reverence for life, especially human life, from its very beginning. People who like to call themselves humanists, on the other hand, are required to put their emphasis on bettering the lot of other people. Are these demands compatible? Is it possible to be both a 'humanist' and a 'Christian'? The question is being asked in this form, not to exclude people of any other allegiance, but to explore the author's own position and defend it against the charges of inconsistency or even disloyalty which some traditional believers hasten to press.

Christians are supposed to have two theological statements to make about developments in embryology, that we must not play God, and that human life is sacred. Both these statements need to be made. We dare not seem to underestimate human hubris, folly, and self-deception. It is not just fearfulness but a contemplative wonder which makes religious people chary of taking liberties with the beginnings of life. They feel that unless we can recover a real reverence for creation as God's handiwork instead of the utilitarian expediency some of our contemporaries seem to take for granted, we shall lose touch with all that really matters. 'As you do not know how the spirit comes to the bones in the womb of a woman with child, so you do not know the work of God who makes everything'.[1]

We do not know; but in all humility we can study. To brandish slogans is to use them as argument stoppers, not vehicles for thoughts but substitutes for thoughts.

First, is it so conclusive that we must not 'play God'? To say that we are made 'in his image' is not a statement about our biological shape. Rather it must have something to do with our human moral, intellectual, and creative powers. In thinking so much about embryos and patients, let us not lose touch with the grown human being, who is most recognizable precisely in 'playing God': in living and loving and carrying out purposes. We are seldom given the chance to say 'the rights and wrongs of this question are not for me to enter into'. On the contrary, if we know anything about our God we know that He is good at

[1] Ecclesiastes 11: 5. RSV

delegating. We are not to set ourselves up in His place; but we are obliged to act in His name, to be His representatives.

Secondly, human life is sacred. Indeed it is, but what does this mean? Those of us who are not pacifists, or who believe that therapeutic abortion can be right, are unable to apply this principle mechanically, translating it straight into prohibitions or permissions. In making decisions we must reckon with honourable convictions on both sides. People of liberal persuasion must honour the intuition, rooted in reverence, that human life however rudimentary is not to be written off for our curiosity or convenience. But on the other hand it is right to acknowledge the equally strong intuition that science too is God-given and that where it offers the alleviation of desperate human misery we cannot fold our hands and play safe, saying 'do not handle, do not touch'.[2] Infertility, sorrowful though that is, is by no means the whole story. How can we face the victims of neurological illnesses like Parkinson's disease or Huntingdon's chorea, if we have refused to do all we can to see whether these dreadful afflictions can be alleviated?

When Christians assume that expediency is wicked one wants to ask, what sort of morality glorifies the *in*expedient? To what sort of God are we witnessing? In Southey's poem 'After Blenheim', old Kaspar's grandchildren kept finding human skulls in the garden, and little Peterkin wanted to know:

> 'What good came of it at last?'
> 'Why that I cannot tell', said he,
> 'But 'twas a famous victory'.

We do not want Christian moralists to win a 'famous victory' over real benefactors of mankind. We must keep asking 'What good came of it at last?'

The argument about problem cases tends to be a debate rather than an exploration, leading to victory or defeat rather than mutual comprehension and the development of insight. Let us try to stand back a little from it. Of course we cannot help keeping half an eye on the practical questions, but we can try to do what was not in the brief of the Warnock Committee. We can look more closely at the notion of 'reverence for life' of which everyone seems to approve, and consider how it is grounded.

Here there is a whole complex of ideas about the soul which needs some disentangling. Christian beliefs can take their rise from the book of Genesis without being naïve about our origins. God is our creator, not our sculptor. To say that we are made of the dust of the earth can be a way of saying that we are made of the same 'stuff' as the physical universe, that we belong thoroughly to the world in which we live. To

[2] Colossians 2: 21

say that God has breathed into us the breath or spirit of life can be a way of saying that we are more than physical because God has endowed us with a spiritual nature. So far, so good. But this is where it becomes too easy to assume that the spirit, the immortal part of us, the sacred part of us, must be a different sort of thing from the body, needing to be attached to it or put into it. This assumption has made it harder not easier to understand our spiritual natures and how we may and may not treat fellow human creatures.

Christians have often been dualists, believing that we are made of mortal body and immortal soul. There is no heresy and much sense in maintaining instead that each of us is a unity, living and dying as a whole. Our creeds affirm the resurrection of the whole person rather than the indestructibility of the soul. To say that people are spiritual beings and candidates for eternal life is a way of saying that they matter; and they matter because they mind: in other words, because they are capable of loving and being loved. This is a practical rather than a metaphysical approach to the notion of the sacredness of life. Far from denying that there are souls, one could define a soul as a 'pattern of lovability': putting the Christian hope, not in our immortality, but in the power of God to recreate whatever bodily frame is needed to express each person's own beloved self.[3] As Professor Dunstan put it in 1970, ' "The soul", we might say, is human personality conceived of relationally.'[4]

It may well be said that in making people as 'patterns of lovability' God entrusts enormous responsibility to other people. We know that this is true of our human bodies. First He lets us bring another human being into existence. Then He entrusts us with the nourishment of the developing human creature. The unborn child is nourished continuously and takes shape in total dependence upon its mother. There comes a point when we say that a fetus is 'viable', by which we mean that it can survive outside its mother's body, but not by any means that it can fend for itself. To lead an independent existence, it will not be 'viable' for many years. Will it ever be truly 'viable'? How viable would any of us be if the human beings known and unknown upon whom we depend were no longer available? It is misleading to say that 'man is born free'. Human beings enter life in total dependence and continue in dependence of various kinds of all their days.

If we are content to say all this about bodies, must we then refuse to

[3] This argument is compressed. I have put it at greater length in *The hope of happiness* (SCM Press, 1983) and in *Looking before and after* (Collins, London, 1988). It owes a great deal to David Jenkins, *The glory of man* (SCM Press, 1967, recently republished.)

[4] Dunstan, G. R. (1970). In *Matters of life and death* (ed. E. F. Shotter), Darton, Longman and Todd, for the London Medical Group. See also Chapter 4 in his *The artifice of ethics* (SCM Press, 1974) pp. 57–74.

say something similar about 'souls'? The human being is not made of two separate parts, a body that other people can feed or starve, and an immortal soul, temporarily attached to it, in God's charge. Our 'personhood' did not arrive fully fledged any more than did our physical frame. We needed the nourishment and warmth of relationships just as we needed the nourishment of food and the warmth of our protective environment.

Had any of this been scanty, we should have been stunted and had it failed we should have perished. An aborted fetus or a girl baby exposed on a hillside dies. But likewise, if in some horrible experiment an infant were merely fed and warmed but isolated from loving care, its human development would be prevented. It is no figure of speech to say that a baby needs parents or foster parents to love it into humanity.

This is a dreadful responsibility, but it cannot be evaded. Is it so surprising that 'pro-creation' includes the making of both souls and bodies? Neither body nor 'soul' need be less real for being shaped in relationship.

Unfortunately, this argument may be thought to lead to merely permissive conclusions. People who are suspicious of metaphysics are deemed to be also morally unreliable. And after all it is no wonder that the traditional notion of the soul as a separate thing dies hard. Without it, the conviction that God has *endowed* us with a spiritual nature loses its tempting simplicity.

Admittedly the most straightforward meaning of an endowment is a 'something' given, and probably given at a particular moment. When we start to look for that moment, the occasion that suggests itself is the beginning of a person's individual existence: when else but the moment of conception? So to people who care about moral integrity, the argument about the soul is apt to seem obvious. We either acknowledge the God-given sacredness of the human being from conception, or we try in various ways to wriggle out of it. We suggest later times for this all-important arrival: implantation, quickening, viability, birth. Or we propound tests by which a being must qualify as a person, like passing an exam, thereby setting ourselves up as judges. Of course, all this looks like special pleading in the name of 'expediency'.

No wonder then that the Marquess of Reading, who would have none of this, swayed the whole debate on the Warnock Report in the House of Lords.[5] In his maiden speech he went back to theological first principles. He rejected the idea that 'personhood' is 'something we achieve sometime after fertilisation' and insisted that 'it is something with which we are endowed from fertilization. Those who say that personhood is

[5] Hansard, 31 October 1984. Vol. 456, no. 180, p. 535.

achieved—for example, at the fourteenth day, or some time later—define personhood in functional terms'.

A 'functional' definition focuses attention upon what a person *can do* rather than what a person *is*; and one can see why this is repugnant. Are we to say, 'that one has failed to qualify: we can treat "it" as a thing'? Or worse: 'that one has deteriorated beyond the limits: we can bring this existence to an end'? Of course not! Personhood cannot be a qualification; so it seems to follow that it must be an endowment; unless the stark contrast is based upon an over-simplification.

Is 'personhood' a gift or an achievement, a bequest or a prize to be won or lost? There is a more subtle way of looking at the creation of a person which disposes of this harsh contrast. Christians of all people have ready to hand a better image than the adding of a spirit to a body. They are used to the idea that what is physical can itself receive spirtual meaning. It happens every time bread and wine are consecrated in the Eucharist. What consecration does is to take material substance and bless it into a new kind of existence so that it becomes holy. Surely this idea can help more than the idea of an 'endowment' to interpret the astonishing development of a child of God from a cluster of cells. Whether there is a 'moment of consecration' is not the point. What matters is that a physical being can be blessed into sacredness, we may even say loved into it. 'Souls' are not granted like charters but, as it were, enabled and fostered. The idea that the world is a 'vale of soul-making' makes good sense.

We can develop this way of thinking about persons with the idea that they can become 'means of grace' for one another. We can call it a 'relational' view, provided nobody thinks that 'person' is therefore 'merely relative' as if it were some kind of fiction or pretence depending upon other people's whim or convenience. Relationships are as real as objects and just as little to be trifled with.

Nor has this argument anything to do with presuming to judge the value of people by the quality of their relationships. It is not working up to a conclusion that unwanted babies with nobody to love them, still less unwanted senile old people, are not really 'persons' and can therefore be painlessly put down. People are not, so to say, 'justified by relationships': they are literally formed by them. A being that has the capacity to become a person actually becomes one by entering into relationships with other persons. To become a human being is not to spring like Athene fully-armed from the head of Zeus, but to enter the human race and grow as a member of it.

This argument needs a lot of care or it will overreach itself. How dare we seem to say that the unwanted child has no soul? Is it like the tree in Ronald Knox's limerick, that

'Just ceases to be
When there's no one about in the quad'?

On the contrary, like Bishop Berkeley, we must take God into account. He 'is always about in the quad'. The unwanted person is His child. The heavenly Father can see all the value and 'lovability' in the most unpromising of His children that the most doting parents could ever see. But on the other hand, the most wanted baby has a long way to go before its potential becomes actual. It is no more a person than a bud is a flower.

Our love for the infant, and God's love, anticipates what it can become. To use a technical term, this is exactly what 'prevenient grace' means: grace that anticipates, that goes ahead of the facts, drawing out what is not yet there, seeing what can be, nourishing and educating, not just appraising. If our love for a new member of humankind fails badly enough, its development into a person will not, humanly speaking, happen. What the power of God can do for His creatures that have no earthly chance to develop is one of the great problems. It is not to be solved simply by defining human life as sacred.

The responsibility with which we are entrusted is a radical responsibility. We are obliged, heaven help us, to 'play God'. In the decisions we have to make we cannot always be on the safe side, even when we are sure which the safe side would be. In particular, we cannot say of the very early embryos that we shall not go wrong provided we treat them as human beings.

The question of what God, so to say, underwrites, is part of the question of what kind of God we believe in. A God who would have us reverence every potential human life as if it were already a person, ignoring the prodigality of nature with such beginnings, or a God who would rather we experimented upon an adult chimpanzee than upon a cluster of cells in a test-tube because *human* life is sacred, is not much like the Creator to which both our studies and our consciences point. It is not special pleading to doubt whether the early human embryo, wonderful as it is, with the potential to develop into a human being, has suddenly a totally different 'sacredness' from the egg and sperm which formed it.

It makes more sense to believe that the arrival of a person is the arrival of 'lovability', inconveniently vague as this idea is compared with conception or birth or even implantation. One is not demanding achievement or qualifications, but looking for the smallest possibility of *response*. A person may not be either beloved or loving, but a person must be a candidate for love; and love, even unrequited love, even God's love for the unlovable, cannot dispense with the possibility of reciprocation.

Although in a way God can love all His creatures as an artist loves his handiwork, not all God's creatures are persons. The question is not, 'who can be excluded from God's love?' as if some of the smallest and weakest might then be rejected. The question is, 'what is, and what is not, a "who" at all?' Surely a 'who', a person, must have some rudimentary capacity for love upon which the love of God and other people can obtain a purchase. 'Capacity' here means much more than 'potential': as we might say that an infant has the *potential* to learn to read, but a five-year-old child has the *capacity* to learn to read. So in a similar way a newborn baby, and maybe already a quickening fetus, begins to have the capacity to be a person. What we are asking about is the dawn of awareness considered as the dawn of response.

The beginning of a nervous system is therefore more important even than genetic individuality when we are looking for a 'soul'. It may seem untidy and unmanageable to say that a person develops in gradual stages, but both biologically and ethically it appears to be the most convincing interpretation of the data.

Does this suggest that before we have 'a person' anything goes? It certainly does not, any more than 'anything goes' when a person has departed at the other end of life. In both cases we have something fully human which claims our respect, even reverence. The honour we owe to an embryo or to a dead body is not sentimental or superstitious. It is 'pious' in a truly human sense, whether we are religious or not. But essentially it either looks forward or back. Neither the embryo nor the corpse is now a person, although every human being has once been an embryo and will be a dead body.

It is easy to become confused, because there are also borderline cases. Sometimes we do have to ask 'person: or not?' because development at the beginning of life is gradual and departure at its end can also be gradual. A fetus, not yet born, is beginning to be a person. Its mother may well claim to love it in a way in which it would be nonsense to claim to love a blastocyst. Likewise a comatose patient, not yet dead but beyond recovery, can be tragically loved and tended. It is certainly not sentimental to call either of these 'persons': yet their 'personhood' has a large element of the forward- or backward-looking about it. If we are challenged we cannot be quite sure that here is a full-scale human being, sacred and inviolable. We are on difficult ground here, a slippery slope. Whatever we do we must not argue that because a creature is unloved it lacks the 'lovability' which makes it a person. An unwanted, handicapped baby whose parents reject him, a senile old lady neither dear nor endearing, are well within the bounds of being persons. Any case for terminating these lives would have to be a case for killing persons, or letting persons die. We should have to say, 'this person would be better dead'; or less murderously, 'this person is dying and we can ease the process'; or, 'our techniques are only prolonging this person's death and should be brought to a stop'.

Because we are doubtful about the border we must draw it generously. We must be very careful not to call 'termination' what ought to be called 'murder': so we must count the borderline cases as persons if we possibly can. We shall probably have to become legalistic, as necessarily legalistic as when we try to measure 'maturity': 16 years for marriage, 17 for driving cars, 18 for voting.

However generously we draw the line, there are still cases we need not try to include. Sometimes we can surely say that there is no person yet or no person any more. The embryo which has not yet begun to develop a nervous system, for all its full complement of human genes, is as much before personhood as a corpse is after it. Neither is now within reach of relationship. But conversely, neither is beyond the reach of the respect we properly owe to what could become, or once was, a human being. Though we cannot and should not promote life or continuing life for every potential or past person, we can still handle such beings with reverence. To buy and sell them would be an indignity; but surely to study them, to let them be a source of great benefit for humankind, need not be.

There is an essential asymmetry, of course: the embryo is alive and the corpse is dead. Yet for Christians this asymmetry is not absolute. It may even go the other way round. Many embryos are never going to be persons, whatever happens. But we believe the person that this corpse was is going to live again. If this is true, surely this will not be by the reanimation of the human remains but by the restoration to life of this particular person's 'pattern of lovability'.

21
The moral obligations of the physician in the rabbinic tradition

J. DAVID BLEICH

THE OBLIGATION TO HEAL

Judaism teaches that the value of human life is supreme and takes precedence over virtually all other considerations. This attitude is most eloquently summed up in a talmudic passage regarding the creation of Adam: 'Therefore only a single human being was created in the world, to teach that if any person has caused a single soul of Israel to perish, Scripture regards him as if he had caused an entire world to perish; and if any human being saves a single soul of Israel, Scripture regards him as if he had saved an entire world' (Sanhedrin 37a). Human life is not a good to be preserved as a condition of other values, but an absolute, basic, and precious good in its own right. The obligation to preserve life is commensurately all-encompassing.

THE ROLE OF THE PHYSICIAN

Judaism views the seeking of medical attention as a moral imperative. Moreover, man is obligated to exercise prudence in preserving health. Thus the Talmud, Sanhedrin 17b, states that a scholar should not establish residence in a community which cannot boast of the presence of a physician.

Despite the obligation on the part of the patient to seek medical care, the concomitant obligation on the part of the physician is somewhat limited. There is no absolute, mandatory obligation which requires any specific individual to study medicine no matter how talented he may be.[1] Similarly, no person is obligated to engage in any specific research

[1] See, for example R. Moses Feinstein, *No'am*, VIII (5728), 9, and *idem*, *Iggerot Mosheh*, *Yoreh De'ah* III, no. 155. Rabbi Feinstein declares that one who refrains from studying medicine for fear that he will later be inconvenienced by being called upon to treat a poor patient, or because he is fearful of committing an error, will be held culpable if a sick person dies as a result of the lack of a qualified physician. This statement should presumably be understood as expressing moral censure of unworthy motives rather than as reflective of an absolute obligation to undertake the study of medicine.

designed to advance medical knowledge. Even after having received extensive medical training and having been licensed to practise medicine, no individual is obligated to enter into the practice of medicine as a vocation or to seek out patients in need of his professional skill and expertise.

However, if a physician is requested to render medical assistance, or if the physician becomes aware of the needs of an individual requiring medical assistance, the situation is quite different. In legal systems based upon common law the relationship between a physician and his patient is a contractual one. Therefore, legally, a doctor has the absolute right to refuse to treat a patient who is not yet under his care. In effect, he may refuse to enter into a contract with the would-be patient. This attitude is reflected in the *Code of ethics* of the American Medical Association which declares, 'A physician may choose whom he will serve'. Judaism, on the contrary, regards the physician not simply as acting on behalf of the patient but as acting in the service of God. He is, in effect, God's messenger and dares not shirk the responsibility thrust upon him. This, quite apart from a general aversion to oath-taking, serves to explain why there is no parallel to the Hippocratic Oath in the Jewish tradition. Jews are considered to be 'foresworn from Sinai' to observe all the tenets of Judaism. For one who has sworn at Sinai to observe the tenets of Judaism in their entirety, a subsequent oath to fulfil any specific religious obligation would be superfluous. Accordingly, the doctor is obliged to render medical care not only in emergency, life-threatening situations, but even when such care is required simply for alleviation of pain or preservation of physical well-being. Man intuitively perceives a social morality which leads to the recognition that man is his brother's keeper. Human society has long recognized that unique obligations devolve upon certain of its members by virtue of their talents, training, and/or unique responsibilities. Enhancement of skills brings in its wake a commensurate increase in moral responsibility.

It is instructive to compare the obligations of the physician with those of the Torah scholar who is requested to impart information or to serve as an arbiter or judge in civil disputes. As a matter of strict obligation, the scholar need not seek out persons in need of his services, nor must he make himself available during such times as he is engaged in earning a livelihood.[2] But, when engaged in study, or in his free time, he must answer questions put to him and render decisions 'for with regard to this, that which concerns his fellow man takes precedence'. The physician, in situations in which the life of his fellow man may be threatened, labours under an even greater obligation. When able to do so, he must act in order to preserve human life.

[2] R. Moses Sofer, *Teshuvot Hatam Sofer, Hoshen Mishpat*, no. 164.

An individual physician might, indeed, sidestep his responsibilities by removing himself from situations in which his aid might be sought. While such conduct would not merit approbation, the physician who acts in this manner would not incur the guilt of a technical infraction of Jewish law. Within autonomous Jewish communities, society's responsibility for promotion of communal well-being is discharged through the *Bet Din* (rabbinical court). The *Bet Din* is empowered to compel the physician to make himself available and to function in his professional capacity. It is the responsibility of the *Bet Din* to assure that the burden of providing medical care is shared equitably by all physicians qualified to render such care.[3]

Physicians possess skills which are not shared by other members of society. In opening a medical office or in accepting hospital appointments, they agree to make their skills available to those whom they serve. Hence, society has a unique claim upon their services and they, in turn, bear a unique responsibility to society. The physician may not, for example, engage in strike action which compromises the health of his patients. He may not fail to attend his patient even if his motive is to effect improvement in health-care facilities or services rather than his own pecuniary self-interest. It is not legitimate for a doctor to shirk an imperative moral responsibility to patients requiring medical attention 'here and now' on the plea that present nonfeasance will ultimately redound to better care for more patients at some future time. An immediate moral claim cannot be set aside in anticipation of future claims which do not as yet exist.

The physician may quite properly refuse to perform 'out of title' tasks, provided such omission does not jeopardize the patient. Similarly, elective procedures which may be deferred without harm or risk do not pose an immediate obligation and may be postponed for good and sufficient reason. But in no circumstances may the real and immediate needs of a patient be ignored.

The physician's right to some form of compensation is clearly evident from the discussion recorded in *Baba Kamma* 85a. A person who has caused physical harm to another is obligated to bear the expenses of medical treatment of the victim. The assailant does not have the option of offering the ministration of a physician who will not demand a fee for his services for the victim may counter, 'A physician who heals for nothing is worth nothing'.[4] While no practitioner may withhold his

[3] See R. Eliezer Waldenberg, *Ramat Rahel*, no. 24, sec. 6; cf. *Aurkh ha-Shulhan, Yoreh De'ah 261:6*.

[4] A survey of halakhic sources which define the limits placed upon the fee a physician may charge for his services is presented by R. Chaim David Halevi, the Sephardic Chief Rabbi of Tel Aviv, in the Kislev 5737 issue of *Shevilin*. This material appears to be based in large measure upon Rabbi Eliezer Waldenberg's discussion of the same topic in his *Ramat Rahel*, nos. 24 and 25.

services because of a patient's inability to pay the required fee,[5] the individual physician is not, strictly speaking, obligated to provide such services on a general basis. However, the community has an obligation to assure that medical services are available to rich and poor alike. The *Bet Din*, as the executive and administrative arm of society, is charged with taking any necessary measures for providing such care. The *Bet Din* may use its coercive power in ordering physicians to treat indigent patients but must see to it that the onus is shared by all available and competent physicians in an equitable manner.

Despite the awesome responsibility placed upon the physician, or perhaps *because* of it, rabbinic writings convey a certain negativism with regard to the medical profession. 'The best of physicians is destined to Hell,' declares the Mishnah, *Kiddushin* 82a. This statement is simply a reflection of the fact that the Talmud recognizes that individual physicians are on occasion quite prone to be remiss or negligent in performing their duties. Such lapses, according to Jewish teaching, occasion the severest punishment.

The physician bears responsibility not only for the physical well-being of the patient, but also for his spiritual well-being. Old time Jerusalemites tell an interesting anecdote about the late Dr Wallach, of blessed memory, the founder and first medical director of Sha'arei Zedek Hospital. It was his invariable practice to visit each newly-admitted patient shortly after admission and to inquire after his or her mother's Hebrew name. Sha'arei Zedek Hospital maintains a synagogue on its premises and has instituted the laudable practice of reciting Psalms on behalf of its patients; thereafter a prayer for the recovery of each of the patients is recited. Traditionally, the prayer for the sick includes the patient's Hebrew name as well as that of the patient's mother. Hence, Dr Wallach solicited this information and transmitted it to the synagogue sexton. Dr Wallach obviously wished to convey a message to the patient: this information is solicited by the medical director himself because he is fully cognizant that all healing comes from God and wishes the patient to be aware of this as well.

Rashi, in his commentary on the earlier cited Mishnah, catalogues the sins of both commission and omission common to physicians. Among them are 'He gives him the diet of healthy persons to eat and does not humble his heart before God'. The latter phrase is conventionally understood as referring to the excessive pride which is, at times, evidenced by physicians who erroneously come to believe that life and death are in their hands rather than in the hands of God. A more grammatically consistent interpretation would render the translation

[5] R. Eliezer Fleckles, *Teshuvah me-Ahavah*, III, *Yoreh De'ah*, no 336; R. Shalom Schachneh, *Mishmeret Shalom*, II, 99; and R. David Katz, *Bet David*, II, *Yoreh De'ah*, no. 306.

'and does not cause him (i.e. the patient) to humble his heart before God'. In failing to impress this awareness upon the patient the physician is remiss in fulfilling the divine trust with which he is charged. In sensitizing the patient to the spiritual component inherent in the healing process the physician bears testimony to the divine purpose underlying all natural phenomena.

INDIVIDUAL AUTONOMY AND THE OBLIGATION TO HEAL

Under the Anglo-Saxon system of law as followed in the United States of America, a physician has no greater obligation to treat or advise a person in need of medical attention than has any other individual. The physician-patient relationship is viewed in common law as a contractual relationship based upon consensual agreement. While it is true that such contracts need not be expressly verbalized and exist even when the physician's services are rendered gratuitously, no obligation exists with regard to the provision of medical care unless the patient wishes medical assistance and the physician offers such treatment. (In the United Kingdom, statutory rights and duties established by the National Health Service Acts have modified the common law.) It is only after a patient is accepted for treatment that certain obligations devolve upon the physician. By submitting to examination and treatment, the patient impliedly grants permission for medical treatment and impliedly agrees to pay professional fees when these are customary and usual. By treating the patient the physician impliedly promises to continue such treatment until his professional services are no longer needed or desired by the patient. Thus the physician–patient relationship is based upon a contract implied-in-fact.

In terms of civil law a physician, despite his skill and licensure, is under no obligation to practise medicine, nor is he under a legal duty to render aid to another in distress. It has been conclusively established that a physician is not legally obligated to accept a patient for treatment. Moreover, except in emergencies, the physician is under legal constraint not to minister to the needs of the sick unless there is a clear indication on the part of the patient that treatment is desired by him. Under common law, freedom from intentional unauthorized touching of the body is one of the basic freedoms enjoyed by every person. While unavoidable trespasses, such as unintentional touching in a crowded bus or elevator or the intentional grasping of a friend's arm in order to attract his attention, are accepted as part of casual social intercourse and do not constitute a personal indignity, medical procedures such as a hypodermic injection, a proctological examination, or the lancing of an abscess constitute an invasion of the integrity of the person, and when unauthorized any such action becomes an act of assault and battery. A patient who voluntarily consults a physician and voluntarily submits to treatment, relying entirely upon the physician's skill and care, gives general consent by implication to at least such operation or treatment as may reasonably be necessary. The patient may at any time withdraw or limit such permission.

Jewish law does not require prior consent of the patient in life-threatening situations. In emergencies, when the patient requires immediate care to preserve life and health, the physician is reasonably privileged to treat the patient. Such action is usually justified on the basis of hypothetical assumption that were the patient competent and were it possible to seek consent without jeopardizing the patient such consent would be willingly forthcoming.

The touchstone of a democratic society is the concept of individual freedom and personal autonomy. Democratic societies are certainly dedicated to the maximization of personal freedom and find it necessary to justify any violation of personal privacy and any intrusion into the personal affairs of their citizens. These democratic traditions stand diametrically opposed to the absolutism which is the hallmark of the autocratic systems of government whose excesses cause so much human suffering.

No one will dispute the claim that personal freedom and individual autonomy are religious values as well. Yet it is readily apparent that, in a hierarchical ranking of values, the values of personal freedom and autonomy do not occupy a position within a religiously oriented ethical system identical to that which they occupy in a secular system of values. That certainly is the case in so far as Jewish tradition is concerned and serves to explain why a patient dares not refuse treatment that is clearly required to preserve life.

Judaism teaches that man has no proprietary interest either in his life or in his body. Man's body and his life are not his to give away. The proprietor of all human life is none other than God Himself. As Radbaz so eloquently phrases it: 'Man's life is not his property, but the property of the Holy One, blessed be He'.

In Jewish teaching it should be recognized that personal privilege as well as personal responsibility, as it extends to the human body and to human life, are similar to the privilege and responsibility of a bailee with regard to a bailment with which he has been entrusted. A bailee is an individual who has accepted an object of value for safekeeping. It is his duty to safeguard the bailment and to return it to its rightful owner upon demand. Judaism teaches that, with regard to his body, man is but a steward charged with preservation of this most precious of bailments and must abide by the limitations placed upon his rights of use and enjoyment. Hence, any claim to absolute autonomy is specious.

This moral stance is reflected in the mores of society at large, although not to the same degree. Despite our society's commitment to individual liberty as an ideal, it recognizes that this liberty is not entirely sacrosanct. Although there are those who wish it to be so, self-determination is not universally recognized as the paramount human value. There is a long judicial history of recognition of the State's 'compelling interest' in the preservation of life of each and every one of its citizens, an 'interest' which carries with it the right to curb personal freedom. What the jurist calls a 'compelling state interest' the theologian terms 'sanctity of life'. It is precisely this concept of the sanctity of life which, as a transcendental value, supersedes considerations of personal freedom. This is implicitly recognized even in the drafting of the Natural Death Act enacted in various jurisdictions; otherwise such legislation would grant its citizens unequivocal authority to terminate life by any means and in all circumstances. Were autonomy recognized as *the* paramount value, society would not shrink from sanctioning suicide, mercy killing, or indeed consensual homicide under any or all conditions.

Jewish tradition certainly recognizes liberty as a value but defines freedom and liberty in a very particular way. The Mishnaic dictum, '*Ve-lo atah ben horin le-hibatel memenah' (Ethics of the Fathers* 2:16) is rendered by the 15th century commentator Isaac Abarbanel, not in the usual manner as 'nor are you free to desist from it', i.e. from obedience to the law, but as 'nor in desisting from it are you a free man'. Freedom is the absence of constraint which would interfere with such realization. Hence casting off the yoke of law is not an act of freedom but its antithesis. This concept is very similar to what the British philospher T. H. Green called 'positive freedom'.

This is true for other religious traditions as well. Liberty, as the term is conventionally understood, is a paramount value only when it does not conflict with other divinely established values. In secular terms, personal autonomy must give way to preservation of the social fabric. The state has an interest, which is entirely secular in nature, in the preservation of the life of each of its citizens. In the absence of other competing interests, it may assert its authority in compelling the preservation of a life against the wishes of a citizen in spite of the deprivation of liberty which is entailed thereby, because public policy accepts the moral thesis that the preservation of life be regarded as a superior value, taking precedence over the right to privacy and the value of personal autonomy.

Jewish law bestows a privileged position upon preservation of human life as a moral value. As a moral desideratum, it takes precedence over virtually all other values. Exceptions to the general rule that preservation of life takes precedence over all other considerations are transgression of the three cardinal sins for purposes of preserving life. These are murder (hardly an exception), idolatry, and sexual offences such as incest and adultery. All other laws are suspended for purposes of conservation of life. Even the mere possibility of preserving life mandates suspension of biblical restrictions, however remote the likelihood of success in saving human life may be.

These provisions reflect the unique position which preservation of life occupies in the hierarchy of values posited by Judaism. Judaism regards human life as being of infinite and inestimable value. Not only is life in general of infinite and inestimable value, but every moment of life is of inestimable value as well. The quality of life which is preserved is thus never a factor to be taken into consideration. Neither is the length of the patient's life expectancy a controlling factor.

As stated earlier, Judaism regards every moment of life as sacred. Hence, the patient must seek treatment, and ritual laws are suspended for the sake of such treatment even if there is no medical guarantee of a cure. Similarly, the physician's duty does *not* end when he is incapable of restoring the lost health of his patient. The obligation 'and you shall restore it to him' (Deuteronomy 22:2) refers, in its medical context, not simply to the restoration of health, but to the restoration of even a single moment of life. Again, Sabbath restrictions and other laws are suspended even when it is known with certainty that human medicine offers no hope of a cure or restoration to health. Ritual obligations and restrictions are suspended so long as there is the possibility that life may be prolonged even for a matter of moments.

In the *Republic* (1,340), Plato observes that a physician, at the time that he errs in treating a patient, is not worthy of his title. When the physician's knowledge fails him, he ceases to be a practitioner of the healing arts. The Sages of the Talmud went one step further: they taught that a physician who declines to make use of his skills is not a physician; they admonished that a physician who gives up his patient as hopeless is not a physician. '*And he shall surely heal*—from here it is derived that the physician is granted permission to heal' (*Baba Kamma* 85a). To this may be added a pithy comment atributed by some to the Hasidic Seer, the *Hozeh* of Lublin, by others to the Gaon of Vilna: 'The Torah gives permission to heal. It does not give the physician dispensation to refrain from healing because in his opinion the patient's condition is hopeless'.

This lesson is also the moral of a story told of the nineteenth century Polish scholar popularly known as Rabbi Eisel Charif. The venerable Rabbi was afflicted with a severe illness and was attended by an eminent specialist. As the disease progressed beyond hope of cure, the physician informed the Rabbi's family of the gravity of the situation. He also informed them that he therefore felt justified in withdrawing from the case. The doctor's grave prognosis notwithstanding, Rabbi Eisel Charif recovered completely. Some time later, the physician chanced to come upon the Rabbi in the street. The doctor stopped in his tracks in astonishment and exclaimed, 'Rabbi, have you come back from the other world?' The Rabbi responded, 'You are indeed correct. I *have* returned from the other world. Moreover, I did you a great favour while I was there. An angel ushered me into a large chamber. At the far end of the room was a door, and lined up in front of the door were a large number of well-dressed, dignified and intelligent looking men. These men were proceeding through the doorway in a single file. I asked the angel who these men were and where the door led. He informed me that the door was the entrance to the netherworld and that the men passing through those portals were those of whom the Mishnah says, "The best of physicians merits *Gehinnom.*" Much to my surprise, I noticed that you, too, were standing in the line about to proceed through the door. I immediately approached the angel and told him: "Remove that man immediately! He is no doctor. He does not treat patients; he abandons them" '.

To depict any human condition as hopeless is to miss entirely the spiritual dimension of human existence. Even were it true that medical diagnoses and prognoses are infallible, the decision to terminate treatment is not a medical decision; it is the determination of a moral question. That the physician possesses specialized knowledge and unique skills is unquestionable. However, his professional training guarantees neither heightened moral sensitivity nor enhanced acumen. He may quite legitimately draw medical conclusions with regard to the expected effects of the application or withholding of various therapeutic procedures. But the decision to proceed or not to proceed is a moral, not a medical, decision. From the fact that a condition is medically hopeless it does not follow that the remaining span of life is devoid of meaning. God has decreed that we must love, cherish, and preserve life in all its phases and guises until the very onset of death. While even terminal life is undoubtedly endowed with other meaning and value as well, subservience to the divine decree and fulfilment of God's commandment is, in itself, a matter of highest meaning.

RISKS INHERENT IN MEDICAL TREATMENT

A moral system which recognizes preservation of life as a paramount value must come to grips with the stark fact that life is fraught with situations in which risks must be confronted and assessed. Most decisions to perform even the most ordinary and mundane acts involve an assumption of some risk. At times, the risks of intervention are as great, or even greater, than those of inaction. A vaccine against a dread disease may be defective and cause the very disease against which it is designed to provide protection. Although exercise is of demonstrated efficacy in the prevention of obesity, physical exertion may well precipitate a heart attack. For reasons which are quite obvious, assumption of such risks presents no moral dilemma. Statistically, the danger of contracting disease through contagion is far greater than the risk of a possibly defective batch of vaccine. Obesity has caused far more fatal heart attacks than has strenuous exercise. Indeed, in situations in which these statistical considerations do not pertain, the approbation of society is withheld. For that reason we require government approval of all drugs administered to patients and recommend that no one embark upon a regimen of strenuous exercise without first undergoing a thorough physical examination.

There are, of course, innumerable occasions in which risks are assumed even though no such balancing act is involved. But there are situations in which the moral dilemma is very real. A patient is afflicted with terminal disease. The only treatment available requires administration of a potent drug which, if successful, will remove all traces of disease and, in terms of anticipation of longevity, restore the patient to the *status quo ante*. However, the drug is highly toxic and in a predictable proportion of patients the drug itself will foreshorten life. Is it morally legitimate for the patient to assume the risks inherent in such therapy? After all, a brief span of human life is endowed with moral value of the highest order. May a patient, in effect, enter into a gamble in which he stakes a limited, but certain, life span against a longer, but uncertain, life expectancy?

Perhaps a moral agent might be required to construct a risk/benefit equation. Let us assume that, in the absence of treatment, the patient is endowed with a life-certain longevity anticipation of one week. Let us further assume that the proposed treatment has a predictable success rate of 10 per cent, with success defined as survival for a period of 10 weeks, but that failure will result in immediate death. If the goal is maximization of human life-quanta, there is no risk/benefit advantage in treatment over non-treatment or vice versa: there is no determinant risk/benefit equation which serves as an objective point of demarcation between prudence and foolhardiness. The net result is that, when confronted by such a decision, there is no morally absolute right or wrong. The *desideratum* is enhancement of life quanta. But in any individual situation it is impossible to determine which choice will yield maximum enhancement. Hence, in such circumstances, the decision to treat and the decision not to treat are, morally speaking, equally acceptable.

The determination that a proposed procedure is therapeutic (i.e. of potential benefit to the patient) rather than experimental is not always obvious. Determination of the existence of a favourable risk/benefit ratio is often even more difficult. If the attending physician's opinion cannot be regarded as unbiased, to whom shall the patient turn for dispassionate evaluation? How can one guarantee the right of infants and minors to a decision based solely upon their best interests?

Over a century ago, Jewish medical ethics developed a *modus operandi* for dealing with this problem. The specific question involved a patient afflicted with an illness which, if left untreated, would have been fatal. A potentially curative drug was available, but there existed a danger that it might cause the immediate demise of the patient. A leading rabbinic decisor was consulted with regard to the proper course of action. He counselled that the risk be evaluated by a number of expert medical practitioners and that after eliciting multiple medical opinions the view of the majority be followed 'upon the acquiesence of "the wise man" of the town.'[6] His role was to assess the reliability and impartiality of the medical advice conveyed and to detect any possible personal or professional bias on the part of the medical consultants. The primary qualification of the 'wise man' was that he had neither a personal nor a professional involvement with either the patient or the treatment and hence he could remain detached and dispassionate.

One might suppose that, under present conditions, such a role might be filled by a hospital's ethics committee. Unfortunately, owing to the manner in which such committees are constituted, this cannot be the case. The requirement for ethics committee approval of all experimental procedures involving human subjects does place certain meaningful restraints upon potentially unethical procedures. But in many situations there is no greater assurance that the ethics committee will arrive at a decision in a disinterested manner than there is that the individual physician will do so. Procedures such as a xenograft are team efforts; success redounds to the glory and benefit of the institution and of all persons associated with it. Although there is community representation on hospital ethics committees, the overwhelming majority of the members of such committees are members of the institution's own medical and administrative staff. Self-interest can be avoided only if the ethics committee is composed of persons with no ties either to the medical facilities whose procedures are subject to review, or to sister and hence 'rival' institutions. Of course, the decisions of such a committee

[6] See Rabbi Jacob Reischer, *Teshuvot Shevut Ya'akov*, III, no. 75.

can be ethically meaningful only if its members are both knowledgeable of, and committed to, the fundamental principles of ethics which should govern all decision.

TRUTH-TELLING

The obligation to tell the truth and to refrain from falsehood is one of the cornerstones of every ethical system. The Bible commands, 'Distance yourself from a matter of falsehood' (Exodus 23:7). Yet, despite the great value placed upon truth-telling, no one would seriously advocate giving a truthful answer to *every* question. Surely a would-be murderer seeking to discover the whereabouts of his potential victim should not be given truthful information. Every system of ethics posits not only a set of moral values, but also a means of reconciling conflicts which must inevitably arise when ethical principles come into conflict with one another. In any hierarchical ranking of values, preservation of human life is certainly far more significant than truth-telling. A lie is most assuredly warranted if that is the price which must be paid for preservation of a human life. The Talmud teaches that a 'white lie' is justified for purposes of promoting tranquil relationships, for obviating pain, embarrassment, or even comparatively mild psychic distress.[7] Promotion of these goals is deemed to be of greater significance than unequivocal pursuit of truth.

In the treatment of terminal patients, the question of whether or not to divulge the nature of the disease and its prognosis is a vexing one. The patient has a certain right to information concerning himself. Indeed, the physician has, in a sense, entered into a contract with the patient to make this knowledge available to him. Often there is a genuine need for the patient to have such information available to him so that he may put his affairs in order, make provisions for his family, or prepare himself spiritually for death.

On the other hand, health-care professionals have an obligation to preserve both the physical and emotional well-being of the patient. An important obligation of the physician is *primum non nocere*, to do no harm to the patient. The physician must be certain that the information conveyed will not have a debilitating effect on his patient. It is for this reason that the third edition of the *Code of ethics* of the American Medical Association, adopted in 1975, states that the physician has a sacred duty to avoid all things that have a tendency to discourage the

[7] See *Pesikta Zutrati, Parshat Va-Yehi*; *Baba Metzia* 23b; and *Ketubot* 17a.

patient and to depress his spirits. In order to prevent this from occurring, some forms of deception are justifiable.

Jewish law is particularly sensitive to the debilitating effects which mental stress may have upon an enfeebled or moribund patient. Since Judaism views every moment of life as sacred, care must be taken not to foreshorten life even by a short period of time.

The question of whether or not it is proper to inform a patient of his imminent demise is discussed forthrightly by the Midrash, *Kohelet Rabbah* 5.6. Isaiah was sent to inform Hezekiah that the latter's sickness was fatal (Isaiah 38:1) Hezekiah is depicted as reproving the prophet, 'Even if [the physician] sees that [the patient] is about to die he does not say to him "Leave a testament to your household" lest [the patient's] mind faint.' Concern lest the patient fall prey to depression or despair, thereby hastening death is cited by the Midrash as establishing the normative principle governing such situations. Not only must the physician refrain from transmitting information which may perchance have this effect, but he must also continue to dispense advice which has the sole effect of reassuring the patient. He must be solicitous and feign medical aid even though there is no medical purpose in his ministrations. The patient must be advised what to eat and drink—and which medicines to take—not because of the therapeutic effect of such measures, but because the significance of removal of dietary restrictions or total withdrawal of medication is not lost upon the discerning patient. The 'placebo effect' of the physician's continued ministrations not only prevents despondency but has a positive psychological value which is beneficial to the patient.

The incident reported in II Kings 8:7–10 has been understood by some commentaries as illustrating precisely this concern. Ben-Hadad, the king of Aram, became sick and sent a messenger to inquire of the Prophet Elisha whether or not he would recover. Elisha informed the messenger that, in fact, Ben-Hadad would die but instructed him to tell the king, 'You shall surely recover'. Gersonides, commenting upon this passage, indicates that absolute candour might hasten the death of the patient. Lack of truthfulness, in such situations, is not merely permissible, or even commendable, but mandatory.[8] The Jewish view in this matter does not parallel the well-publicized recommendations of Dr Elisabeth Kübler-Ross.[9] Kübler-Ross based her conclusions upon information obtained through highly subjective personal interaction with some two hundred dying patients. Dr Kübler-Ross's scientific

[8] See Rabbi Betzalel Stern, *Teshuvot be-Tzel ha-Hokhmah*, II, no. 55; and *She'arim ha-Metzuyanim be-Halakhah* 191:2.

[9] Kübler-Ross, E. (1969). *On death and dying*, Macmillan, New York; see also Kübler-Ross, E. (1974). *Questions and answers on death and dying*, Macmillan, New York.

objectivity and the validity of her conclusions have been challenged by a number of her colleagues.[10] Other researchers have reported markedly different findings.[11]

Nevertheless, whether or not Kübler-Ross's methods were scientifically sound is essentially irrelevant to our concern. Jewish teaching with regard to this issue is based on considerations which do not necessarily contradict the data upon which Dr Kübler-Ross's findings are based. The five stages of dying, culminating in the ultimate acceptance of death without adverse physical effects, as described by Kübler-Ross, may well have been manifested by the subjects of those studies and by countless others as well. However, no universal generalization may be drawn with regard to the reactions of all patients. Not all patients react in the manner she describes. The devastation experienced by some patients and their consequent loss of a desire to live is a repeatedly observed phenomenon. The physical effects of such psychological phenomena do not readily lend themselves to clinical analysis. The *possibility* of adverse reaction is sufficient reason for eschewing a policy of full disclosure. Jewish law is concerned with the foreshortening of even a single human life. Accordingly in this, as in other areas of Halakhah, the possibility of hastening death in at least some patients must be the determining consideration.

Despite the growing tendency of health-care professionals to advocate that the terminally ill be made fully aware of the gravity of their condition, medical science is well aware of the adverse effects which may result from a policy of full disclosure. The halakhic consideration that *tiruf ha-da'at*, i.e. acute medical anguish, may cause or hasten death has some empirical confirmation.

The fear of hastening death must, however, be carefully balanced against the patient's need to settle his affairs and to repent before death. Accordingly, the *Code of Jewish law*[12] rules that a patient should be instructed to turn his attention to his affairs, to make appropriate arrangements in the event that 'he has lent or deposited money with others or others have lent or deposited money with him', but adds that the patient must explicitly be told that such instructions should not be construed as an indication that death is imminent. Similarly, a patient should be told to repent and to confess his sins, but must be counselled

[10] Schultz, R. and Alderman D. (1974). Clinical research and the stages of dying, *Omega*, V, 137–43; and Branson, R. (1975). Is acceptance a denial of death? Another look at Kübler-Ross, *Christian Century*, (7 May 1975), pp. 464–8. See also *Time*, 12 Nov. 1979, p. 81.

[11] See Hinton, J. M. (1963). The physical and mental distress of dying, *Quarterly Journal of Medicine*, XXXII, 1-21; and Achte, K. A. and Vaukkonen M. L. (1971). Cancer and the psyche, *Omega*, II 46–56.

[12] *Yoreh De'ah* 335:7.

that 'many have confessed and have not died, while many who have not confessed have died'.[13]

The way in which information is imparted, the language, tone of voice, and facial expression, are as significant as the message itself. The physician must never convey the feeling that there is no hope. Indeed, such a message constitutes an untruth, for remission and even recovery have occurred even in the face of the gravest prognosis. There is no need to convey a precise diagnosis to the patient, when such information can reasonably be withheld, if the patient will identify the diagnosed condition with a terminal malady. When the patient is aware of the gravity of his condition, the physician should always be encouraging and positive in his approach.

[13] *Ibid.*, 338:1.

22

Authority, social policy, and the doctor–patient relationship

PETER BYRNE

The declared aim of this collection of essays according to the editorial opening chapter is to enable doctors themselves to expound the ethics of their practice. In that chapter claims are made on behalf of the doctor as the true locus of moral responsibility and authority in the practice of medicine. The author of that chapter recognizes that these claims cannot be made good unless a number of other propositions are accepted, propositions which run counter to accepted fashions in what has come to be called 'medical ethics'. For example, the authority of the doctor cannot be affirmed unless experience (here the experience of those who actually make medical decisions) is given some primacy over theory (particularly ethical theory as articulated by philosophers). This authority cannot be maintained unless we are also prepared to go at least part way in recognizing some relationship of dependence or subordination between patient and doctor, and this goes against much recent thought about the role of informed consent in medicine.

The philosopher may be said to occupy the role of villain in G. R. Dunstan's argument, for it is from the ranks of philosophers that the professional 'ethicists' are drawn who are responsible for questioning and diminishing the proper role of doctors as authoritative moral agents in medical decision. Despite this opprobrium, I, as professional philosopher, can see much to welcome in Dunstan's argument and to bemoan in my colleagues' intervention into medical ethics. The attempt to make ethical dilemmas into an occasion for the construction and application of moral theory is a noted feature of the modern moralist's intervention in this area. If taken to extremes, and it often is, it has the effect of subordinating the experience of moral agents to the over-simplified demands of consistency and abstraction. It makes us suspicious of our experience of the reality of moral choices, whereas in fact it is this experience which we must rely on if we are to adjudicate between competing theoretical concepts in ethics. It attempts to reduce the terms of moral reflection to those expressible through some favoured, selected concepts (current theory tends to offer an unattractive choice between rights and utility) and thereby makes us jettison aspects of ethical experience. All in all it will not do to pretend that it takes a philosopher to recognize a moral distinction (cf. Williams 1985). If we give primacy to moral experience, then in medical ethics we must attach some importance to the moral experience of doctors.

Fondness for ethical theory promises, if taken to extremes, to eliminate altogether the need for ethical judgement on the part of physicians, for if the job of theory construction were completed we would have a decision procedure for ethics which would need only to be fed with factual data to produce conclusions. A similar result would be reached if we followed another philosophical obsession to its limits and so stressed the autonomy of patients that we eliminated the need for clinical decision at all. This has been done, with the consequence that the doctor's role in relation to his patient is portrayed as one of supplying information. The patient is to be informed as to diagnosis, prognosis, and the merits and demerits, including risks, of possible treatments, and it is for the patient then to decide what treatment is to be undertaken and to invite the doctor to use his professional expertise to carry it out. It is not for doctors to make medical decisions (cf. Culver and Geert 1982). Such a conclusion is the logical extreme to which some talk of the evils of medical paternalism might take us. It is contrary to the experience of doctors (and patients) as the chapters of E. J. Dunstan and S. Spiro make clear. It ignores the facts of weakness and dependence which frequently accompany being ill and it sets at nought the expertise of doctors which ought to come from their training and experience. If they are not better qualified to make medical decisions than patients, they are unfit to practise. Their experience and training is, or ought to be, not such as to leave them simply as *technicians*, suppliers of information and skilful executors of others' instructions.

Granted, then, that much can be said for stressing the authority and experience of doctors in medical ethics, how far are we to take this authority and how normative must their experience be reckoned? These questions relate to others that are important in considering the contributions to this book. How do we structure the doctor–patient relationship? What role do we give to the experience of others (non-doctors) in the formation of an ethics for medical practice? Where do we bring in the reflections of moralists and the contributions of law and social policy? Professor G. R. Dunstan recognizes the importance of these questions, for the authority of the doctor is for him a conditioned and relative one. It is dependent on a larger moral community whose values inform it and it is exercised in the service of that community. These questions are all the more important because, as the essays in this volume abundantly testify, medical decisions are never simply that. They involve or shade into other sorts of decisions—about how to use society's resources or about how to manage people's lives or about what kind of lives are worth living.

Taken to one extreme 'authority' implies 'empire': free and unfettered control over others. An extreme reading of clinical authority along these lines puts us in mind of the famous tag about the professions: that they are organized conspiracies against the public interest. G. R. Dunstan is not for a moment supporting a clinical empire, in which the public is wholly subject to the medical profession. One of the thoughts that prevent us from supposing that clinical authority can properly take this form is articulated by R. Gillon in Chapter 10 and rests upon the idea that the doctor–patient relationship is a moral one. Dr Gillon draws from this the conclusion that decision-making in the relationship can only proceed via a respect for the values, interests, wishes, etc. of each party to it. Out of this demand comes one of Gillon's four principles defining the ethical practice of medicine (respect for autonomy). More formal characterization of a moral relationship can be given by suggesting that it is one made possible (that is, is partly constituted by) a whole-hearted trust between those party to it. A moral relationship is one governed by certain conventions, constraining the actions of the parties involved, and in which there is a shared acceptance that these conventions are to be followed, regardless of the separate interests or changing projects of the different parties (Harrison 1984). Friendship is an obvious example of a moral relationship which exhibits this whole-hearted trust and readiness to abide by the demands of conventions which govern and inform the relationship. One fact which the moral relationship of friendship does display applies to other forms of moral relationship. Moral relationships are non-manipulative and shaped by a certain reciprocity, facts which flow from their being structured by trust and the acceptance of the restraints of conventions. They have in consequence what has been described as an 'aimless' or 'purposeless' character (Scruton 1980). Friends might, for example, unite in the pursuit of a common purpose, but the way any one of them acts as an individual in pursuit of that purpose will be limited by the wishes of the others. The desire to achieve the purpose will be limited in its authority by the demands that grow out of the conventions of mutual respect that inform the relationship itself: 'A certain reciprocity arises, and the absolute authority of my aim—as the sole determining principle of what it is reasonable for me to do—must be abandoned' (Scruton 1980). If the doctor–patient relationship is one of this sort then the authority of the doctor within it has to be qualified by the patient's own understanding of the terms and limits of the relationship. The relationship would appear to be one that paradigmatically has an end in view: restoring the patient's health. But if it is a moral one, then what is done to bring about that end will not necessarily be what is most efficient in securing it.

The last point brings us on to the troubling issue of informed consent. A number of the medical essays in this book show a concern with the amount of information patients should be given about their condition and its treatment. Contributors recognize that consent to treatment is a requirement of sound medical practice and that consent is made real only if patients know to some real degree what they are consenting to. However there is also a recognition that informed consent is a barrier in the efficient pursuit of medical goals. The most sensible means of tackling the dilemmas surrounding the requirements of informed consent to emerge from these essays is to move away from trumpeting and the abstract demands of either clinical authority or patient autonomy. If we consider the doctor–patient relationship as a moral one, then each instance of it must be seen as important in itself and as the unique source of convention-backed claims that define trust within it. It would be a violation of any particular instance of the relationship if the patient concerned were either forced to be an active participant in treatment decisions against his evident wishes and in violation of his anxiety *not* to be informed of the details of his condition, or forced to be a passive, ignorant subject in the face of the doctor's designs. There are two evident evils to be avoided: on the one hand, forcing all patients to be the kind of autonomous moral hero who stalks the pages of works in moral philosophy, and subjecting all patients to the professional's perception of what is in their best interests, on the other.

The remedy for avoiding the two evils described above is clearly presented by E. J. Dunstan in Chapter 18. It is that of tailoring the amount of information to be given about condition and forms of treatment to the expectations of the particular patient concerned. The wisest course on informed consent is that which corresponds to the general verdict on good doctoring confirmed by the experience of the clinicians contributing to this volume, namely that good practice should respond to the unique needs and demands of individual patients. If we relate this position to the description of informed consent in the medical ethics literature we see that it corresponds to a 'subjective' or patient-orientated standard of proper disclosure, but not a standard which reflects some a priori determination of what a patient ought to want to know. In this respect it is significant to note that the judicial committee of the House of Lords has made some strides in its consideration of the recent *Sidaway* case toward the acknowledgement of this standard as normative in English medical law (see Scarman 1987 and Lee 1988 and cf. comments in Chapter 1 of this volume).

How does allowing a patient-orientated standard of right information in informed consent conform with the idea of the doctor's authority? Let it be noted first that it does suggest possible limits to the doctor's pursuit of the overriding goal of health where an individual patient is one who wishes to be informed of his condition and possible treatments in some detail. However, such a limitation is part of what we have seen to be the essence of acknowledging the doctor–patient relationship to be a moral one and can hardly be objected to in itself. In an instance of the relationship in which there is a strong desire to be informed on the part of the patient, clinical authority is still present in the fact that the doctor will still be the 'senior partner' (see Kennedy 1986). The relationship will not function properly unless the doctor's expertise and judgement are acknowledged within it. The seniority of the doctor is present in his claim, implicit in the practice of his profession, that he has a trained judgement to offer his patient. Seniority need not entail manipulation or coercion, any more than leadership in a friendship or the necessary exercise of parental authority entails that these relationships are manipulative.

Problems mentioned in the earlier parts of this book may now be commented upon. In the chapters by Dr Spiro and Professor Baum attention is drawn to the limitations in a surgeon's knowledge of the effectiveness of forms of therapy for various cancers. This fact of ignorance is an obvious threat to the perception of clinical authority. It is thus understandable that both authors hint at a reluctance fully to inform patients before entering them into randomized trials of new forms of therapy. But this hardly measures up to the thought that surgeon and patient are partners in a moral relationship. The public may need to be more fully educated into a perception of the limits and fallibility of medical knowledge, but prior to that educative process the consequence may have to be accepted that certain improvements cannot be pursued as quickly as desired while the demands of a proper doctor–patient relationship are respected. It can hardly be a proper reason for not disclosing the random basis of treatments that, if it were done, patients would not consent to receive them, for that implies that compliance can only be gained by deceit. Compliance is then condemned.

The sketch of a doctor–patient relationship offered here allows an obvious place for the notion that patients' confidences are to be respected. This notion reflects an intrinsic, defining convention of the relationship, one that makes possible the patient's disclosure of his medical and personal history to the doctor. This disclosure in turn makes the doctor's offer of his judgement and skills in the restoration of health a useful one. If I were prepared to tell my doctor only what I would be happy to let anyone else hear, the peculiar relationship of doctor to patient would be impossible and the doctor's prospective services nullified. But we must distinguish between saying that confidentiality is an intrinsic good within sound medical practice and saying that it is an absolute good. The latter implies more than that there is always some intrinsic reason from within the doctor–patient relationship to acknowledge an obligation to respect confidences; it implies that where this obligation conflicts with other compelling ones it is always to win out. In the preceding essays we see a clear case (I do not say it is overwhelming) for allowing the obligation of confidentiality to give way in the circumstances of the disclosure of possible HIV infection to third parties and the protection of others from the mentally deranged. There are no easy solutions to dilemmas of this sort, but it should be noted that it is hard to endorse the conclusion that confidences should in no circumstances be communicated to others (contrast Dr Mindel's chapter above), simply because it is easy at least to imagine cases where one patient was a mortal threat to others and from whom others could rightly expect protection.

The weight to be given to the obligation to respect the demands of the doctor–patient relationship as against the weight to be given to other obligations in which the doctor is enmeshed is something we might expect to be illuminated by the general moral context in which the doctor operates. Social morality and policy may have a role to play in informing a conscientious decision to betray confidences, because they have something to say on the mutual importance of obligations owed to particular patients and obligations owed to society at large. (In the case of conditions covered by the infectious diseases legislation the law certainly has something to say). In regard to the role played by confidentiality we might with good reason expect to see the authority of the doctor limited by a larger moral context. So too might we expect to see it limited over the crucial matter of which individuals in society are to be afforded the opportunity to enter into the doctor–patient relationship and thus be offered the protection of the peculiar obligations it lays down. This I perceive to be the import of the Department of Health and Social Security (DHSS) and General Medical Council (GMC) guidance on a doctor's treatment of children without parental consent. I take it that, since this is a matter of important social policy (in part adjudicating the dispute or overlap between the parent–child and doctor–patient relationships), the doctor cannot be allowed to be the sole judge of who is fit to be a patient in his own right (cf. John Hare's chapter; similar issues are raised in Maurice Lipsedge's discussion in Chapter 14 of when to accord the mentally deranged the privileges of the whole range of conventions of the doctor–patient relationship). Social regulation of physician autonomy and limitation of clinical authority is surely in order in this case, otherwise authority *will* tend toward empire.

The relationship between clinician and the moral values and norms of society at large is particularly important in those areas of medical practice described in this book where decisions are taken about the termination of life. A high proportion of the chapters by clinicians mention or describe such decisions, including the chapters by Campbell, Wilkes, Hare (in the matter of abortion) E. J. Dunstan, Branthwaite, Spiro, and Shinebourne. Two things in the treatment of such decisions are initially worthy of comment. First we must note the unanimity of the doctors in rejecting implicitly the type of ethics of life-saving and homicide outlined in Rabbi Bleich's chapter. They do not endorse a practice based on the premise that each and every moment of a life is of infinite value and that life is accordingly to be extended whenever medically possible and at all costs. The clinicians are implicitly using the principle of non-maleficence mentioned in Gillon's chapter and reasoning that in many cases it would do positive harm to the patient to fight for an extension of life. The second point to note is the manner in which the doctors testify to the belief that it is properly within the sphere of clinical judgement (and thus beyond the need, for example, for detailed regulation by the criminal law) to determine when it is no longer worthwhile fighting to extend the life of a patient.

The use of clinical autonomy in making these decisions about the termination of life is worthy of further exploration. In the varied cases assembled in these chapters, relating to treatment of children at the margin of life, adults suffering from fatal disease, and the aged, no absolute clinical autonomy is claimed. The decision to refrain from extending life or to terminate life is conscientiously reached in the light of the wishes of relatives and/or the known or presumed wishes of the patient himself. Yet the essays collectively leave the responsible doctor with a large power of decision. This measure of autonomy and authority might seem natural and at the same time decidedly odd. It appears natural if we consider that a clinician's training and experience necessarily accustom him to making decisions about the balance of benefit and harm accruing to human beings from proposed courses of action. This fact reflects one of the obvious reasons why ethical decisions are inherent in medical practice. If this training and experience did not bring with it a certain wisdom in the making of decisions about the balance of medical benefit and harm, then something would be seriously amiss. Yet, on the other hand, it might appear strange to suppose that the practice of medicine gives any authority at all in the particular decisions we are now concerned with. They relate to how far the harm of not prolonging life, or the harm of shortening life, is outweighed by the harm of whatever suffering or disability is a consequence of continued life. To make such a decision would appear to involve placing a certain value on life itself and finding a means of measuring that value against distress, discomfort, handicap, etc. Here we seem to have something which is primarily a matter for social morality, perhaps as expressed through law, to pronounce upon. How can the question of the value of life itself in relation to the quality of life be left to the authority of doctors to determine?

There is a certain artificiality in the presentation of the above dilemma. For in some measure clinical judgement in the matter of life-saving and life-terminating decisions can be seen to be the application of a pre-existing social morality. Clinical authority in that case can be seen to be a proper autonomy in the detailed working out of values already implicit in the ethical life of society, a task for which clinical training and experience *do* fit the doctor. However, while this reply may eliminate part of the dilemma, it is not wholly satisfactory. In part it is also possible to see clinicians in this book as extending, or forging new elements in, social morality. We shall not necessarily condemn this aspect of clinical decision. Ethics is properly extended or reshaped by the experience of responsible moral agents, and in this context (of questions about the worth of human life) the experience of doctors may be vital testimony. But I shall argue that where the extension of social morality is in question, clinical practice cries out for social endorsement at least *ex post facto*. This in turn calls for the need for greater involvement from law, philosophy, and the like.

Further exploration of these matters can proceed by focusing on Professor Campbell's chapter on the treatment of premature neonates, because of the clarity and thoroughness with which he raises questions about life-saving and life-terminating. Reference to these themes in other chapters will be made as necessary.

The area where decisions not to strive any further to extend life seem least problematic is illustrated in Campbell's discussion of those infants whose death is imminent, or at least expected shortly. Professor Campbell describes a range of cases where acts of commission or omission may be undertaken whose anticipated result is that the sick infant will die sooner than if the commission or omission had not been undertaken. Rabbi Bleich's principles would appear on the surface to forbid any decisions of this sort, but we do acknowledge in ethics outside medicine that sometimes our normally stringent obligation to preserve human life must give way to our obligation not to inflict otherwise needless suffering. A classic case would be on the battlefield where it would be a licit act of mercy to shorten the dying agonies of a soldier for whom absolutely nothing else can be done in the circumstances. If we accept that our obligation to protect and preserve human life can be limited in this way, it might appear that we are endorsing an ethics which says that human life is not intrinsically valuable in itself. It is only a certain quality of life that is valuable and we have no obligation to preserve and protect life unless it manifests this quality (however defined). But we need not give up our belief in the intrinsic worth of human life, or in the intrinsic evil of homicidal acts, to make this kind of judgement. We can conclude merely that necessity in some cases permits us to set aside the good of life and the evil of taking it. We have a clash of intrinsic evils: taking life (or not preserving and prolonging it), versus permitting very great suffering or pain or distress. Where death is near anyway, the one evil can be permitted to outweigh the other. We can have an ethics (and I think as a society we have this ethics) which makes all homicidal acts wrong until justified or mitigated, but which allows ending pain and distress in some circumstances to be a sufficient plea of necessity properly to justify or mitigate (cf. Devine 1978).

It is in these terms that we might see the doctor's decision to give therapy or withhold it where such giving or withholding is expected to hasten death. Note that I do not place any great stress in this account on the mitigation or justification which might come with saying that the expected outcome of clinical decision (hastened death) was the result merely of an omission or was only the indirectly intended consequence of the doctor's act. (These pleas can be found in a number of the clinical papers in this book. But it is noticeable that the clinicians disagree themselves over their force: Campbell and E. J. Dunstan defend the importance of the difference between hastened death through commission and hastened death through omission; Branthwaite doubts this distinction). It is a matter for great philosophical scepticism whether the elements of omission or indirect intention in action can serve to justify or mitigate foreseen consequences of acts, where those consequences are otherwise impermissible (see Kuhse 1987 for a detailed critique of omission and indirect intention as pleas to mitigate homicide). There is no need to rely on such doubtful pleas unless one accepts the kind of ethics of homicide which need to state that homicide, suitably qualifed, can *never* be performed. An ethics which allows necessity as I have described it to create at least some justified homicides requires no such absolutist principle. It is probably clearer all round to recognize that the kinds of commission and omission described by our clinicians share a vital common element with acts we would normally count as homicidal: they are undertaken with the clearly foreseen or expected consequence that the subject will die sooner than if they had not been undertaken and the bringing about of this consequence is freely and voluntarily accepted. It is this element which gives them a homicidal thrust and at least indirectly a homicidal intent. This common element is that which requires mitigation or justification, granted that we do recognize an inherent obligation to preserve and protect human life. The strength of the homicidal thrust (however precisely described) of at least some of these decisions is clear from the following statement in Campbell's paper: in some circumstances, he tells us, 'Once a decision is made that death is preferable to continued life of this kind [that is, 'vegitative' life] I believe that anything, including feeding, that prolongs this artificial existence is wrong for the infant, wrong for the family, and wrong for society'. Where a plea of either omission or indirect intention to cause death would substantially deflect the homicidal thrust of an act would be where the hastening of death were uncertain, though foreseeable to some extent. In that case it might be described as a 'mere side effect' of the act which does not at all tend to give it a homicidal thrust. In E. J. Dunstan's decription of the use of analgesics in the care of the elderly dying there are indications that it is on this ground that he thinks the licitness of doing something which may shorten life is grounded.

If we do not allow the element of omission or of indirect intention to cause hastened death to qualify our view of the nature of these acts, then we have indeed a problem in distinguishing the licitness of these acts from what might classically be termed 'mercy killing' in medicine. The experience of the clinicians recorded in this volume implicitly testifies to a sense of distinction between such things as no longer fighting a mortal infection, or refusing to treat a secondary infection that appears alongside some mortal or incurable condition, and the direct giving of, say, poisons to shorten life. This may be ground for examining the philosophical arguments against the importance of omission and indirect intention again, or for seeking some new, perhaps pragmatic, distinction between the licit area of clinical non-treatment and use of analgesics on the one hand, and the illicit area of 'mercy killing' with lethal agents on the other. Our readiness to allow some latitude to the hastening of death in the case of those whose life expectancy is very limited is witnessed by the great reluctance we feel to conclude that the doctor in these cases is the cause of the patient's eventual death. This, we commonly judge, is the underlying mortal condition. The doctor has merely chosen to manage this condition in a certain way, that is not to eke out the patient's last days with it.

So far we may see the clinician's decisions concerning life-prolonging and life-shortening to be the proper application of an accepted ethics of homicide. Yet there are decisions relating to both the treatment of the new-born and of the aged recorded in these papers which do not fit that ethics as described. These are cases where, if the patient has an otherwise mortal condition, its thrust can be deflected by available treatment. He can be given some reasonable life expectancy. After the contemplated treatment he would not be described as 'dying'. However, clinical autonomy and authority demands the liberty to judge that the degree of the patient's likely handicap, disability, or dementia is such that he is not to be offered the contemplated treatment. His death is the foreseen result of this refusal (and may even be hastened by other means, as indicated in Professor Campbell's description of withholding nutriment from an infant in this condition). The language of the clinical papers is not altogether clear on this point, but there are clear statements in Campbell's and Shinebourne's chapters of withholding life-saving measures from infants on the ground, not that their death is imminent whatever happens and so they should not have their distresses needlessly prolonged, but because the quality of continued life they would enjoy after life-saving treatment is so low that it is not worth having no matter how long it lasts. There are hints in E. J. Dunstan's description of some types of non-treatment of the aged sick which are justified by similar forms of reasoning (see p. 189).

There is no reason to suppose that the clinicians who describe such treatment decisions in this volume are in any sense out of line with accepted and usual medical practice in this country, but it is important to see that these decisions do not quite fit with the ethics of homicide constructed for the non-treatment of the dying and that no appeal to omissions or the indirectness of the intention to cause death will take away their homicidal thrust. The latter point is easily made good. If one's reason for withholding some treatment is to prevent a life continuing that is so low in quality that it is not worth living (because, say, it contains no real prospect of relationship with others), then the bringing about or hastening of death is an essential part of one's commissions or omissions. One is using the occasion of non-treatment of some underlying or secondary mortal condition as the means of preventing the spinning out of some mode of life which is considered worthless. Death has been judged preferable to continued life. That this is different from the defence of acts homicidal in thrust on the plea of necessity mentioned so far is seen when when we remind ourselves that that plea depends on two factors, neither of which need be present in the cases of non-treatment on account of expected handicap, disability, or dementia. These factors are, first, imminent death whatever is done and second, considerable distress, suffering, or discomfort, which may be relieved or shortened in duration by non-treatment or use of analgesics, etc. What principally appears to be involved in the cases now under consideration is the hastening of the death of those, infant or aged, who are not otherwise in imminent danger of death and whose future life is expected to be at such a low level of consciousness that they cannot be said to be likely to suffer unduly.

Medical judgement thus appears to be introducing a fresh dimension to the ethics of homicide. Consider, for example, what could honestly be entered on the death certificate of one of the infants who dies as a result of the regime described on p.59 of Professor Campbell's chapter. In general, necessity in justification of homicide is in place where self-defence, or an absolutely unavoidable choice between lives, is in question, and, I believe, where merciful relief of the suffering of those dying in any event is contemplated. There may be other categories not mentioned here, but it is hard to see how a plea of necessity is appropriate in the case of preventing worthless lives (because too severely handicapped or too low in consciousness) continuing. Judgements of this latter sort do look as if they fit in more easily with the type of philosophical view which holds that human life in not inherently worthy of preservation in itself, but that only worthwhile life is so worthy. 'Homicide', on this philosophical view, is not the label for an act which is forbidden unless otherwise justified. The obligation to preserve life arises only when life is the occasion for a certain quality of life. In fact it is possible to hear echoes of philosophical theories which produce such consequences in the language of some of the clinicians writing in this volume (a fact to be expected if they operate in a society currently debating within itself the ethics of homicide).

Some of the decisions relating to not prolonging or terminating life appear, then, to be no more than the tacit application of accepted notions about justified homicidal acts. The decisions taken on 'quality of life' considerations I have judged to be against 'traditional' social morality. It could be argued that they are not so new. Doctors, it might be said, have for years been making clinical decisions of this sort without hindrance or social condemnation. Any novelty lies only in the public attention and discussion this category of life/death decision has received. But it must be pointed out that medical ethics as written up by moralists has tended to favour governing homicidal acts within clinical practice by some version of a sanctity of life principle, and in this it may be judged to reflect more closely established legal principles on homicide. The radical nature of the new ethics of homicide suggested by these clinical decisions, backed by some philosophical ethics, is clear when we reflect that the ethics and the decisions appear to make a nonsense of the laws governing homicide in this and similar jurisdictions. Murder is not a crime defined relative to the actual and expected quality of life of the victim nor upon his age. This is perhaps why something like the case of Dr Leonard Arthur in 1981 appears inevitable in retrospect and why, as a matter of law, his aquittal on a charge of attempted murder still seems odd (Linacre Centre 1982). As noted above, the radical character of clinical judgements about the ethics of homicide does not condemn those judgements. We may feel in the light of the facts that the experience of doctors is rightly leading them in the direction of extending or modifying traditional social morality on these issues. What is clear is that clinical decision cannot operate in a vacuum. That is to say, clinical judgement cries out for confirmation by social morality, even if this confirmation comes about through clinical experience modifying existing social morality and policy. It will not do simply to plead that medical training gives doctors no expertise or authority in deciding who should live and who should die. This is naïve. As reflective moral agents with unique experience of the making of decisions concerning life and death doctors are at liberty to reconsider the ethics of such decisions. It may well be that the greatly enhanced power of medicine to interfere with life is the very thing which calls for society to rethink homicide and related matters, and it may be that clinical experience will be a force in shaping this rethinking. (This is in part the argument of Kuhse 1987). But we cannot have decisions relating to life and death being governed by one set of values in one area of social life and a conflicting set of values in another. This is why the ethics of current medical practice need wider endorsement. The experience of society as a whole (for example of parents if we consider the ethics of the termination of infant life) is relevant to the ethics of life-saving and preserving. This is why I cannot condemn in all respects the 'Baby Doe' rules in the USA or the recourse in that country to committees to consider life and death decisions in paediatric care. Professor Campbell's cautionary comments on these developments are no doubt justified by the matters of detail concerning the rules and the paediatric committees. But the general notion of bringing social policy to bear on medical practice and of surrounding clinical authority and autonomy with well-developed social policy is right. This point is surely in accord with Dunstan's opening remarks. Clinical authority and autonomy is in place in the reflective application of social policy and, equally importantly, in the deposit of unique and thoughtful experience it offers for the formulation of social policy, but it cannot operate independently of such policy.

I have tried to describe the apparent conflict between traditional ethics, and social policy, and some of the clinical decisions described in this book, in as neutral a fashion as possible. I leave open the question of what should give most ground: whether the ethics of homicide as previously cast or what I have suggested is the new, or at least newly publicized, clinical policy of not preserving the existence of those with too low a quality of life. The main points I have wanted to make concern the need to bring general and clinical ethics into harmony and the necessity of avoiding a false over-simplification of the doctor's relationship to general ethics and social policy. He is neither to be seen merely as one who applies an ethics worked out independently of his own practice (no clinical autonomy and authority), nor as one who dictates to society what is licit and illicit in his practice (complete authority and autonomy). There must be instead a mutual informing between general ethics and clinical ethics, between social policy and clinical practice. What should concern us is the manner in which medical ethics (something that grows out of this mutual informing) is made. Because of the fact of the connection and interpenetration between clinical practice and wider social policy and values we cannot leave these medical ethics to be made entirely by the profession, vital though its contribution to them are. Yet the means we have of bringing wider values to bear are manifestly imperfect. Parliament's interest is spasmodic. Governments introduce legislation only when need absolutely forces them. Private members take up some matters but again spasmodically and often in response to public pressure rather than to the areas of greatest need. Judges, as in the instance of the House of Lords' decision in *Sidaway*, may give medical ethics a push in one direction or another, but that will be in response to the haphazard matter of who chooses to litigate about what and when. Some better means is required to ensure a continued, intelligent, and reflective engagement between medical practice, and the values it prompts, and the wider values of society.

How can the medical and non-medical experience of moral realities be brought into more sustained, systematic, and reflective engagement with one another? It is at this point that the suggestion is offered of a standing national commission on medical ethics, analogous to the various Congressional and Presidential commissions that have served to shape medical ethics in the USA. The merest suggestion of such a body raises medical hackles in this country, largely because it appears to match perfectly the vision of the replacement of informed medical experience by the theories and slogans of professional 'ethicists' that Professor Dunstan castigates in the opening chapter of this book. Whether such a commission need fulfil these nightmare visions is another matter. This might appear to depend on how it was staffed and how it operated, especially how it made use of the experience of the medical profession itself (see Capron 1988).

In relation to the obligations owed to embryonic life we have had, of course, an *ad hoc* body (the 'Warnock' committee) to produce a reflective determination of the future shape of medical ethics. But, as Dr Braude notes in his chapter, the manner in which this task was tackled reveals again the limited nature of our attempts to reflect on clinical and general ethical experience. He points to the prima facie oddity of seeking complicated legal and quasi-legal means to protect the embryo *in vitro* while the embryo *in vivo* is deemed by social policy to be capable of sacrifice in large numbers and on no very stringent grounds. The oddity is strengthened when we consider the practice of abortion at later stages of the conceptus as revealed in Mr Hare's chapter. Medical practice, as there described, may offer terminations to adolescent mothers on social rather than medical grounds: (recall that Hare makes a point of playing down the medical risks of coitus and pregnancy for adolescents). In this it is endorsed by social policy and the very liberal interpretation of a loosely worded Abortion Act. Even current attempts to lower the time limit for legal terminations will presumably not affect these facts very greatly. In this context it appears even more odd to agonize over the possibility of pre-embryos being manipulated in laboratories to the point were they can no longer be re-implanted into a woman.

This kind of hiatus in the way profession and public forge medical ethics could be the result of some deep insight, if, for example, it reflects the practical, legal difficulties in offering protection to *in vivo* pre-natal life, as opposed to the ease of controlling what laboratory scientists do with *in vitro* embryos (for this argument see Eekelaar 1988). However, it would be naïve to suppose so. It looks more like muddle: the result of failure to take what clinical experience of ethical decision in medicine offers and relate it in a vital way to the larger social morality which must in the end cohere with it and support it. We need a mutual support and enrichment from these two sources for a complete system of medical ethics. Only then can we have an autonomy and authority invested in the doctor which is not an empire over society at large, not a declaration of independence from social morality or the larger experience of mankind, and not a lonely moral gesture without anchor or grounding.

REFERENCES

Capron, A. (1988). A national commission on medical ethics? *Health, rights and resources* (ed. P. A. Byrne), pp. 177–94. King's Fund Press, London.

Culver, C. M. and Geert, B. (1982). *Philosophy in medicine*. Oxford University Press, New York.

Devine, P. E. (1978). *The ethics of homicide*, Cornell University Press, Ithaca.

Eekelaar, J. (1988). What legal duties does a mother owe to her unborn child? *Health, rights and resources*, (ed. P. A. Byrne), King's Fund Press, London, 55–75.

Harrison, B. (1984). Moral judgement, action and emotion, *Philosophy*, 59, 229, pp. 295–321.

Kennedy, I. M. (1986). The doctor-patient relationship, *rights and wrongs in medicine*, (ed. P. A. Byrne), pp7–21, King's Fund Press, London.

Kuhse, H. (1987). *The sanctity of life doctrine in medical ethics*, Clarendon Press, Oxford.

Lee, S. (1988). Medical Law 1987, *Health, Rights and Resources*, (ed. P. A. Byrne), pp. 35–54, King's Fund Press, London.

Linacre Centre (1982). *Euthanasia and Clinical Practice*, London.

Lord Scarman (1987). Law and medical practice, *Medicine in contemporary society*, (ed. P. A. Byrne), pp. 131–9, King's Fund Press, London.

Scruton, R. (1980). *The meaning of conservatism*, Penguin, Harmondsworth.

William, B. (1985). *Ethics and the limits of moral theory*, Fontana, London.

Index

THE URBAN ENVIRONMENTAL SYSTEM

THE URBAN ENVIRONMENTAL SYSTEM

Modeling for Research Policy-Making and Education

PETER HOUSE

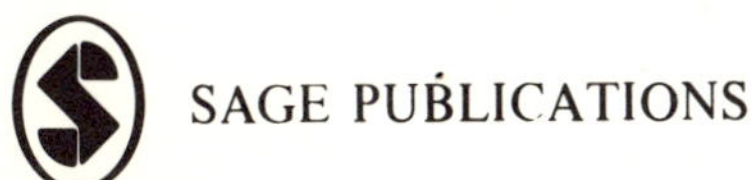
SAGE PUBLICATIONS Beverly Hills / London

For information address:

SAGE PUBLICATIONS, INC.
275 South Beverly Drive
Beverly Hills, California 90212

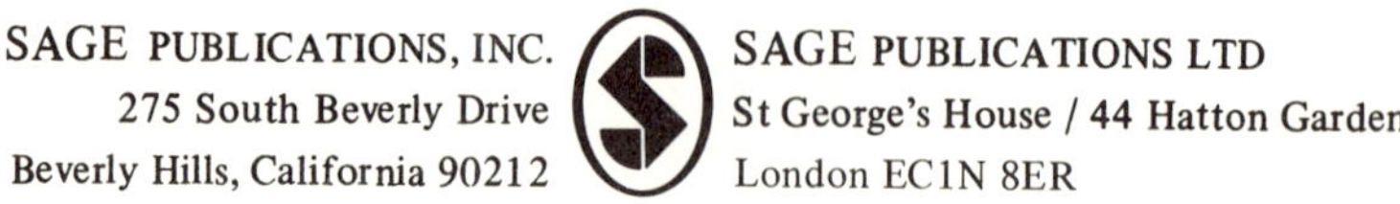

SAGE PUBLICATIONS LTD
St George's House / 44 Hatton Garden
London EC1N 8ER

Printed in the United States of America

International Standard Book Number 0-8039-0182-8

Library of Congress Catalog Card No. 72-98034

FIRST PRINTING

Dedicated to
the girls

ACKNOWLEDGMENTS

The day of single authorship for complex models is at an end. With the advent of the computer, the advances in the complexities and sophistication of models has become so great and the number of disciplines represented in a single model so numerous that it is beyond present training capabilities for any individual. All of this is a roundabout way of stating that the model described in this book belongs to a large number of people; however, space will only allow me to list a few.

Regardless of how long one has been publishing and giving papers, the moment of his first book is almost religious. As he comes to write a section such as this which will make it clear to the reader that he is merely a conduit through which his ideas and those of many others have been filtered, he finds that his debt to others is so great that a recitation of the total ledger would be embarrassingly long.

The only solution I found to this dilemma is to acknowledge the debts which are directly tied to this work and particularly to the time of Envirometrics. My professional debts to the past must at least include three men: Don Fixler, who oriented my ego toward an intellectual payoff matrix; Fritz Stocker, who introduced me to the realities of the research world and steered me back to the womb of the academic community for further seasoning; and Allen Feldt, whose love for people coupled with an astonishing ability to teach, introduced me to a most interesting field, human ecology. The fires ignited by these men are in no small way responsible for the model ideas in this book.

Envirometrics was a fun place in which to create. Throughout its lifetime, it had a reasonably large number of members, all of whom have been different but have had one ideal in common—freedom. The group was oriented around the hope of talented adults being able to produce high quality research because they liked their milieu. Except for the output expected from each person, there were few explicit rules. I liked the place, and it was certainly the only atmosphere in which I could have evolved the enclosed theory.

Before enumerating some of the more influential model designers who have worked on the CITY model series, I must acknowledge a couple of particular actors in the drama. Phil Patterson and Janice Cooper are the only two professionals who were with me from the very beginning. I have no idea how the group could have functioned without them.

Phil, besides being a good friend and invaluable colleague, provided a perfect balance for the group with his unbelievable patience, willingness to listen, and intuitive grasp of details and empirical reliance. It would be difficult to find a portion of this book that did not bear his stamp or guidance.

Jan grew to be the "keeper of the keys," the main contact between the designers and the programmers. She was the harbinger of delays and difficulties and usually made up for these with personal sacrifice. Although not often part of the public side of Envirometrics, these people are the ones who led the continuing day-to-day evolution of the model.

On the programming side, the debts are many but not as easily noted. A young man, Paul Schauble, was the backbone behind CITY I and taught us a great deal about the operation of a computer. A small company, Language and Systems Development (LSD), worked like animals to help us meet impossible deadlines or accomplish equally impossible design demands. Finally, Greg O'Connel, a philosopher in the true sense, took to the computer and to our type of problems with unusual zest and today is responsible for the smooth operation of the model and many of its more sophisticated computer systems.

Ed Northwood and Tom Mierzwa aided in the design and carrying out of the Wisconsin experiment, and Bob Pickett, Jerre Manarolla, and Nancy Adler are among those who helped mount the operational phase of the model. Bill Furr did a great deal of work with the model test for this book, and he and Sam Ratick assisted with the macro equations in the Appendix.

Not to be forgotten are the support staff, including Bill Arnold, Joy Gail Raywid, Marilyn Shockey, Sharon Fitz-William, Patricia Minson and Lynne Atherton (who edited this book), all of whom gave up the idea of "business" and joined our crusade to effect social change through education.

To cut this short, let me add the expected comment, that all of these people helped considerably in one way or another with this manuscript. Some portions or ideas were fleshed out by several of them. However, I have gone back and imposed my stamp on those parts throughout.

Many times in life a person stands alone; birth and death are the most touted–but publication must also be included. Therefore, all of the above must take credit for the ideas in this book. Only I will answer, however, for the presentation and form they now take.

CONTENTS

LIST OF FIGURES AND TABLES

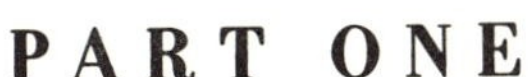

PART ONE

Chapter 1

INTRODUCTION

This book is about a model; more specifically, about a modeling process, its results and its uses. The uniqueness of this model lies in many areas but starts with the purpose for which it was built.

Most models are built to satisfy a specific need. Often they are built as an analytical device for management and planning studies. Others are constructed by educators as teaching aids. Still others are developed out of intellectual curiosity and then built to demonstrate a theoretical construct. The General Environmental Model (GEM) and its present derivative, Envirometrics' CITY, are unique in this realm in that they were not restricted to satisfying any one use, but were built to serve four general purposes: education, training, research and policy-making.

The model went through various stages, and in a sense can be conceptualized as having progressed or evolved from simpler end goals to ones which were more complex. In the early phases, the CITY models were only meant to be used in the classroom or for pedagogical purposes, and consequently, many of their functions were discussed mainly in terms of general direction of decision inputs and probabilities. As the use of these models spread and as the audiences became more involved with individual aspects of the social, economic, or governmental systems, the model[1] was expanded to include those areas, making it more realistic.

A research model required even more sophistication and more attention to summary statistics. This richness and complexity increased to the point where the model appears to be useful to researchers for answering general questions about the effects of alternative theoretical structures on the various aspects of the social system. (The last chapter of this book notes the use of the CITY model in this mode.)

Finally, it was suggested by numerous users that GEM might be useful for policy makers, a step which took it in the direction of becoming an ever more realistic and sophisticated model. (Research in this area has begun and is reported in the next chapter.) In essence, therefore, we can say that the GEM model has evolved from a model for education to one which stands on the threshold of research/policy-making applications. This track from simplistic to complex did not, however, result in the specialization of the models. In fact, the latest CITY model is in some ways even more useful for educational purposes than its predecessors.

The research technique used to build GEM leads to some interesting conclusions from the point of view of model building today. Both those who are attempting to construct models for policy makers and those who are evolving models toward this goal are, in effect, attempting to build the same model. The difference is that policy model builders do not usually proceed through the path of theoretical structure but by collecting data and building data banks. These models, when finally constructed, are often an attempt to relate numbers to each other in some systematic fashion. The models, then, are usually forced to be unnecessarily restrictive for the sake of "realistic" and available parameters.

On the other hand, the method of evolving a model turns the above process upside down. The principal research used for GEM is based on the structure of the social system. Little work is done with data bases. This feature, combined with the fact that, in our case,[2] the model is built independently of any specific project and not for a certain city or state, has made the GEM concept a most general model for education and policy decisions.[3]

GENERAL FORMAT

The book is divided into two major parts. The first is a discussion of the concept of a model in general form. The framework of a model is delineated into five categories: data base, executive routine, input, operating programs, and output. Examples of the use of this structure from the CITY model are cited.

This section also focuses on the problem of structuring social science theory for computer modeling. Our typology, system sectors, evolved after the design of the CITY model and solved the problem of making social science theory adaptable for computer applications.

The system sectors are a decision-making way of looking at an environmental system. The three sectors are divided into economic, social and government. The system framework is the most convenient for the user of the model since it clearly delineates the resources of the local system and indicates their sector control over the evaluation and use of these resources.

With the first half of the book providing a modeling framework along with the structural basis for collecting the social science theory and data, as well as some information on the usefulness (validity and predictability) of GEM/CITY, it remains for the second part to present the more technical aspects of the model most recently evolved—the River Basin Model (CITY IV). This part includes a more precise description of the specific model seen from the Sector theory framework.

The resultant format, just described, is such that it will often be particularly irksome to some who are specializing in modeling or urban theory as they would like more detail in their specialty. Since this book has a very global viewpoint, the attempt to satisfy all of these very understandable desires would have led to the production of a tome. This result is not in itself to be considered undesirable. However, the strategy would have frustrated the purpose of this book. The purpose of this treatise is to demonstrate how a complex and holistic environmental-urban theory can be developed which is useful for quantification and of a form for computer programming.

Further, the reader is presented with a stylized description of a structure for describing any model which is designed for computerization. This paradigm was of enormous use to the evolved design of the GEM model and has been used many times by various federal agencies to reduce complex models to subsets which are clearly understandable both to the disparate hard and soft scientists, and

FIGURE 1.1
EXPANDABILITY AND FLEXIBILITY OF A GENERAL MODEL APPROACH

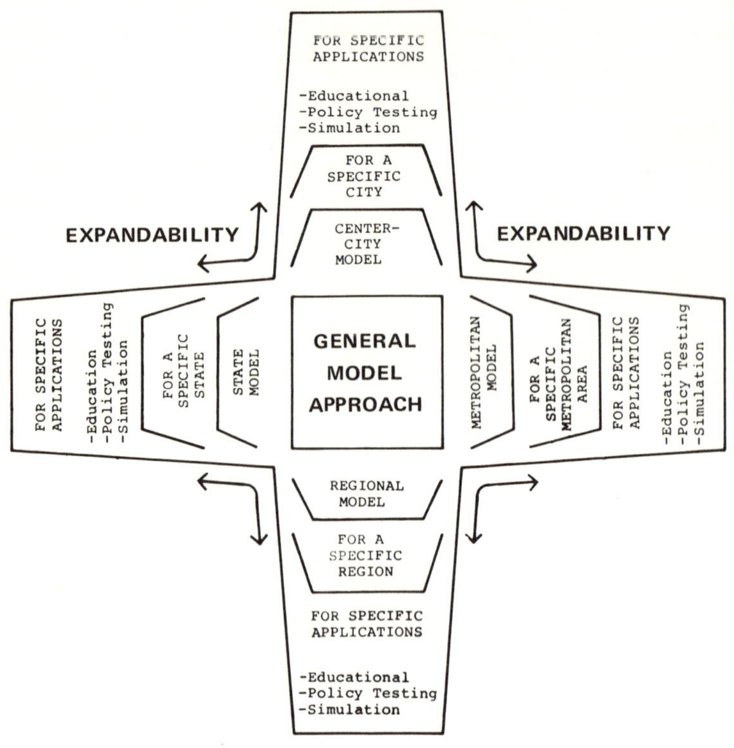

politicians preferring the data and models, and the system analysts and programmers who must put it on the machine.

Then, theoretical structures are used to describe the CITY model, which has been used for a large variety of purposes in an even wider variety of institutions. This section is meant to take the highly esoteric nature of a general theoretical structure and subject it to the rigor of a working model. Finally, this model is presented in operational form to give the reader some idea of how these theories, in the form of an operating model, can be used to handle day-to-day problems of the nature normally assigned to computer modeling.

The General Environmental Model (GEM) developed at Envirometrics was designed to allow as many theory inputs on the part of the user of the model as possible. GEM is therefore, a versatile computer-assisted decision-making model. It is environmental in that it can be used to represent economic, social and governmental decision-making entities within the regional, metropolitan, city, or subcity geographical areas. The model is general in that it can be used to represent any such environmental system and can be used with a wide variety of purposes: education, training, research, policy formation, and policy testing (Figure 1.1).

GEM is also holistic in that it deals with the whole system and is not a partial model that is simply concerned with transportation, public budgeting, housing, or a number of other issues looked at in an isolated fashion.

It is my hope that this work will be of use to several groups of people: first, to my colleagues in the research world, who are called upon to design the computer revolution; second, to the policy makers who must order and lead the revolution by establishing both a basis for clearer understanding of the total human habitat system and the framework required to successfully use the computer in the understanding and decision-making of this system; third, to those who are presently undergraduates and graduates who will have to take the techniques proposed out of their birthed stages toward maturity; and fourth, to the general reader who is interested in an exciting approach to the study of the urban area in which he lives.

Chapter 2

MODEL STRUCTURE

The CITY series of models built by Envirometrics often were designed in an intuitive and evolutionary fashion rather than systematically. The conventional model-building guidelines and techniques as outlined by Lowry and others were not followed.[4] Two major reasons account for this. First, the techniques were not searched out or explored by the staff because we always considered modifying or adding to a basic model that we knew would work. Second, and more importantly, the models under construction were not thought to be conventional and the designers were wary of using modeling techniques that were not evolved out of experience with the decision-making models themselves.

THE CONCEPT OF A MODEL

"A model is something–a physical object, a living organism or a social system–it is a physical or symbolic representation of that object, designed

> to incorporate or reproduce those features of the real object that the researcher deems significant for his research problem. The term model, as used here, refers to a scientific tool. It does not connote that the representation is an ideal or a 'good model,' worthy of emulation. Brody points out that 'developing a model involves abstracting from reality those components and relationships which are hypothesized as crucial to what is being modeled.' The choice of essential aspects of the reality being modeled depends upon the purposes for which the model is being constructed [Guetzkow, 1962].

Everyone builds models. The world and each of its component parts is more or less complex. At some level of detail this complexity exceeds the ability of people to comprehend and act. Consequently, decision makers (and educators and researchers) are often forced to aggregate, to simplify, and to make limiting assumptions in order to make a situation or problem comprehensible. This reduction of problems to basics has numerous obvious advantages but leads us back to our original statement, "everyone builds models."

There are various types of models, and all are abstractions: the blueprint of the architect, the mock-up of the builder, the mathematical formulations of the scientist, the dress designer's mannequin, and the programmer's algorithms. We shall restrict our attention here to the abstraction of the social system. More specifically, for the purposes of this book, we are mainly interested in two types of models: the models of the social scientist, and the adaptations of these theoretical structures to the computer in the form of a computer model.

Functionally speaking, Figure 2.1 describes almost any type of computer model. It simply says that such a model is designed to accept data from a source, and add it to the data already available to the model, perform a series of specified operations on the data and produce an output. The whole process is a cycle.

Perturbing or exercising a model requires the modification of the simpler model diagram to represent a complete iteration. This cycle includes the addition of inputs or newer information to the given or existing data base. The inputs can be of three forms:

(1) Pure machine, in which the model, after accepting the data base, cycles according to present relationships which are part of the model itself, then continues operating without human interferences until it arrives at a solution.

(2) Man-machine, in which the model may operate in a manner similar to the pure machine but which at some point in the model's operating

procedure, requires inputs from a human decision maker in order to proceed to a model solution.

(3) Gaming, in which the model is so designed that it allows a number of entries into the model operation in order that players can affect the model system according to an overall strategy determined by players of the game.

Actually, in a model of the type described in this book (GEM), there is really no difference among the various models. Whether from a machine simulation, a human decision maker or a player, all inputs serve the same purpose—that of providing data or parameter weights to the operating parts of the model (Figure 2.2).

These inputs when added to the data base provide the parameters to be operated on by the model itself. The functional relationships described by the Operation Section of the model can be of several forms. This book will focus on only one of these but the general paradigm offered here for the concept of model is by no means limited to the behavioral functions discussed later.

Finally, the parameters, after being related to each other by the relationships described by Operations, produces a new data base. The point from which the model can again be executed to another cycle. At the same time, the model user is fed information on the results of the model iteration in the form of computer output. The timing of the output (in terms of real or actual time; i.e., seconds, days, months, years, etc. and the specific format of the output) is also immaterial to this discussion.

This total iteration produces data changes which have been preordained by a model designer and, theoretically, will give him information which is useful for his specific purpose.

The concept of a "model" has gained widespread acceptance in the social sciences. Partially as a result of this, the use of paradigms has gained even greater stature as these theories and structures have been demanded by policy makers. The theoretical models of the researchers have moved from the scholarly journals to uses in the solutions of day-to-day policy problems. The need to use models in the arena of reality has tended to force model design into two directions: toward eminently detailed specific models of individual system features, and toward holistic models of the system at large.

It is the latter model form, holistic, which interests us here.

FIGURE 2.1
DIAGRAM OF A MODEL

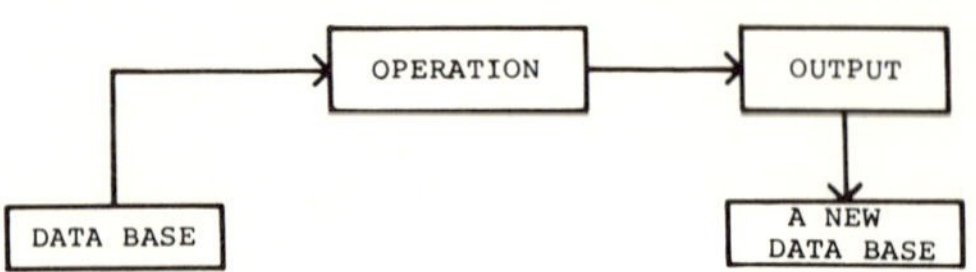

FIGURE 2.2
ONE ITERATION OF A MODEL

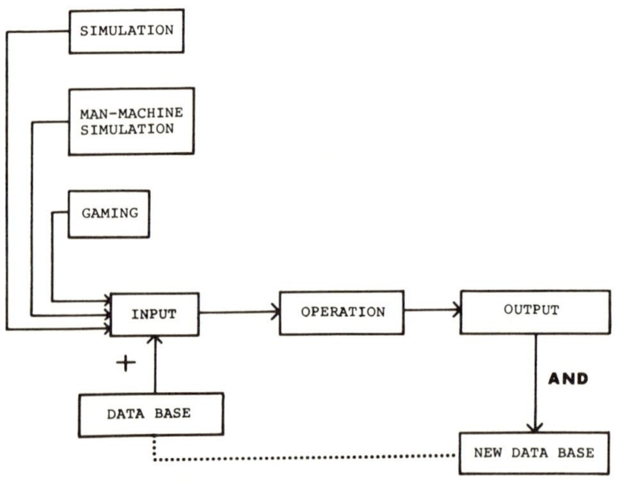

THE CITY MODEL AND ITS ELEMENTS

Throughout our total model building experience, the effort did not proceed in a straightforward fashion during its design stages. However, when the written specifications for the various subroutines or modules were finally solidified for presentation to the systems analysts, the model had to be in a form suitable for computer programming.

When building the more simplified models, our instructions to the programmer were described in self-contained sections for program components. The instructions detailed a whole concept, from what data would be needed to how the routine worked and what the output should look like. Consequently, the programmer responsible for, say, the education portion of the model had to look at only the design specifications related to education to understand all of what was required for that particular routine.

As the models progressed through the various stages, from initial design to redesign and reprogramming, we noted that many of the separate routines as originally conceived and programmed were quite similar in the end product, except for specific parameter values. Further, even some functional differences in otherwise identical subroutines could many times be made more alike by simple changes in basic algorithms. This recognition resulted in our redoing model specifications in the form of computer phases instead of (or sometimes, or as well as) by functional portions of the total environmental system these computer phases are referred to as elements. The following description represents some mix of the actual and idea implementation of this conceptualization.

The building of a model in five parts has distinct advantages and gives the model builder a clearer perspective of how to approach computer-oriented modeling. On the other hand, it does not describe what goes into a model and how the component parts relate to one another. The Sector Theory discussed in the next chapter evolved to fill this gap. The two theories together form a description of a specific kind of model; a model of a general social system, and provide the design of what became the General Environmental Model (GEM) and its derivative, CITY (see Figure 2.3).

DATA BASE

The Data Base parameters can be visualized as a description of the area being simulated. The programs in this section allow the user to change the basic starting description of the system and therefore allow a very large number of initial configurations for training purposes and, of course, allow the loading of a data base for a real area.

Lowry (1965) distinguishes between the theory part of a model (the logical coherence and generality) and the model part of a particular model (the application of the theory to a concrete case). This also holds for the GEM model: the model relationships (Operating Programs) reflect part of a theory and the Data Base elements (or Executive Routines discussed next) are equivalent to applying the relationships (or theory) to a specific geographical area.

There are also theory implications involved in the way the model cycles and generates new data bases which represent subsequent years. Likewise, implicit or explicit theoretical assumptions are a part of the design decisions with respect to (1) the level of aggregation of the model's elements, (2) the handling of time (sequencing, dynamics, time lags and the real time and play time length of a cycle), (3) the concept of change, (4) inputs to a model, and (5) the algorithms used to process data, make assignments, and generate probabilities (Figure 2.4).

Data Base Programs

As the data base programs are used to feed the computer the descriptive information needed for simulation, the deciding of which parameters to use in describing particular portions of the environment often becomes quite complex. Let us look, for example, at the concept of water. Water has, among others, the following characteristics: a measurable quantity; variation in amount due to evaporation rate; direction of flow; rate and volume of flow by time of year; color and taste; contains organisms and minerals. It also has sources such as lakes, river, runoffs, sewers, dams, and harbors; freshness or salinity; force which can be converted to power; and so forth. The designer must choose which of these is relevant to his particular model and how they will be represented.

One of the ways of defining the scope of a model is through the Data Base routines, since they determine what data are loaded and prepare the descriptive parameters and their interrelationships. Attempts to achieve all-inclusiveness in the Data Base and model capability result in a need for sufficient flexibility so that any conceivable feature of each part of the natural or social environment

FIGURE 2.3
MODEL OPERATION

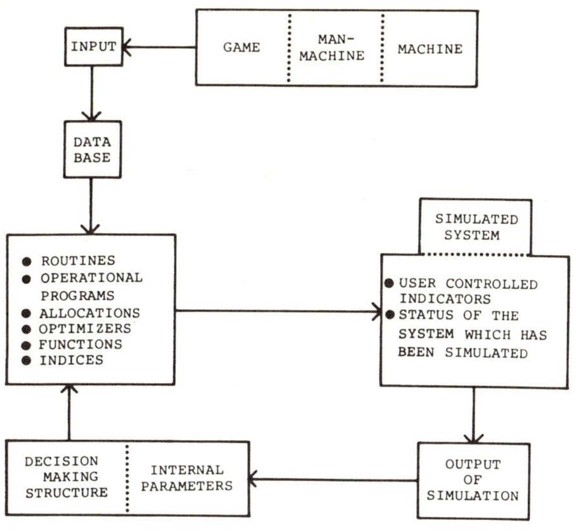

FIGURE 2.4
THE GENERAL SECTOR AND MODEL OPERATION

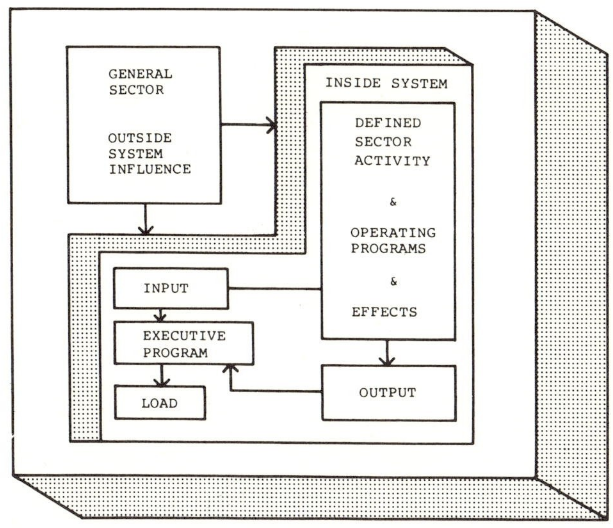

may be added. Deciding to produce as complete a picture of the environment as possible requires that each parameter be loaded so that it can be related to other parameters. The more parameters loaded (or derived), the more complex the model. As a means for proving for this flexibility in an interrelated and complex model, GEM was built in a modular fashion.

Modularity is the ability to change parts of a model without disturbing or redoing the other parts, or restructuring the whole model. This feature led to an emphasis in the design of GEM whereby the program could be changed after the model was developed; general equations could be defined to allow the inclusion or omission of variables, and the weights and parameters of each routine could be user-specified. In essence, this design allowed a user to substitute, say, a mathematical simulation for a particular routine used in the GEM model or to replace a portion of the GEM model with a specific routine, without extensive systems work. In most cases, substitution could be carried out without any reprogramming at all. The practical use of the concept of modularity is made possible by the use of Executive Routines (Figure 2.5).

EXECUTIVE ROUTINES

A number of procedural and model alternatives, called executive routines, provide the user with a means by which he may choose the scope of the modules used. He might have a choice of a detailed or simplistic school sector, a limited or wide variety of manufacturing types, small or large population units, etc. He might also choose the type of module used, e.g., a migration module that responds to welfare policy versus one that omits such considerations, or the mix of modules, to operate with or without certain subsystems being explicitly represented.

The ability to cope with this degree of flexibility proved to be very difficult to accomplish in a digital computer. Although this had always been our aim, each of the various stages of the evolution of GEM-CITY either required a complete reprogramming job or an often unsatisfactory and inefficient patching of the current model. CITY I was programmed on the IBM 1130 and the features required to expand the model forced the CITY II expansion to a larger computer (GE 635). The design of this model was not sufficiently flexible and so the next stage, the CITY III model was programmed on the Univac 1108.

The latest evolution moved the model to the IBM 360/370 series (40 and above) and included a complete redesign and rewrite. Included in this rewrite was a method of facilitating more complete modularity through building a generalized file handling procedure. In earlier models all design parameters (i.e., those which are not changed when a new board configuration is run) were data items in the program which used them. Every time we wished to change a design parameter (e.g., the number of workers in a population unit), we had to update and recompile all programs requiring that parameter. The task was frequently quite complicated, lengthy and expensive. With the development of a general model like GEM, we designed, as an alternative, a flexible program structure which would enable us to modify parameters with minimum cost and inconvenience.[5]

Building Blocks

In addition to the computer file handling structure, all models required that a number of basic decisions be made by the users of the model as to how data, relationships, change, and time are to be handled. These issues are part of the complementary decision as to the level of aggregation and the scope of the model. What are called model building blocks are the results of aggregation decisions being applied to the data, such as the physical environment, population units, business activities, government functions, time, and so forth.

The physical environment is comprised of the land, water and climate of a particular system. The land component consists of all of the descriptors associated with it, such as soil type, fertility, slope, availability of minerals, petroleum zoning, present uses, and so forth. Examples of the various characteristics of water were noted earlier. They would include characteristics of quality, quantity and location. The climate of the local system would have to handle such parameters as mean temperature, rainfall and snow, and air quality.

Population

Just as the physical environment has to be described to that it represents a particular locale, so must the population be defined. The categories in which people are sorted can be simplified to the point of three socio-economic classes, as they are in the CITY model, or refined to something similar to the five classes used by the Census

Bureau. On the other hand, the class concept could be ignored completely and the populous described in terms of size, sex, race, and skills. It might also include other descriptors such as church affiliation and union membership.

The first method of sorting the populous into preconceived categories requires that assumptions be made about the people and about how the individuals become members of a specific group. The model then handles the population groups (P1's) in terms of these categories and, regardless of the size of the P1, addresses the person as a member of that group with the group's average characteristics. The second method handles P1's individually (remember a P1 can range from a family to any number of people) and ascribes to this P1 each of a series of attributes. The model than addresses itself to the specific attributes that it is interested in and does not consider the rest of the features of the people.

The latter method of assigning values to P1's is the most accurate and yields the greatest amount of information for the user. It is significantly more difficult, however, to keep track of the P1 attributes individually. The model itself, of course, does not depend on how the information is kept, although the finer detail in the case of individual P1 characteristics requires more careful design as one is no longer able to depend upon averaging to match population attributes to the rest of the model. Consequently, it depends upon the intended use of the model and the amount of time and money available as to which path is chosen.

BUSINESS ACTIVITIES

Population and business activities are the two non-government building blocks that have to be loaded in a model of the GEM type. The decision as to how to handle them also defines most of the rest of the model. The details of defining business activities (MOD categories) are related later in this book. Note will be made here only of the concept.

All business activities (industrial, commercial and residential) are included in the model. The categories are defined from the Standard Industrial Classification Codes (SIC) of the Bureau of the Census. The categories used by the Census are grouped into a number of MOD classifications and each of them is defined as having given average characteristics.

As a rule, the fewer MOD categories defined, the grosser the findings of the model based on the assumption that the wide diversity of business types available in a community would be more or less homogenized. If, on the other hand, there were only one or a few industry types, the average would then represent a specific industry type or be close to it.

Residences are handled differently in the GEM model than industrial and commercial properties, as they are not assigned to workers to produce revenue nor do they produce physical output. Therefore, the number of distinct categories possible is determined by a combination of building type (i.e., single family duplex, multifamily), structure quality and present condition. This methodology allows for a number of categories.

Government Functions

The public sector provides a large number of necessary services for any system but the government organizations are usually the same in any area. The relation between public and private is often unclear. For example, utilities can be provided by either sector or both. Bus, rapid rail, and hospital services fall into equally unclear situations.

The setup of individual government organizations is also individually determined by each municipality. Therefore, the model has to be able to load various combinations of functions to accommodate the richness of real life. Designing it to do this also allows the user to choose several levels of aggregation for government detail. If the user is able to assemble the various departments of a government into any form he desires, he can choose to handle each function separately, designate all functions under the heading of government, or anywhere in between.

Time

In addition to questions regarding the building blocks noted above, there are questions about the aggregate money unit and the concept of time. The users when deciding on monetary and population units have to keep both of these constant throughout the model. The feature of time, however, is somewhat complex.

Time implies not only many dimensions in a model but is also tied to the concept of organization. A realistic model of the social system would have to take into consideration the day-to-day or year-to-year activities which result in changes within the system. Not only does the model have to be prepared to accept these feedbacks, but it has to be set to log them in an appropriate manner. In effect, every decision has a feedback on the next iteration.

On the other hand, some decisions cause effects which are more long-run in nature. These decisions require that the computer keep track of their effects over, or until, a given time period. For example, a decision to devote resources to improving educational quality might have no obvious effect on model output in the short run, but would be expected to improve the efficiency of workers over the long run. Consequently, a model should account for these effects so that decisions in one time period can be reflected at future time periods.

Real Time

The length of real time as represented in the model refers to the simulated period under consideration; i.e., the period of time represented by a cycle of the model. The decision schema is a complex of the choices being made overlayed with the results obtained from earlier actions. However, sorting them out for modeling purposes is a gross simplification, regardless of how short the time span being simulated.[6]

It appears that the decision as to which specific time frame is to be used depends largely on the model scale itself. A model of several regions or of the nation lends itself more easily to decade by decade iterations than does a model of a single household budget. On the other hand, while an hour to hour simulation of the day (or days) of one individual is within comprehension, similar analysis of a whole metropolitan area is mind staggering.

Our research only evolved to comparative static iterations of relatively large aggregations of people on a yearly time scale. Research into more dynamic time frames not only requires more information than is generally available, but the continued use of a computer which is kept running throughout the time the model is used in order for human decision makers to get continuous feedback on the results of their decisions.

Time in Sequencing of the Model Operations

The concept of time influences the sequence in which the designers of a model perform the various operations of the simulation. Not only is reality continuous, but everything affects everything else and does so simultaneously. At present there is no feasible computer method available for accomplishing this feature. Although strides are being made to identify the various system components and specify the "how" of their interrelationships, little has been done to specify the "when." For the sake of having an operating model, a designer is therefore forced to decide which operations are done together and which are to be sequenced first, second, and so forth. The larger the model and the greater the number of variables considered, the more important the sequencing.

Although time sequencing is the most practical method for dealing with simultaneous relationships in a complex system, it introduces some distortions (i.e., period T data being used for some calculations, T–1 for others, and T+1 for still others).

An example from the CITY model (1108 version) will illustrate this. Table 2.1 was provided to the user in order for him to determine the temporal factors involved in the simulation-produced maps. The players' output is assumed to be for Round T; thus, the previous round's data base is indicated by T–1. The columns A, B, and C represent the status map factors produced by: (A) the execution of the simulation (CITY) on the previous round's data base (normally altered by EDIT); (B) the execution of MAPS after EDIT and before CITY on the altered Round T–1 data base, and (C) the execution of the MAPS after CITY (in this case MAPS operates on the unaltered Round T data base). If there were no inputs for any round, CITY would be run anyway to produce new output and data. MAPS executed prior to this simulation reflects the same factors' status as case B.

Relating the Data Base to Executive Routines

The Data Base Programs make available to the model the necessary parameters and values for the functions in the model. The Executive Program assembles a particular level of aggregation for the model user and allows him to highlight specific portions of GEM. A simple example of a program might make the use of the Data Base and Executive Programs more clear. Imagine three computer tapes. Tape 1 contains the general program and relationships of the model. Tape 2 contains the data for the Data Base and Executive Programs. When tapes 1 and 2 are combined, the resultant tape (3) is the specialized model describing the environment in a fashion of particular interest

FIGURE 2.5
MODULAR CONCEPT OF A GENERAL MODEL

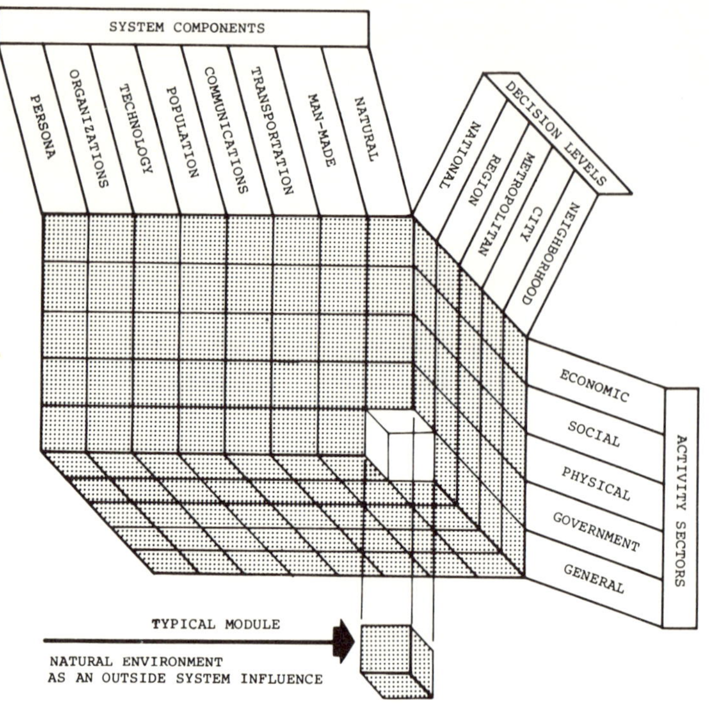

TABLE 2.1
EXAMPLES OF TIME EFFECTS ON DIFFERENT MAP OUTPUTS

Facts	A	B	C
Social decision maker control for round	T	T	T+1
All land uses (except UT and RAIL) construction projects completion status through round	T	T	T+1
UT and RAIL construction projects completed through round	T	T	T
Land use demolition projects completed through round	T	T	T
Land use value ratios after depreciation for round	T	T–1[a]	T[a]
Land use value ratios after maintenance for round	T	T–1	T
Migration for round	T	T–1	T
Property ownership for round	T	T	T
Utility service for round	T	T	T
Zoning for round	T	T	T

a. The effects due entirely to depreciation can be seen only on the Demographic Status Map generated by the execution of CITY (column A). Columns B and C refer to value ratios which have been "maintained." Only where there has been no maintenance will the value ratios apparent in these last two cases be equivalent to the value ratios which are entirely due to depreciation.

to the user. In essence, the method is reminiscent of a computer compiler, where the programmer (and the system software) decides which part of the general compiler is needed for his routine.

The Data Base and Executive Routines have evolved to the point where it is difficult to conceive how they could be made more general or user-oriented. They allow the specific loading of any Data Base, changes in many kinds of parameter generalities (building blocks) and replacements of whole sections of code by different programs, without extensive redesign and reprogramming. The same level of evolution can be noted in the description of the Input Programs and Output Section. Consequently, most of the evolution of GEM remains in the Operating Programs.

The next section, Input, is very much like the original loading of a Data Base in conceptual terms. However, since this change in the model parameters has to be accomplished during the run of a model, the computer design has to be different.

INPUT

The Input Programs allow the user to change given parameters in the model. There are two types of Input Programs. The first allows a user to selectively modify all data values without program interference and it closely resembles the Data Base Programs. This form of the program is useful only to those who understand the model very well, as there is no check on the Input to see if it makes sense. For example, if a user should wish to change an average salary from \$10K to \$100K, the model would not prevent the decision but would accept the input as valid and the rest of the program would act on it. Further, if a desired decision required crediting or debiting accounts (as in a land transfer) the user would have to be sure to do all of the necessary accounting. This form is quite impractical for most uses, except possibly for research.

The second form of Input Program is that which processes participant decisions. This program checks for internally related decisions, such as the availability of resources and the legality of a decision. This form of handling participant input is the one found in our present CITY model and in every one of the CITY submodels where we have chosen a particular path through GEM.[7] The basic principle to be used is similar to that of the Executive Program described earlier, where all of the possible checks are noted and the user defines which are applicable to his needs.

To some extent, even in this latter form, there is very little difference (from the point of view of computer program) between Inputs (decisions) to the represented area, which alter its status, and the Data Base, which contains the initial status of the represented area. It is useful to maintain the distinction, however, since the former represents the policies which are made by a person acting as a system decision maker while the latter represents the empirical findings of a researcher who fits an actual or hypothetical area to the model.

OPERATING PROGRAMS

Operating Programs are the mechanisms by which the various processes of the model are carried out. The Operating Programs act not only within each sector, but among all three sectors and with other Operating Programs. These programs can be allocators (including the satisficers and the optimizers), processors (including the transactors and the generators) and can perform accounting.

One type of operating program is an Allocator, which involves a market mechanism. An Allocator Program is carried out partly by the computer in the form of an optimizer or a satisficer. Inputs to an Allocator usually come from more than a single sector. The Employment Allocator is an example of this type of program in that it contains machine-programmed satisficers and requires inputs from all three sectors (Economic, Social, Political) in order to allocate workers to jobs.

A second type of operating program, the Processor consists of a set of functions and interrelationships which carry out a defined operation. The inputs for a Process originate only from the sector which is using the particular process at that time (although indices which are generated indirectly by other sectors may also be used). The Production Process is an example of this type of operating program. It is used to calculate the production output for a given industry type. The Process acts on direct inputs affecting that industry (level, equipment, etc.) along with indices provided by other sectors or operating programs (depreciation).

A third type of operating program, Accounting, is a simple transactor of numbers in files (including all necessary input checks). A cash transfer would be an example of this type of program, which would transfer the stated amount of dollars from one specified computer account to another.

To illustrate this section of the element structure, let us briefly examine the Operating Programs used in the CITY model.

Computer Operations in the CITY Model

The CITY model has nine major computer operation sections that follow the processing of user inputs:

(1) Migration
(2) Assessment
(3) Depreciation
(4) Employment
(5) Transportation
(6) Government Allocation
(7) Time Allocation
(8) Commercial
(9) Bookkeeping

To some extent these categories are highly misleading as each of these computer programs contains several subroutines. For example, migration contains the programs that measure housing dissatisfaction, personal dissatisfaction, etc., and it uses sixteen subprograms to accomplish the many calculations necessary to move P1's into, out of, and around the local metropolitan system.

The following verbal description of each of these major subroutines which make up the Operating Routine in the CITY model are arranged in the order that they are processed by the program. As noted earlier, the sequencing introduces a systematic bias on the output of unknown form and proportions.

Rather than tracing through the details of all of these calculations via the use of a programming flowchart, the following verbal description of the sequence of flow is presented to show the major factors involved in a cycle of the model.

Sequence Flow for Major CITY Model Programs

(1) Migration.–Calculates various forms of dissatisfaction indices to be used to generate movers. In local migration, it develops a pool of movers comprised of a percent of the most dissatisfied of the population displaced by housing demolition, a percent of the total population (random movers), natural population growth, and the inmigrants. It then moves the members of this pool into housing that has adequate capacity and quality. In terms of outmigration, it

allows a certain percentage of each income class that are either unemployed to outmigrage from the local system. Other movers who cannot find adequate local housing also become outmigrants. Finally, it allows depending upon local condition a marginal percentage of each of the socio-economic classes to inmigrate.

(2) Assessment.–Calculates the assessed value of land and buildings taking into account new purchases, new developments, and assessment ratios. It also selects parcels of land up for auction and generates their market value.

(3) Depreciation.–Buildings and roads depreciate in value and utility each year as a function of the passage of time (obsolescence), the amount of use they receive (wear and tear), and the quality of local municipal services (especially police and fire protection). Local decision makers may choose to maintain a constant value for their developments by expending the required amounts of money for maintenance. This routine depreciates all developments and calculates maintenance expenditures.

(4) Employment.–All P1's in the local system compete with one another for jobs in the local labor market. Likewise, all employers compete to hire workers with the highest qualifications. There are two types of employment: full-time and part-time.

The full-time employment routine assigns population units (high income first and best educated first) to full time jobs based on the assumption that workers will attempt to maximize their net salary (salary received minus transportation costs using last year's transportation cost figures). A new job must offer a 10 percent salary increase to cause a P1 to change jobs. P1's will take jobs in the next lower class if none is available in their class. The part-time employment routine assigns part-time workers (80 time units in part-time work equals one full-time job) to part-time jobs (fixed by businesses, variable for construction industry and schools for adult education teachers) on the basis of best education first. The number of time units allocated to part-time jobs is set for each group of P1's on a parcel by the social decision makers. If time allocated for part-time work, but not enough part-time jobs exist, the dissatisfaction of the P1's is increased.

(5) Transportation.–Taking the origins (homes as determined in migration) and the destination (jobs as determined in employment), this allocator assigns workers to transportation mode and routes in an effort to minimize total transportation costs (dollar costs plus the dollar value of time spent) subject to the constraints imposed by public transit capacity, road congestion, and transportation boycotts.

(6) Government Allocation.—Assigns students by class to public schools or private schools based upon school quality criteria (value ratio, teacher mix and student/teacher ratio ratio) and capacity of the school serving their district; and assigns time units spent in public adult education to the available public education program. Other routines assign the functions of police, fire and sanitary services (aggregated under the title of Municipal Services or MS). Each of the land use is assigned an average useage (loading) on an MS plant. The number and type of land uses serviced by a particular plant determines the quality of service from that plant. Heavily loaded plants feed back in the system in terms of poorer service, causing greater building depreciation and higher personal and environmental dissatisfaction.

(7) Time Allocation.—For each population unit grouping, time spent in transportation is deducted from a total of 100 units; then time spent in part-time employment and public adult education time is deducted; private education costs are determined and the time is deducted; voter registration is changed as a result of the time spent in politics and the time is deducted; time is deducted for time spent in recreation; and the remaining time is labeled "involuntary time."

(8) Commercial.—The various purchases of the population groups are allocated to personal goods and personal services establishments using the criteria that establishments have a limited capacity and shoppers attempt to minimize total costs as determined by a standard consumption function where consumption is a function of income, sales price, and total shipping costs; the purchase of businesses (including personal goods and personal services establishments) for normal operation and for maintenance are allocated to business goods and business service establishments[8] based upon the same function as above. Terminal users are also allocated to the nearest terminal that has adequate capacity.

(9) Bookkeeping.—This routine makes all the final calculations of incomes and expenditures and of indicators for use in the detailed computer output to the economic activities and teams, the social decision makers, the government departments, and the summary statistics. The program operates in the sequence shown and outputs from one program become inputs to the later ones. Some of the operating programs that are early in the sequence receive their inputs from the results of operating programs run in the previous cycle (each cycle represents a year), thus creating some lagged relationships (see the section on Time in the discussion of Data Base).

The individual Operating Programs underwent considerable evolved change throughout the total design period. It might be interesting to follow one module in GEM that is concerned with employment to illustrate this point.

This module has been part of each phase of the GEM evaluation but has changed considerably with each redesign. The following discussion is meant to point out the various forms of this module without exhaustively documenting each of them.

Briefly stated, in the CITY model, the Employment Allocator grew from a relatively simple optimizer in CITY I to a multiphase optimizer in CITY II and III, to a satisficer in GEM which matches lists of employer and employee work objectives.

In CITY I a worker, if he qualified by income class, would work for the employer that offered him the highest net income. In CITY II and CITY III, the optimizer process was enlarged so that an employer, in hiring each round, would also look for a worker's educational level, whether or not he worked for the employer the last round, and if the worker was on boycott. In the GEM model, neither the employer nor employee is looking for the best conditions, only those which will satisfy a list of given conditions.

The original method used to allocate people to jobs or customers to commercial establishments was derived from Allan Feldt's CLUG. In that model, employment matches were made by players who swapped pseudo-money with each other to simulate transactions. In REGION we had those financial transactions handled by an operator who used a matrix in which monetary sums were added and subtracted from the acount of each player, but the players still made the assignments based upon negotiations. By introducing the computer in CITY I, we were able to release the players from that bookkeeping chore.

The CITY I employment optimizer assigns employees to the employers that offer the highest net salary. In doing so, the routine (1) compares employee lists of net salary (net of last round's transportation expenses to that employer location) for ten employers; (2) assigns employees to employers so that those employees with the highest net salaries are assigned first; (3) when all the obvious solutions have been derived, the computer assigns employees with equal net salaries on a random basis.

In each round of CITY I, the employment optimizer operates four separate times with four socio-economic classes of workers. The high income class is matched to jobs first. If the number of high-income positions equals the number of high-income residents, there is an even match. If there are too few high-income residents in the system, the needed high-income employees are imported from outside the local economy at twice the average salary level for that class. (This is to show the effect on the net income of the local employers if the local economy has to import workers.) If there are too many high-income workers, the surplus gets the first choice of middle-income jobs (and receives middle-income salaries). This sequence of job assignments tends to push all unemployment down to the slum residents, as the optimizer aligns the four income levels with available jobs.

After the job assignments are made, a computer subroutine surveys them to note travel-to-work over various road sections. These commuting journeys are part of the calculation of the amount of congestion on, and depreciation of roads. These congestion and depreciation figures are used to calculate present round travel costs for the whole system. Thus, workers are assigned to jobs using last year's estimate of travel costs but end up paying this year's travel costs, which may vary significantly from that of the previous year if new roads or more users have materialized.

In the CITY II model, employment is still optimized. However, employees are not part of the Economic Sector, as in CITY I, but are part of the population units in the Social Sector. The population units "belong" to the Social Sector (a third decision-making division of the CITY II model). The employment process takes population units in order of descending income class and matches them to the extent possible with the employers that require high-income workers. In each round, all population units (P1's) have the opportunity to switch jobs. There is, however, a built-in bias in favor of keeping the job held last round, accomplished by assigning a shadow transfer cost to changing jobs.

The social teams making decisions for population units can influence which jobs P1's consider by making decisions about work boycott, transportation mode boycott, and/or the value of time index. Thus, a P1 may rule out working at some locations because of a job boycott, refusal to use bus or rapid rail service, or the high dollar value that it assigns to a unit of time of travel.

In both CITY II and III the employment assignment allocator considers the transportation costs of the previous round. Therefore, each P1 is trying to maximize his actual salary offered this round minus the transportation cost to get to that job based upon the lowest cost route given last year's modes, routes, and congestion. Once all P1's who have found work are assigned, the process calculates new and actual transportation costs based upon current modes, routes and congestion.

For CITY II and III the first step of the employment process takes the most educated high income class P1 and assigns it to the highest net salary high income job. In this manner, those population units that are more educated tend to get paid more than less educated units. The first step ends when either high income class P1 or jobs are exhausted.

The second step of the employment process takes the most educated middle-income P1's and high-income P1's (if any were not employed in step one) and assigns them to the best middle-income jobs. In this manner, high-income-class P1's tend to find lower-class jobs if not enough higher-income-class jobs exist. The number of P1's employed in a lower-income-class job is a measure of the under-employment in the system. If there is a deficiency of workers in a particular class, the employers do not hire from the outside system as in CITY I but instead have their production levels or capacity levels reduced to reflect the labor shortage.

The third step repeats the process for low-income-class and unemployed middle-class population units. The fourth, fifth, and sixth steps of the employment process follow the same class sequence by matching those P1's who allocate their time for part-time jobs with those employers offering part-time work. In the part-time assignment process, however, P1's never take jobs at a lower level. To the extent that jobs are available, all P1's who allocate at least ten units of time are assigned ten units of part-time work in the first cycle. The second cycle takes the second ten units of time for all P1's and so on. This allows all P1's, regardless of economic class, to have somewhat equal opportunities for part-time work.

A General Employment Allocator

A General Employment Allocator is to be introduced in the GEM model and is a significant departure in composition from its predecessors. The optimizer approach has been replaced by the satisficer. By implementing sets of minimum standards which both the employer and the potential employee must meet—or satisfy—we have suggested that there is a tendency for the best educated and trained employees to obtain the highest salaried and otherwise most appealing job openings. However, the allocator no longer guarantees this situation.

In order to evaluate a job opening, some standard criteria are applied. In addition to salaries, an employment location's index includes measures of fringe benefits, accessibility, an indicator of working conditions, and an indicator of employment stability. The introduction of these factors produces a more complete employment picture. Moreover, recognizing that working conditions, for example, may be more important to a higher-class population unit, different weights are applied to each factor for each class of population unit. Consequently, each population unit can possess a relative measure with each potential employer, thereby enabling a meaningful allocator condition.

Likewise, the attractiveness or potential productivity of all workers is measured. This index (measure) is comprised of such factors as years of education completed, an indicator of work experience, and a feed from training functions. Thus, to obtain a position, a population unit must have a minimum acceptable education level which may vary by employer or employment type.

While transportation as an element of the employment process has been deemphasized (as will be illustrated later), many other aspects have been added. For example, during any one round, a maximum of one-third of the total labor force will seek new employment locations; correspondingly, approximately up to one-third of the total jobs will be vacant at the start of any round.

Job applicants include the previous round's unemployed, those highly dissatisfied with their previous job (as determined by a low employment index), those fired or who lost their jobs due to layoffs, and a small random selection. In addition to those vacant jobs, openings will accrue from the previous round's unfilled jobs and expansion of plants and departments.

OUTPUT

The final section of the model is the Output phase. The model has three specific sector outputs: economic, social and government; plus some general and summary statistics common to all sectors. Through the use of the Executive Programs, each of these outputs is made more or less specific, depending upon the needs of the user.

Added to these sector outputs are those of general interest to the whole system, such as the Outside System, the physical environment changes, the summary statistics from some of the computer allocators and processes and a series of indices which help to measure the relative position of various sectors in the system The final version (CITY IV) added a time series to allow the users to do trend analyses.

For GEM the procedure for obtaining printed output is designed for maximum flexibility so that the user can determine what information will be printed and how it will be grouped. For example, the user can specify what information he wants displayed by a graphic technique and whether it is to be grouped by parcel or by jurisdiction (i.e., a map showing population density by parcel). In the Government Sector, he can indicate which department's revenues and expenditures he wishes to have summed and on whose output and summary is to appear; e.g., the user might wish to add police and fire budgets into a single Public Safety Output.

Another aspect of output flexibility is illustrated in the Government Sector where certain types of information are printed only if relevant to a particular department. For example, the model is designed to allow a great deal of the flexibility in government revenue alternatives; i.e., a tax not in effect is not listed on any department's output; when a new tax is instituted, it appears as a separate item in the appropriate department's list of revenues.

In addition to the more generalized forms, the four types of printed output are: function level descriptors, visual and mapped output, summary accounting sheets, series data and indices.

These outputs would be derived for all of the sectors. They would be unique in those cases where specific measure were applicable. As noted earlier the executive programs are so structured that they can pick both the decision and function levels that will be simulated on a particular model path.

(1) Functional Level Descriptors—Each of the function units (service provided) has a general format for its output. The first type of information describes the parameters used by the decision maker which relate to land areas. The summary output shows various indices for each subarea; as an example, school districts. The general organizations for school districts are topic headings without subdivisions as follows: the district in a column with the level of students served and those not served; employment, with each class delineated by salary; workers requested, workers hired and their average productivity; equipment quantity and quality; building quantity and quality; capacity to provide service; demand for service.

(2) Visual and Mapped Output–There are two alternatives for printing mapped output for the GEM model. Because the model makes use of a rectangular coordinate system, it is easy to incorporate such generalized graphic routines as the Harvard Computer Graphics Center's SYMAP and SYMVUL programs. One variation of these programs takes raw data of a ranked nature, divides it into deciles, and displays it in squares (as one form) of different shades. This form of mapping does not specify the absolute parameter values but ranks the value in its place in relation to all other values of the same kind. As a result each map only discusses one parameter at a time.

As an alternative to this form, we designed a map which gives the user a great deal of information in one output. This form (in reality, four varieties of one form) allows the user to specify what he wants to see in a map and the model displays this information as part of the total output. For example, a map related to educational facilities might include such features as the location of the school plants, the school district boundaries, the number of students in attendance and where they live, and the condition of the school, all in one map.

(3) Summary Accounting Sheets–The Accounting Sheets are divided into three general areas: (1) Income: capital and current appropriations; (2) Expenditures: capital and current; and (3) Asset Sheet.

The income and appropriations section include all of the revenue sources of a business, government department, and population unit (P1). It would include such things as salaries and welfare for a P1; revenue from the sale or rent of property, loans or loan payments received, subsidies, interest or dividends, and other numerous items for a business; and appropriations (capital and current), special revenues, bonding, and fees for the public sector.

The expenditures would include maintenance or purchase of a plant and equipment, and services: purchase of land, salaries and bond payments for government departments; for the private sector, purchase of land, construction, maintenance, or demolition of structure, loans or loan payments made, salaries, purchase of goods and services, taxes, and other cash transfers or investments; and rent,

FIGURE 2.6

COMPONENTS OF THE QUALITY OF LIFE INDEX

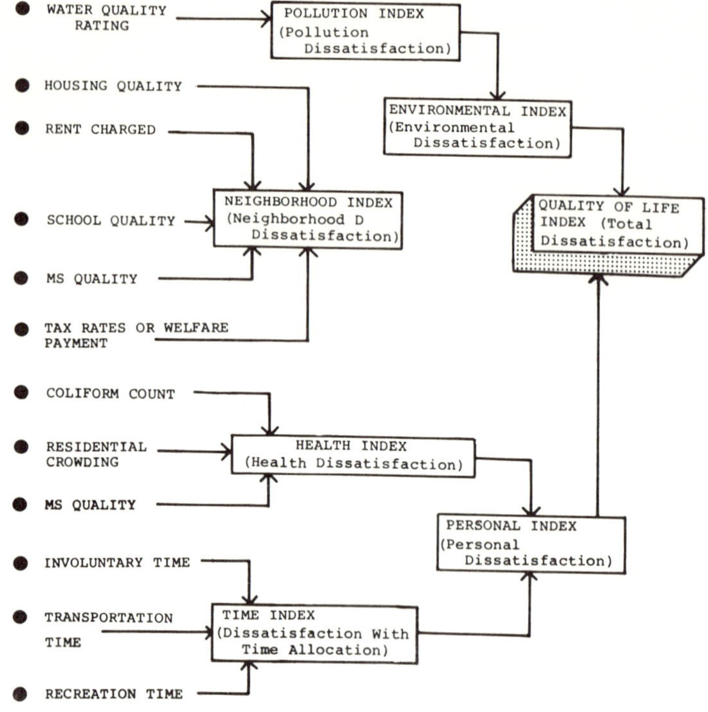

transportation costs, purchase costs for goods and services, education costs, various taxes, and other items for the P1.

The Income and Expenditure items are subtracted from each other and the residual added to previous cash-on-hand or debts to get current liquid assets. These are then arranged in a standard asset and liability balance sheet showing the liquidity of the sector.

(4) Time Series Data and Quality Indices—The latest improvement in the output phase of the model has been the introduction of time series data and quality indices. The time series numbers make it easier for the user to relate summary data from the various sectors over a period of several years, thereby adding the feature of historical perspective to his decision-making.

The appearance of quality indices resulted from incessant demand on the part of users of the model for measures of performance. Of course, the indicators developed leave much to be desired from the point of view of immediate real world use. On the other hand, the real need for, and the present lack of, comprehensive environmental indicators might be mitigated by research in the direction of the GEM indices. (This refers to research of a conceptual nature, not on the limited surrogates chosen for use with the present version of the model.)

All of the dissatisfaction indices and quality of life indices are calculated in such a way that a high value indicates large dissatisfaction or low quality of life. In Figure 2.6, the components of the Quality of Life Index are illustrated. For each of the indices, the corresponding dissatisfaction term is provided in parentheses. These dissatisfaction are used as feedbacks throughout the Operating Programs.

Note that both of the components of the Environmental Index are indices which are based entirely upon locational quality factors outside the direct control of the social decision makers. For example, they can only indirectly affect water quality, school quality and local tax rates.

The Personal Index, on the other hand, is comprised of two indices, one of which is based on locational quality factors while the other is population oriented.

Interrelated Output: Two Examples

The total output of the CITY model is quite interrelated, for example, the following figures relate CITY map to various other outputs in the public and private sectors (see Figure 2.7):

HOUSING OUTPUT

TWOCITY
ECONOMIC DECISION MAKER B — RESIDENCE OUTPUT

LOCATICN	8828
TYPE AND LEVEL	RA 4
QUALITY INDEX	85
MAINTENANCE LEVEL	85
MS CISTRICT	1
UTILITY DISTRICT	1
DEPRECIATICN (%)	
MS	1.0
FIRE	0.5
FLCOD	0.0
WATER CONSUMPTICN (MGD)	
MUNICIPAL	0.30
CUTSIDE	0.12
OCCUPANTS	6M 0H
PERCENT OCCUPANCY	100
RENT/SPACE UNIT	159000
INCOME	
RENT	1272000
EXPENDITURES	
MAINTENANCE	98CC0
UTILITIES	160000
WATER	78840
PROPERTY TAXES	143410
INCOME TAXES	256750
SALES TAXES	3240
NET INCCME	531760
RATE CF RETURN	14.37
ENVIRCNMENTAL INDEXES	
LOW INCCME	204
MIDDLE INCOME	147
HIGH INCCME	139

INDUSTRY OUTPUT

TWOCITY
ECONOMIC DECISION MAKER G — BASIC INDUSTRY OUTPUT

LOCATION	9828
CONSTRUCTED LEVEL	TE 1
OPERATING LEVEL	TE 1
VALUE RATIO	100
MAINTENANCE LEVEL	100
MS DISTRICT	3
UTILITY DISTRICT	2
DEPRECIATICN (%)	
MS	5.0
FIRE	3.2
FLCOD	0.0
WATER QUALITY	0.0
WATER CONSUMPTION (MGD)	
NORMAL SOURCE	2.80
OUTSIDE	5.20
PERCENT WATER RECYCLED	0
EFFLUENT TREATMENT	
TYPE AND LEVEL	0
SALARY (PER WCRKER IN 100'S)	
HIGH	105
MIDDLE	55
LOW	26
EMPLOYEES	
FULL TIME (IN P1'S)	
HIGH	25
MIDDLE	22
LOW	15
PART TIME (IN UNITS)	
HIGH	80
MIDDLE	80
LOW	80
EMPLOYMENT EFFECT	1000
UNITS PRODUCED	1000
PRICE/UNIT OUTPUT	196800
INCCME	
SALES(PRIVATE)	196800000
EXPENDITURES	
GCODS	20000000
SERVICES	17400000
MAINTENANCE	20800000
UTILITIES	2000000
WATER	
RECYCLING	0
INTAKE PROCESS	0
OUTFLOW TREATMENT	0
MUNICIPAL SUPPLY	1274000
TRANSPORTATION	21860984
SALARIES	61320000
PROPERTY TAXES	1635000
SALES TAXES	1746000
INCOME TAXES	17974750
NET INCCME	32063266
RATE CF RETURN	17.81

MUNICIPAL SERVICES OUTPUT

MS	LCCATICN	LEVEL	MAINTENANCE LEVEL	VALUE RATIO	EFFECTIVE CAPACITY OF SERVICE	LOADING	EMPLOYMENT LOW	EMPLOYMENT MIDDLE	M.S. USE INDEX
2	94-30	1	80	80	440	2335	3	3	530
3	98-26	1	85	85	467	1180	3	3	252
TCTALS					0	3515	6	6	436

EMPLCYEE SHORTAGE LCW 6; MIDDLE 0
SALARY OFFERED LOW 2500; MIDDLE 5200.

WELFARE PAYMENT PER UNEMPLCYED WORKER IS 1600.

SCHOOL OUTPUT

SCHOOL UNITS

SCHOOL	LOCATION	LEVEL	MAINTENANCE LEVEL	VALUE RATIO	STUDENTS HIGH	STUDENTS MIDDLE	STUDENTS LOW	TEACHERS REQUESTED HIGH	TEACHERS REQUESTED MIDDLE	STUDENT/TEACHER RATIO	USE INDEX
1	9030	1	90	91	6240	11480	700	5	5	13	64
2	9032	1	90	91	8710	3920	0	5	4	10	48

CITY MAP

PARCEL KEY
TOP LEFT: OWNER
TOP RIGHT: ZONING
MIDDLE: LAND USE AND LEVEL
BOTTOM LEFT: UTILITY LEVEL
BOTTOM RIGHT: % UNDEVELOPED LAND

PARCEL EDGES
.. .. BOARDED
-- ll TYPE 1 ROAD
== HH TYPE 2 ROAD
WW TYPE 3 ROAD
00 00 JURISDICTION BOUNDARY

INTERSECTIONS
+ TYPE 1 TERMINAL
X TYPE 2 TERMINAL
* TYPE 3 TERMINAL

ZONING	LAND USE	ZONING	USE
--	ANY USE	33	PS
10	ANY BUSINESS	34	PC
20	HI,LI,CI	35	PS
21	HI	40	RA,RB,RC
22	LI	41	RA
23	CI	42	RB
30	NS,RG,RS,PC,PS	43	RC
31	NS	50	PARKLAND
32	RG		

Figure 2.7: ILLUSTRATION OF CITY MODEL OUTPUT AND RELATED CITY MAP

(A) The single-family housing on parcel 94-22 is located on the outskirts of the city. It is served by the First Municipal Service District and the school age children living there are in the Second School District. Figure 2.7 shows the characteristics of the people living in this housing.

(B) The Heavy Industry at 96-28 is located toward the center of the city. It attracts workers from many parts of the city (shown in still another output). It is served by the Second Municipal Service District.

(C) The School Department operates four comprehensive schools located at the specified sites. Each has school boundaries which define its service area. The map showing these districts is a separate piece of output.

(D) The Municipal Services Department has spatially located facilities which provide fire, police and health services. A use index above 100 for these facilities means that less than national average service is being provided.

A second example illustrates the interrelatedness of the output of the Social Sector to the other output printed by the model.

Population units (P1's) which live in the represented area attempt to find jobs, purchase goods and services, receive education, etc. Figure 2.8 is an illustration of how the computer output for the two PL's (low-income-class population units) on parcel 94-22 is related to the output generated by the major operating programs of migration (dissatisfaction), employment, transportation, commercial, and taxes (final accounting):

First, the dissatisfaction index of 113 places the two PL's in the middle-range of dissatisfaction for that class (120 PL's are more dissatisfied with their housing quality, rent paid, quality of schools and municipal services, etc. and 75 PL's are less dissatisfied).

Second, the two PL's are employed in jobs paying $3800 and $3500 per worker at the National Services at 94-28 and the Heavy Industry at 96-28, respectively.

Third, as a result of the availability and cost of public transit, the dollar value of time for the PL's, and highway congestion, both PL's travel to their jobs by private auto and consume four units of time and spent $220 annually for home-to-work transportation. The actual route traveled is also indicated.

Fourth, the consumption by the 2PL s on 94-22 for personal goods is made at the PG located at 90-24. As the commercial detail shows, 42 units of PG consumption were purchased at a price of $420,000, and transportation to shopping increased the total expenditure by $8,064.

Fifth, the students of the PL s on 94-22 attended the public schools in district #2 (see Figure 2.7).

Sixth, the population paid federal, state and local taxes. The local tax rates and the total revenue received as shown on the tax summary for the local jurisdiction.

In summary, the output section of the model has the highest visibility to the user or potential user. It had to be designed in an understandable, flexible, and convenient format so that users might easily grasp the status of the area being represented, relate problems to one another, and see the effects of the decisions they enact.

The CITY Model Subroutines Seen in the Form of the Elemental Framework

To illustrate the use of the elemental framework in the GEM series, we have divided subroutines of the CITY III version of the model into the five areas, (1) Data Base, (2) Executive Routines, (3) Input, (4) Operating Routines, and (5) Output (Figure 2.9).

A SIMULATION COMPILER

As model designers become more and more proficient at building models, they begin to notice, as we did, that certain operations which they are required to perform to produce a simulation are repeated time and time again. This realization has led to the formulation of various computer languages of which SYMSCRIPT, DYNAMO, and GPSS are probably the best known.[9] These three have one feature in common in that they are designed to make the modeling task easier for mathematicians and computer programmers. Provided the user will organize his data in a given fashion and be satisfied with the output format, he can use one or more of these languages when the problem with which he is confronted is of the correct form.

On the other hand, the logical extrapolation of the modeling form discussed in this book is not a language but a simulation compiler which, although useful for the mathematicians and system analyst, really almost obviates the need for consulting these specialists before models can be designed by the researcher and educator for computer usage.

If the end goal of GEM is realized, then the model will be able to load in data base and set the building blocks, be able to change not only any functional parameters in the model, but replace whole

SOCIAL SECTOR OUTPUT

EMPLOYMENT OUTPUT

EMPLOYMENT SELECTION INFORMATION FOR LOW INCOME CLASS

RESIDENCE LOCATION	EMPLOYER LOCATION	POPUL. UNITS	SALARY	TIME UNITS	AUTO COST	BUS COST	RAIL COST	ROUTE					
9422	UNEMPLOYED	0											
	9630	2	2800.	15.0	440.0	0.0	0.0	9529	9527	9525	9523		
	9432	2	2800.	20.0	540.0	0.0	0.0	9531	9529	9527	9525	9523	
	9832	1	2500.	22.5	615.0	0.0	0.0	9731	9531	9529	9527	9525	9523
	9432 (FSE)	2	2600.	20.0	540.0	0.0	0.0	9531	9529	9527	9525	9523	

COMMERCIAL ALLOCATION OUTPUT

CUSTOMERS

PERSONAL GOODS ASSIGNED TO	LOCATION	CLASS OR LAND USE	DECISION MAKER CONTROLLING	CONSUMPTION UNITS	TRANSPORTATION COST	PURCHASE COST	TOTAL COST
1	6828	RA	B	6	0.	78000.	78000.
1	8828	MID	A	171	0.	2223000.	2223000.

LOCAL TAX REVENUE

DISSATISFACTION OUTPUT

		NEIGHBORHOOD INDEX							
LOCATION	POLLUTION INDEX	CLASS	RESIDENCE QUALITY	RENT	MS	SCHOOL	WELFARE OR TAXES	TOTAL	ENVIRONMENTAL INDEX
9422	-7	LOW	13	30	100	0	32	175	168
		MIDDLE	33	0	100	0	26	158	151
		HIGH	43	0	100	0	26	168	161
9622	-15	LOW	44	0	100	44	16	204	189
		MIDDLE	64	0	100	44	26	234	219
		HIGH	74	0	100	44	26	244	229
9822	-7	LOW	10	0	100	44	16	170	163
		MIDDLE	30	0	100	44	26	200	193
		HIGH	40	0	100	44	26	210	203
10022	0	LOW	5	3	100	44	16	168	168
		MIDDLE	25	0	100	44	26	195	195
		HIGH	35	0	100	44	26	205	205
9424	-7	LOW	30	45	100	0	32	207	200
		MIDDLE	50	0	100	0	26	176	169
		HIGH	60	0	100	0	26	186	179
9624	-15	LOW	40	0	100	44	16	200	185
		MIDDLE	60	0	100	44	26	230	215
		HIGH	70	0	100	44	26	240	225
9824	-7	LOW	40	0	100	44	16	200	193
		MIDDLE	60	0	100	44	26	230	223
		HIGH	70	0	100	44	26	240	233
10024	0	LOW	35	0	100	44	16	195	195
		MIDDLE	55	0	100	44	26	225	225
		HIGH	65	0	100	44	26	235	235
10224	0	LOW	10	45	100	44	16	215	215
		MIDDLE	30	0	100	44	26	200	200
		HIGH	40	0	100	44	26	210	210
8826	0	LOW	0	78	100	0	32	210	210
		MIDDLE	9	22	100	0	26	156	156
		HIGH	19	1	100	0	26	145	145
9026	0	LOW	0	75	100	0	32	207	207
		MIDDLE	17	20	100	0	26	163	163
		HIGH	27	0	100	0	26	153	153
9226	0	LOW	9	9	100	0	32	150	150
		MIDDLE	29	0	100	0	26	154	154
		HIGH	39	0	100	0	26	164	164
9426	0	LOW	39	0	100	0	32	171	171
		MIDDLE	59	0	100	0	26	184	184
		HIGH	69	0	100	0	26	194	194
10026	0	LOW	50	0	100	44	16	210	210
		MIDDLE	70	0	100	44	26	240	240
		HIGH	80	0	100	44	26	250	250
10226	0	LOW	10	0	100	44	16	170	170
		MIDDLE	30	0	100	44	26	200	200
		HIGH	40	0	100	44	26	210	210
8628	0	LOW	0	9	100	0	32	141	141
		MIDDLE	5	0	100	0	26	131	131
		HIGH	15	0	100	0	26	141	141
8828	0	LOW	0	72	100	0	32	204	204
		MIDDLE	4	18	100	0	26	147	147
		HIGH	14	0	100	0	26	139	139
9028	0	LOW	9	60	100	0	32	201	201
		MIDDLE	29	10	100	0	26	164	164
		HIGH	39	0	100	0	26	164	164
10028	-7	LOW	44	0	100	44	16	204	197
		MIDDLE	64	0	100	44	26	234	227
		HIGH	74	0	100	44	26	244	237
10228	-7	LOW	24	21	100	44	16	205	198
		MIDDLE	44	0	100	44	26	214	207
		HIGH	54	0	100	44	26	224	217
8430	83	LOW	0	63	100	0	32	195	278
		MIDDLE	0	12	100	0	26	138	221
		HIGH	10	0	100	0	26	136	219
8630	83	LOW	0	99	100	0	32	231	314
		MIDDLE	0	36	100	0	26	162	245
		HIGH	10	8	100	0	26	144	227
8830	83	LOW	0	78	100	0	32	210	293
		MIDDLE	15	22	100	0	26	163	246
		HIGH	25	1	100	0	26	152	235
9030	83	LOW	0	9	100	0	32	141	224
		MIDDLE	10	0	100	0	26	136	219
		HIGH	20	0	100	0	26	146	229
10030	-15	LOW	39	0	100	0	16	155	140
		MIDDLE	59	0	100	0	26	185	170
		HIGH	69	0	100	0	26	195	180
10230	-15	LOW	19	9	100	0	16	144	129
		MIDDLE	39	0	100	0	26	165	150
		HIGH	49	0	100	0	26	175	160
10830	0	LOW	0	75	100	0	16	191	191
		MIDDLE	0	20	100	0	26	146	146
		HIGH	10	0	100	0	26	136	136
8432	166	LOW	0	93	100	0	32	225	391
		MIDDLE	0	32	100	0	26	158	324
		HIGH	9	6	100	0	26	140	306
8632	166	LOW	0	90	100	0	32	222	388
		MIDDLE	0	30	100	0	26	156	322
		HIGH	10	5	100	0	26	141	307
8832	166	LOW	0	36	100	0	32	168	334

Figure 2.8: SOCIAL SECTOR OUTPUT

FIGURE 2.9

THE ELEMENTAL FRAMEWORK AND THE CITY MODEL

AREAS	NAME	DESCRIPTION
	BIGCITY	
	BLUECITY	
	DOTCITY	
	LARGECITY	
	MADZOOONE	
	MADZOOTWO	Data Bases
	SMALLCITY	
	TELECITY	
	THREECITY	
	TWOCITY	
	TWOFLE	data base of inputs for TWOCITY
3	ACAUC	makes decisions on auction land bids at end of EDIT
3	ACBLD	actualize builds and demolitions
3	ACRID	actualize redistricting at end of EDIT
3	AS	assessment input (\$ASMNT)
5	ASMAP	routine to print assessment maps
4	ASSESS	main assessment driver
4	ASSES1	called by ASSESS to do assessment for each parcel
4	ASSES2	prints assessment data
4	ASSES3	picks up data from assessment input file
4	ATTACHF	adds records when needed for GM
4	ATTCHF	adds records when needed for GT
4	AUCTN	generates parcels up for auction and sets values for all unowned land
4	AUCTN1	called by AUCTN to find distances
1	BCINT	subroutine of LOAD for boycotts, GS-BS contracts
3	BLDRR	actualize rail build called by RAIL. Input program
1	BNDNTY	enters bonds into files
4	BNDPAY	calculates bond payment
3	BRIAN	initializes file for FSA requests
	BUILD	main build input program. Accepts or rejects and enters those accepted on constr. table. (\$BUILD) or (\$OUBLD)
5	BUSOUT	bus output entire. Financial and maintenance calculations
3	BYCT	boycott input (\$BYCT)
3	CASHT	cash transfer input (\$CASH)
3	CCHEK	input check on owner of land, amount available, jurisdiction, and CI
3	CHECK	used by vote
5	CHMAN	chairman output, called by PBOUT
3	CHPVT	(\$CVPT) general input change
2	CITY	main post-process routine
4	CLNATTM	called by MIGRAT to update attachment records
5	CNTRCT	list BG-BG contracts calledby SCHOUT and PWSRPT
2	COLAPF	cleans attachment records
4	CONAC	process construction files and determine status of builds after employment. At end of CITY, through ACBUL, actualizes builds.
5	CONIN	lists construction contracts for contractor and contractee. Called by PRYOUT.
4	CONTRC	maintains schools and MS's and determines amount of BG-BS required and allocates it if there are contracts. Called by OPTCM.
4	COTRN	return cost for transportation construction site.
3	COUNTR	called by VOTE
4	DEPREC	depreciation of all but BUS,RAIL, and roads.
2	DFIXUPM	adjust list of residences in order of dissatisfaction Called by MIGRAT.
4	DHISTM	called by MIGRAT. Builds histogram matrix.
2	DLTEF	deletes an entry from attachment records.
4	DPRTAX	calculate property tax. Called by PRYOUT.
4	DSORTM	called by MIGRAT. Sort Pl's by dissatisfaction.
5	ECBOY	economic and social boycott printout. Called by PRYOUT and TELOUT.
2	EDIT	main input. Decodes input stream according to formats.
4	EMP	employment
2	ENTAF	enters data to attachment records
2	EXFND	find item in an array
2	FILCKRF	dummy called between each routine in CITY, used in debugging.
2	FILDEFF	define file structure
2	FILZROF	zero files
5	FISTA	economic financial output in PRYOUT
3	FSA	FSA input
3	FSAAMT	calculate amount of FSA available on build. Called by BUILD.
3	FSAID	FSA input (\$FSA)
4	FSMAX	determine maximum level of FSA available
1	GARY	initialize assessment input. Has assessment constants. Called by Load.
2	GDATA	data statements basic to many programs.
2	GETMAP	generate MS map, UT map, park map, zoning map, SCH map, HY map and beginning maps.

AREAS	NAME	DESCRIPTION
5	HSTPRNM	print histogram scales
5	HWYMAP	highway map. Called by CITY
5	HYMAP	highway output
1	IANNP	annual payment on loan or bond
1	IASGL	called by LOAD. Sets boundaries
2	IBCOR	transforms coordinates
2	IBIN	random number getter in binary
2	IBLIN	transforms coordinates
2	IBLOCK	block input user
2	IBNPY	annual payment on bonds
4	ICROWD	degree of residential crowding. Called by MIGRAT.
5	IDEMEC	summary output. Zeros files for next round.
2	IEF	effective capacity of SC or MS
2	INDATA	data statements used by input. Like GDATA.
2	INROAD	returns two parcels bounding a given road.
3	INRTN3	($QUERY)
2	IOCF	generates cost of UT operation.
2	IPRIN	calculates principle payment for loan or bond.
2	IRLIN	transforms intersection coordinates.
4	ISTRESM	called by MIGRAT. Finds best residence available.
2	ITOTP	calculate remaining principle on loan or bond.
1	JUCNML	called by LOAD and determines UT level required.
3	JURWRDV	called by VOTE.
5	LANDO	land summary output.
2	LDIST	straight-line distance between parcels.
2	LINT	4 parcels surrounding an intersection.
1	LNDPARL	called by LOAD to process government cards.
4	LOADMS	determines drain on MS.
4	LOADSC	assign children to schools.
2	LOANS	enter loans and generate loan and bond interest rates.
5	LOSTA	loan statement on economic output (PRYOUT).
2	LUAMT	called by LOAD. Determine land requirements.
2	LUTS	level of UT necessary given land use.
5	MAPA	5 maps at beginning of output. Prints.
5	MAP3	print public maps.
2	MARGIN	suppress or restore output margins.
2	MEDIT	main EDIT driver.
3	MFSA	called by FSA. prints information at end of EDIT.
5	MGSTATM	migration statistics.
4	MIGRATM	main migration driver.
2	MINT	used by EMP in transportation.
4	MOVINM	called by MIGRAT to alter attachment records.
4	MOVOUTM	called by MIGRAT to alter attachment records.
5	MPGEN	generate maps for public information, like MAP3.
5	MSMAP	print MS map.
2	MVOTEV	main vote driver.
2	NCODDCOD	simulate FORTRAN encode-decode.
2	NEAR	find intersections adjoining parcel.
3	NEWBR	input to change routes ($ROUT).
5	NEWCON	print government contruction tables.
2	NEWJOB	determine # new jobs available based on new construction. Used by IDEMEC.
4	NSPACK	load night school.
2	NUMEDT	insert commas in #s.
2	NWBND	determine amount of current bonding necessary.
4	OFPTRC	computes time cost of travel.
4	OPTCM	main commercial optimizer. Calls CONTRC. Renovates buildings.
2	PAYMNT	interest and principle remaining on loan or bond.
2	PBDEBT	figure amount of outstanding principle owed by a department.
5	PBOUT	main output driver for MS, UT, PZ, CH.
4	PCTAB	table of commercial establishments. Called by OPTCM. Has outside costs.
3	PEOPLE	Called by VOTE.
4	PKOPT	park optimizer and time allocation and update voter registration and education level.
5	PLINE	prints line for maps. Called by MAPA.
3	PRBND	prints bond list for department.
2	PREMP	main CITY driver thru employment.
5	PRIBONT	print bonds for teletype output.
5	PRKLOC	park location -- use map.
5	PRYOU	main economic output driver.
2	PSTEMP	main CITY driver past employment.
3	PU	($PU) land purchase input program.
3	PUNC	alter character set used in input ($PUNC).
5	PWSRPT	MS output.
5	PZONMP	PZ map.
5	PZRPT	PZ output.
3	QUERYT	used by teletype and INRTN3.
3	RAIL	build rail and station input ($RAIL).
2	RANGUS	generate random number given mean and standard.
2	RDATTM	read and write residence attachment for MIGRAT.
2	RDMISC	read miscellaneous file for MIGRAT.
5	RDSET	road matrix for MAPA.

AREAS	NAME	DESCRIPTION
4	RDWEAR	road depreciation for highway. Also maintains.
2	REDEJT	read GT files.
2	REDERITE	random read-write.
3	REDIST	redistrict input for MS and SC ($REDIST)
2	RETER	decrease term of loans.
5	RROUT	rail output.
5	RTBMAP	bus and rail route map.
5	SCHMAP	school map.
5	SCHOUT	school output.
3	SHEMPT	called by QUERY to produce shopping and employment detail.
3	SORTEMV	used by VOTE.
2	SPLIT	coordinate transformation.
2	SPROB	probability function.
3	STARTV	used by VOTE.
3	TALOC	time allocation input ($TIME).
3	TAXES	taxes input ($TAXES).
5	TAXSUM	print tax summary on chairman output.
2	TELEOUTT	main driver for teletype output.
2	TELETOTT	debug for TELEOUT.
4	TERMS	terminal optimizer.
4	TINIT	off-peak transportation initialization. Generates road costs for OPTCM.
2	TMF	team letter to # conversion, and vice versa.
4	TRAFIC	employment transportation optimizer.
4	TRTRC	trace route used to work.
4	TSCAN	transportation optimizer used by OPTCM.
4	TSRCH	find least cost for transportation for EMP.
2	TSTRT	test route map. Main driver.
5	UNDVLT	print undeveloped land for public in teletype version.
5	UNUSE	print undeveloped land for public.
5	UTMAP	print utility map.
5	UTRPT	print utility output.
3	VALUE	dollar value of time input ($VALUE).
2	VDATAV	data statements used by VOTE.
3	VOTESV	used by VOTE.
4	WEIGHTM	used to generate dissatisfaction based on overcrowding for MIGRAT.
5	WRHEAD	write heading.
5	WRITM	print charater manipulation.
5	WRPOPM	write population tables for MIGRAT.
2	ZERO	zero elements of an array.
3	ZNCH	keep track of new zoning changes.
2	ZRRESM	generate list for MIGRAT.

modules. The user will be able to set his own indices (performance standards) and format his output to his own needs. This suggests a level of model flexibility which has heretofore been impossible.

The final evolution of the output stage would be in the form of a "list processor." A list processor would allow the user to add to, delete from, or reformat data before each model run. Further, it would allow the calculation of simple indices, etc., and other tests to be run on the existing data base, in addition to whatever calculations were already part of the ordinary output.

However, once such a framework is completed, the money spent for modeling can be focused toward refining the model relationships, rather than continually diverted toward structural handling. This might prompt more use of models, as the researcher, educator, or policy maker does not have to add large amounts of expensive programming to his cost estimates each time he wants to use modern analytical techniques to attack or illustrate a problem.

The next chapter focuses on a theoretical structure which allows one to organize concepts and data on the system into a form for insertion into the framework.

Chapter 3

SECTOR THEORY

The terms model and theory are so intertwined in many people's minds that in discussions about the GEM model, the subject of its root theory inevitably comes up. Until the sector theory evolved, the queries were all met with the disappointing response that there was no single theory nor was there a particular blueprint being developed.

The CITY series of GEM began its development as a gaming simulation. Its original construct was as an economic model relating man to his physical environment, but dealing mostly with his role as an entrepreneur. The fact that the model did not represent many other parts of the system prodded expansion of the model and each function of the system became a separate sector. The first addition was the area of government, representing the land uses, functions and resources of a city administration. About halfway through the project we envisioned time as a resource and also added a social sector. Each potential function to be carried out in an urban area was noted and then combined into various decision roles so that each game player had about the same amount of resources at his disposal.

FIGURE 3.1

INTERRELATIONSHIP OF COMPONENTS IN AN URBAN SYSTEM

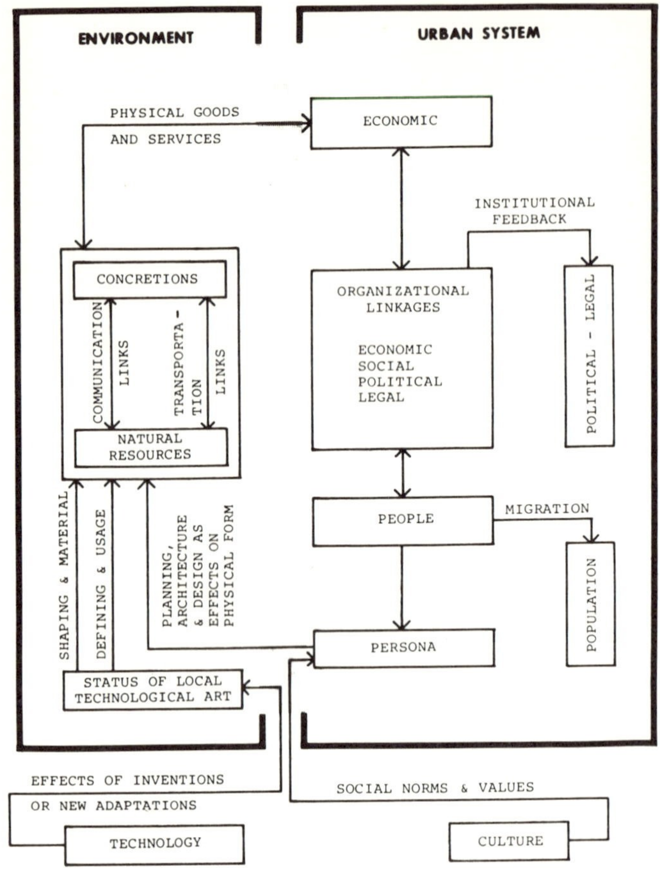

This concern for the role of each of the game players led to the first approximation of a descriptive theory which dealt with resource allocation.

COMPONENTS OF THE URBAN SYSTEM

The following description of an urban system (see Figure 3.1) is designed to show the interrelationships of the system's components. It is not meant to be an operational theory but a framework for organizing relationships which are not now precisely known or quantified.

Four of the urban system's components are physically oriented aspects of the environment and consist of: natural resources, concretions (man-made physical structures), internal connectors (transportation and communication linkages), and technology. The last three components are people-oriented: population, organizations, and persona.

The last component–persona–provides the character, ethos, culture, and style of the local system. Although the concept of persona, or personality, of an area may seem obvious when mentioned, it is easily overlooked.

The component typology was not a sufficient explanation of our model which participants could understand and use. We had to devise a way that would open it up meaningfully. The concept of sectors answered this need. It provided both an effective way of dividing the resources of the model for game participants and also seemed to describe the system more clearly for those programming the model for computer use.

A SECTOR CONSTRUCT OF URBAN COMPONENTS

A sector is a theoretical construct which includes a series of relationships and their concomitant data to describe some portion of a total system[10] (see Figure 3.1). The three sectors we derived to describe the sector concept, economic, governmental and social, allowed us to focus our research into relatively tidy areas, even though we clearly recognized that the divisions were largely artificial. This framework for looking at the GEM model as consisting of three sectors is fitted into an overall structure of the urban system as a representation of the relationship between people and their environment. It also takes into consideration the relationship between a local and extralocal, or outside, system.

THE TOTAL SYSTEM TO BE MODELED

The Outside System

Assuming that we can define a particular system in a geographic and functional sense, we must then define the larger system within which it functions.[11] For a neighborhood, the larger system might be a city; for the city, a metropolitan area; and so on through a regional area, a megalopolis, a nation and finally the world. For our purposes, we will assume that the larger system is the totality of all the systems outside the specific one under consideration.

The outside system provides several major functions. We will discuss four for illustrative purposes:

(1) The larger system determines the political, legal and social institutional limits within which the local area will operate and develop. For example, the local area is legally bound by national and state laws. In addition, the larger system dictates and influences the social customs which become internalized within the smaller system.

(2) The larger system defines the technological framework in which the local system operates. The local system is both an innovator and receptor of changes to and from the outside system. Technical changes made on the larger system eventually filter down to local systems. This can be seen in the case of Robert Fulton's steamboat, which was developed in one subsystem and eventually had repercussions throughout all local areas. The larger system's role was that of a receptor of a particular invention made at one local area and subsequently acted as a clearing house for the innovations of local areas.

,(3) Factors at the larger system level affect the population growth of a local system. The outside system supplies inmigrants for local areas and in turn receives people who move out of the local area. Two of the more striking examples in this country were the migrations of people out of the rural areas and into urban areas at the turn of the century, and out of the cities and into the suburban areas after World War II.

(4) The existence of the larger area provides an economic network for the smaller system and allows it to specialize. Most local systems have a comparative advantage in producing particular types of goods and/or services. They are therefore able to produce these items relatively cheaply

and trade them for those produced by other subsystems in the outside system. Thus, the larger system provides both the organism and the organization for economic exchange.

In addition to using the larger milieu for exchange purposes, the local economic system is also affected by such things as the business cycle, monetary policy, and fiscal policy of the larger system.

The Inside or Local System

Although the ultimate simulation would probably handle both the outside and local systems in equal detail, at present this is not possible. We will therefore focus mainly on the local system, as represented in our models, and show ties to the outside system only to the extent needed to provide local closure.

The local system consists of two parts, the natural environment and society.

The Natural Environment

The earth, air, water and climate are natural resources and nature's endowment to a particular area. Their characteristics include such factors as terrain, slope, soil type, mineral content, weather and climatic conditions and amount of available water. The climate and natural foliage affect the style and living patterns of the inhabitants. The presence of valleys, rivers, mountains or plains influences the use and type of buildings, the size of the city, the placement of streets, and even the number of people. The availability of sufficient potable water alone often proves to be a significant limiting factor on present and future urban forms.

The economic base of a regional system, for instance, is greatly affected by the type of natural resources in the area. The presence of a deep water harbor allows the operation of particular industries which require bulk raw material import and bulk shipment export. These features, and others, help to explain many major American seaports. Natural resources, such as large nearby deposits of coal and iron, plus good transportation access, permitted the growth of a steel industry in Pittsburgh and allowed other related types of manufacturing to develop nearby. The field of economic geography documents numerous cases of localities whose original structures were defined by the physical environment. In summary, while not the only defining feature, the natural environment both limits and sets potentials for the locale.

A large part of man's environment is self-created. These man-made structures include homes, stores, factories, roads, plazas and the like. For simplicity's sake, we will call these man-made creations, "concretions."

Prior to the construction of any structure at all, the early settlers had broad freedom to design and shape their locales. They were limited only by the building techniques available at the time, their imaginations, needs, funds, materials, and most of all, the natural landscape. However, as an area grows in population, the importance of the natural landscape begins to diminish and the new construction desires of the inhabitants become more limited by the concretions already existent. Generally, developments in a growing area not only follow the natural terrain, as it is the easiest for the settlers to deal with, but later developments also follow the path of least resistance demarcated by existing man-made structures. Telephone lines, water and sewer mains, streets, sidewalks, overhead lights and many other capital improvements are invested in the present city form. These, not to mention stores, homes and office buildings, tend to limit the number of alternatives open to expanding or changing the face of a community.

In short, the environment is a limiting and shaping factor on all urban growth and development. The more developed an area is, the more set it becomes with each subsequent construction. In this way, the concretions themselves become a major shaping force of an area, and even more so as the amount of natural environment shrinks. As a result, the larger and more developed an area is, the more difficult it is to overhaul it.

If we were to consider the environment as merely made up of a landscape dotted with concretions, we would be hard pressed indeed to understand how humans could function in the milieu. In truth, our mental image of this area is one in which some sort of order has been imposed by the intercession of such things as streets, roadways, railways and water courses. The entire mechanism of moving goods and people in, out, and around a local system is referred to as a transportation network and is one of the two connectors which made the environment a cohesive whole.

These connectors have an interesting two-way relationship to the local area. They are created where access is needed to move people or goods and, therefore, can be said to follow the demands of the locale. On the other hand, once created, they allow the formation of new clusters of concretions and so can be thought of as demand creating. The most obvious current example is the development of interstate highways and large city beltways. This duality of purpose results in transportation acting as both a cohesive force, defining and delineating an area, and as a major determinant of areal growth.

The second type of internal connector is communication. These links, which include radio, TV, newspapers, telegraph, telephone, magazines and the like, are not as structurally visible as the transportation links but are vitally important as descriptors and definers of local communities.

Society

The society, or people, portion of our model structure includes the relatively static portion of the human environment, the composition of the society itself. As with the physical environment, these individuals, unless connected by linkages, are not able to be thought of as a functional whole. Population, in this context, would include the number of people in a local system and their associated characteristic: their spatial distribution and density, their rates of growth, and their composition in terms of age, sex, race, and social class.

Population characteristics, such as social class, race, and age composition help determine the basic work force, the potential work force, the types of service and entertainment industries and other labor-related factors. They also yield the social and political institutions and forces of a local system.

We have described the linkages between the natural landscape and man-made structures in terms of transportation and communication. Similarly, we find that there are linkages within the population and between the population and the environmental structure. These linkages evolve functionally and necessarily through the increasing complexity of the system. They create more or less permanent slots which individuals fill. This is the essence, for example, of a bureaucracy, one of the many organizational structures. For convenience, we will break these into two broad categories: organizational structures which relate people to people, and those which relate people to their environment.

The organizational channels which relate people to people can be either formal or informal. Formally, for example, portions of tort law are largely concerned with injuries to persons instead of damage to property. Informally, all of our manners and customs which

FIGURE 3.2
RESOURCE FLOW IN THE ECONOMIC SECTOR

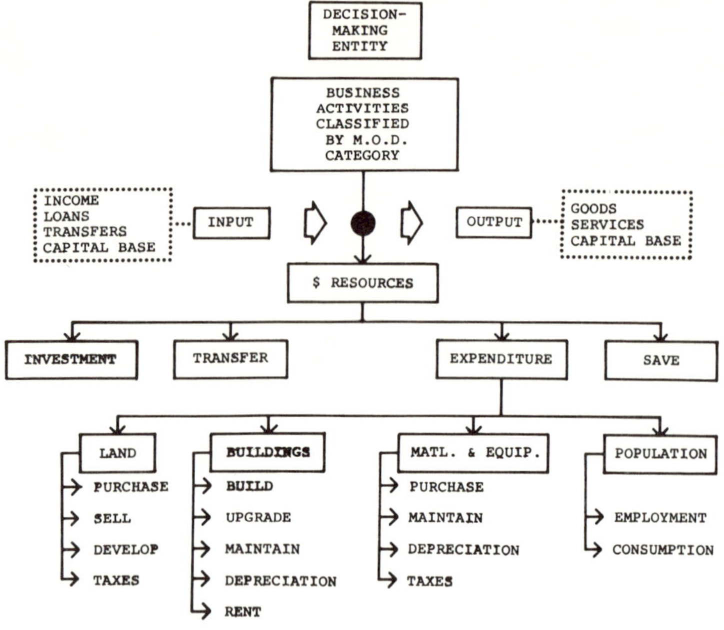

prescribe what we wear, what we eat and drink, what we say to each other, or organizational linkages, too. They provide continuity and change relatively slowly over time. Our political structures and forms, at local and national levels, along with the style of politics which we prefer, are manifestations of our system's attempt to organize itself so that its population can function smoothly. The business community with its formal structure and methods of operation shows similar arrangements, including hiring and firing policies, number of working days, coffee breaks, and the like.

There are just as many organizational linkages set up between people and their environment as there are among people themselves. Simple mathematical calculations like profit and loss, of supply and demand concepts, or even the business organizational structure itself, are artifacts set up by man to score and to organize himself in the business community. The business community, in turn, is organized so that it can operate in and within the larger urban system. It seems that even the concepts of public and private are designed to relate man to the natural and man-made environment.

These relationships can be used to define the Data Base of GEM but only begin to explain how the model is interrelated. It is not until the system is divided into Sectors and their respective resources manipulated that the behavioral feature of the various decision makers begins to become clear.

RESOURCE FLOWS IN THE ECONOMIC, GOVERNMENT AND SOCIAL SECTORS

Economic Sector

The Economic Sector includes all of the private business-type institutions in the system It is broken down into industrial, commercial and residential divisions with all the related decision-making possibilities (Figure 3.2).

The various economic activities are allocated financial resources which they can save or spend. The method and amount of expenditures of these resources affect other parts of the system and feed back to change the resource base for the next time period.

Figure 3.2 indicates the schematic flow of resources in the Economic Sector. Resources are specified in items such as income, loans, etc., which are available for input and distribution in the

FIGURE 3.3
RESOURCE FLOW IN THE GOVERNMENT SECTOR

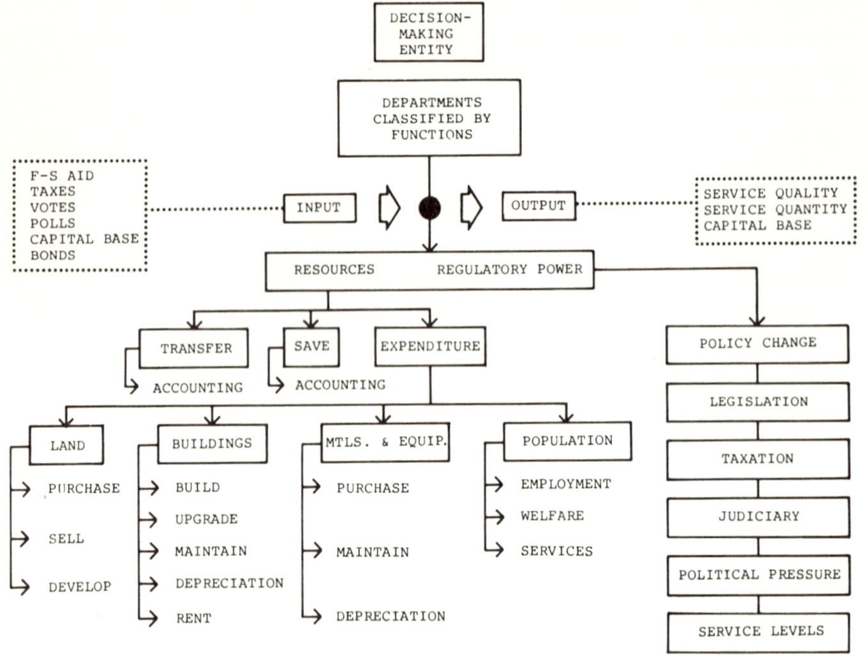

system by a decision-making entity (e.g., a business activity). The decision entity thus acts as a control valve on the distribution of resources throughout the system. Once a decision is initiated, the resource is then allocated and routines perform an accounting of the resulting effects. A response to these system effects is fed back to the decision entity after each iteration cycle in the form of an output or status report. This output is expressed in both qualitative and quantitative resource units.

The typology at this point proceeds to describe the categories of resource expenditure. The resource, capital, (liquid and fixed) can be invested either inside the system in the form of intangible assets or outside the system in any form. The capital can also not be utilized (spent) at all and therefore (in the Keynsean sense) is assumed to be saved. If the capital is transferred between sectors, it is largely a system bookkeeping function. For example, liquid assets are transferred from the private to the public sector through the expedient of taxation. Finally, the resource of capital can be spent. The expenditure can be in four areas (as in micro-economics) of land, buildings, materials, equipment and people.

The expenditure of capital on land is of a binary nature. Either the land can be developed or left as undeveloped land. If left undeveloped it can be sold or purchased or rented.

The act of developing land moves it to the category of buildings. These buildings can be built, upgraded, maintained, sold, or rented.

Buildings, particularly when used for commercial or industrial purposes requires the addition of materials and equipment. These factors of production can also be maintained, purchased or rented.

Finally, there is an expenditure of capital for people. Usually, this expenditure is in the form of employment. However, it can also be in the form of welfare payments or for services. The concept of people and capital also means consumption of goods and services.

Government Sector

The Government Sector is the public area which supplies municipal goods and services to the citizenry; i.e., police and fire protection, utilities, schools, highways (Figure 3.3). The resources available to the system are both financial and regulatory. The end results of these government decisions have repercussions throughout the environment.

Figure 3.3 indicates the schematic flow of resources in the

FIGURE 3.4
RESOURCE FLOW IN THE SOCIAL SECTOR

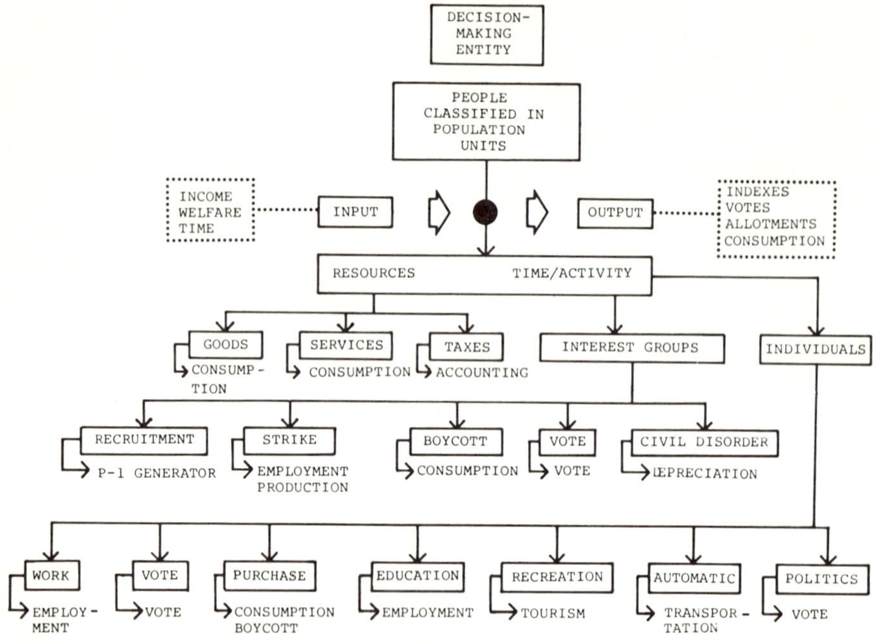

Government Sector. Resources are specified in items such as federal-state aid, bonds, etc., and are available for input and distribution in the system by a decision-making entity (e.g., a government department). As in the Economic Sector, the decision entity distributes the Sector resources. Once a decision is made, it is interrelated to the rest of the system. The model then reports the quantitative and qualitative effects of this interaction.

The last resource, power, is dispersed throughout the sectors (economic, social, and political). The power can be used to get a policy change, to enact legislation, to initiate and levy taxes, to perform a judicial function, to apply political pressure to gain other ends, and to provide and maintain service levels.

Social Sector

The Social Sector is the only sector in which participants can be concerned with people. It is largely quality-oriented (quality of life) and provides a quantifiable response to the subjective reactions of citizens to the inputs from the other sectors.

Figure 3.4 indicates the schematic flow of resources in the Social Sector. Resources are specified in items such as income, time, etc., which are available for input and distribution in the system by a decision-making entity (in this case, population units). Again these decisions are meshed with those of the Economic and Government Sectors and the current data base. These are all fed into the computer and then distributed to each sector in the output phase.

Time is the principal resource of people. When people act in groups the time is used to recruit members, to strike or boycott, for training and policing, for voting or, as a last resort, for civil disorder. The individuals' use of time (part of which is to join an organization) is divided between work, purchasing, education, recreation, politics, traveling and leisure.

Sector Resources Flows

We have at this point described the concept of a sector, a decision-making unit; and an element, which is a system's functional unit. Both of these conceptualizations have the common trait of being descriptive features of the overall system. It is the responsibility of the typology designer or builder to define them and to make his decisions known as part of his overall assumption.

FIGURE 3.5
RESOURCES

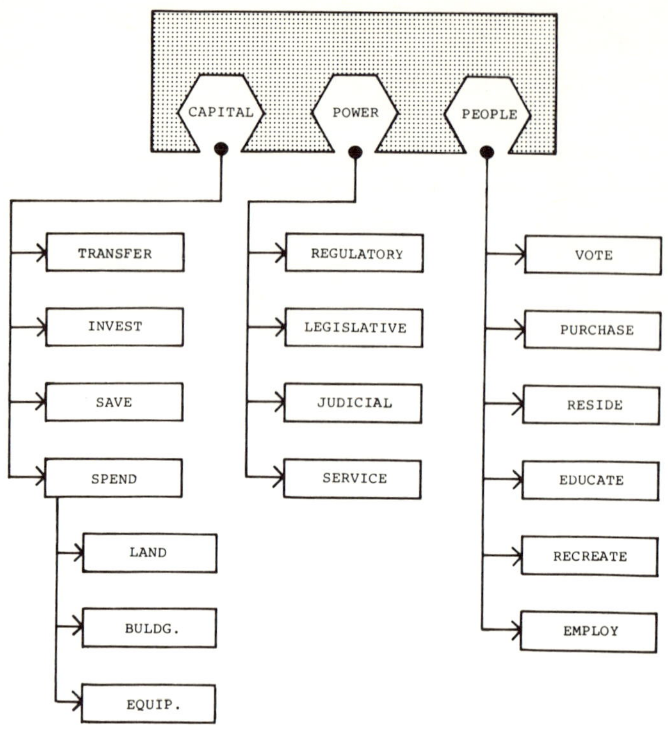

In order to see the interaction that takes place within the total system, the GEM model is better viewed as a resource allocation device. As such, it is based on a series of assumptions and decisions made by humans, machine simulations, or a combination of both, to allocate various types of resources among a number of alternative uses. The three general types of resources considered are capital, power and people.

The concept of a resource includes both qualitative and quantitative measures. The relationship between quantity and quality is the prime determinant of the supply of a resource, whereas the relationship between the supply and demand of an asset for any use determines its actual value. Counting the resource in quantitative terms of capital, power, or people is relatively easy. The determination of quality, however, is highly subjective. Consequently, the model is structured so that the user is able (by changing parameter values) to set his own quality factors.

Capital, Power, People

Capital—A resource which consists of physical assets, such as the plant and equipment of a business, and money; or intangible assets, such as the potential productive power of a labor force. The tangible capital resource base is first considered as a given amount of land and/or number of buildings. These assets are transferable into cash value depending upon a number of factors such as their quality and final demand (Figure 3.5).

Power—Usually thought of as an intangible asset and associated with any form of business, political, or institutional activity. In terms of GEM, the concept of power is only used explicitly when the "win" strategy of a particular sector is measured.

For example, it is normally not possible for a department of the government to serve the people of a system with a particular service and have the same profit maximization matrix as a business. Since the need for resources is theoretically a function of the system's needs for a particualr service and there never seem to be sufficient funds for all the departments to provide these services, the only possibility for getting a larger share of the budget is to take a portion from another department. This is one exercise of power.

Government is formally the seat of regulatory power in the system and the final arbitrator of all disputes. Its function is to apportion

FIGURE 3.6
RESOURCES ALLOCATION

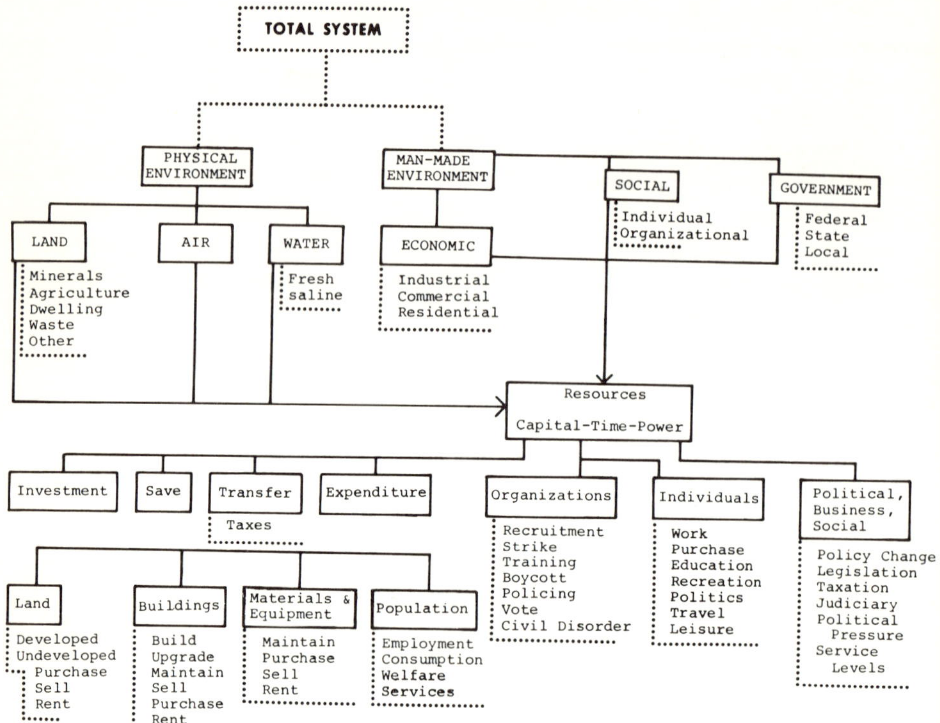

power so that it is able to perform the services required by its citizens most efficiently and so that other sectors are free to handle their responsibilities with a minimum amount of friction. They do this through the mechanizm of laws and regulations, which they enforce in a court through legislative procedures which this sector sets up and maintains. These processes are another type of power which can be quantified and are recognized by the system at large.

People—Their changeable desires and the amount of time they have available are a system resource which is often ignored in many models. Decisions by people as to how they value their surroundings and allocate their time[12] have pronounced effects on the outputs of the general system. For example, a decision on the part of a large segment of the population to spend more time in leisure or educational activities and less in work-oriented pursuits, usually forces the other portions of the system to adjust their resource allocations to meet these desires. Personal time budgeting has been under careful study lately as more and more researchers discover the importance of this resource as a system commodity.

Allocation of Resources

The diagram in Figure 3.6 ties in the above concepts and represents the resource allocation flow of the General Environmental Model.

The actual methods of handling these allocations are not specified; however, the general categories can be noted. In terms of capital, the owners of this resource can take the money available and save it, invest it, transfer the capital to others within a sector or to other sectors, or spend capital resources to acquire or improve such items as land, buildings, materials, and equipment. The power resource is expended through a control mechanism which provides legislative, judicial, service, and regulatory functions for the system Finally, people allocate their time to voting, shopping, living, education, recreation, work, and other activities.

This method of looking at activities and resources in a system allows us to explain a number of factors about the model. The resource base of a total system, for instance, assumes that at any given period of time the total amount of resources available to different decision makers in each of the sectors comes from a given known amount; i.e., the resources available in the base year. The model's iteration through a single cycle takes into account not only this base amount, but the changes to this amount as influenced by human or machine inputs. Consequently, charting resources and their allocation can be viewed both as a description of the resource base of the system and, at the same time, as a description of all the possible areas in which change can occur within the system.

A resource allocation model of the environment, divided into the major sectors which control these resources, provides a form of system analysis which allows for a relatively clear series of networks through which the various mediums of exchange can flow and be traded off. Although each of these sectors is more or less clearly distinct from the others, as they interact in the allocation of their various resources bases the distinction often becomes blurred. This model form also appears to be most useful as a take-off point for the construction of a computer model of the environment.

The use of the descriptive forms presented as the Sector theory requires that each of the major components of man's social system, the Economic, Political, and Social, be thought of as having distinct (although obviously overlapping) resources which can be allocated in definable ways to achieve measurable ends or to acquire concrete ends. The success of this methodology will require that we begin as a science to attempt to measure such things as power. This resource, along with other input and output variables, has long been relegated to the area of the nonquantifiable. Early theoreticians argued that such factors were not measurable in an ordinal sense but only in a relative one. Unfortunately, the economist took this warning to mean that these parameters represented forbidden ground. In recent years the sorties into welfare economics and full scale cost-benefit analysis have weakened this doctrine. Numerous techniques are evolving to attempt to deal with data of relative form (as well as numerous behavioral writers who are beginning to question the fact that such parameters are inherently unmeasurable). It is only when the social sciences have learned to deal with the full range of resources that meaningful holistic models will be able to be developed.

Taking the resource flows and adding the various sectors to these flows in the framework of a total system we arrived at Figure 3.6. The typology not only provides us with a descriptive framework for building a model such as GEM but is the basis for a complete theory of a social system regardless of the level of abstraction.

However, since the focus of this work is the GEM model, we will shift our attention to the actual modeling methodology used to relate these factors to each other in a fashion that they could be utilized.

Chapter 4

MODELS AND MODELING METHODS

SOME COMPARISONS

It is all but impossible to realistically discuss the similarities and differences between models. Yet, some comparisons with other models is inevitable, for no other reason than to put the model in a general frame of reference.

Probably the most striking feature of the GEM-CITY model, from a designer's point of view, is the combination of detail and scope. The detail is evident from the number of activities represented and the sophistication of the relationships that tie those activities together. The scope of the model is evident in the number of decisions that may be made by the user in the economic, government, social, and outside system sectors.

To illustrate some of the detail included in the model, it will be compared with a number of other models in terms of the number of elements it contains. Further, to allude to the scope of the model, CITY will be compared with different classes of models. Thus, the land use detail in the model is compared with other land use models.

TABLE 4.1

COMPARISON OF THE CITY MODEL WITH OTHER LAND USE MODELS

	Other Land Use Models	CITY Model
Number of Types of Private Land Uses	CATS – 6 EMPIRIC – 4 UNC – 1 PITTS – 5 PJ – 10 SFCRP – 27+	40 (12 agricultural, 11 manufacturing, 3 retail, 5 services, etc.)
Number of Types of Residences	CATS – 1 UNC – 9 EMPIRIC – 2 PITTS – 1 PJ – 6+ SFCRP – 114	40 (5 income classes, 2 races, and 4 household categories)
Elements in Attractiveness of Parcel	CATS – 2 UNC – 55 EMPIRIC – 5 PITTS – 2 SFCRP – 5	9+ (tax assessment, intraparcel and interparcel transportation indices, zoning, land code, quality of government services, etc.)
Size of Parcels	CATS – ¼ sq mi UNC – 23 acres (2.5 acre subparcels) EMPIRIC – irregular PITTS – 1 sq mi PJ – ¼ sq mi SFCRP – 2 acres	Variable (ranging from a portion of a census tract to an entire county)

CODE: CATS = Chicago Area Transportation Study
UNC = University of North Carolina Model
EMPIRIC = EMPIRIC Model
PITTS = Model of a Metropolis
PJ = Penn-Jersey Model
SFCRP = San Francisco Community Renewal Program

Table 4.1 shows four characteristics of six land use models along with the same characteristics for the CITY model. Most of these six models were developed for transportation to create travel parameters (origins and destinations as well as amount of traffic generated). The theoretical basis for many of these models is a gravity approach which takes one of the basic laws of physics and applies it to the area of human interaction. The models assume that the attraction of particular modes (areas) to each other is directly proportional to the mass at each point but is inversely proportional to the distance between them. As is true for the CITY model, most of these models did not have land use as their primary focus. The comparison, however, is quite illustrative. Diversity in land uses was not very important in these selected models. The type of manufacturing or residential development, in most cases, was not considered because in the minds of the designers, the purpose for which the model was developed did not require such detail. The CITY model, on the other hand, was developed as a general purpose model in which the employment requirements, land consumption, pollution generated, transportation requirements, and local service requirements of manufacturing industries are important. A more detailed discussion follows.

Input-Output Models

Input-Output is a detailed account of flows between sectors of the economy. The inputs and outputs of all of the areas under consideration are measured in terms of some least common denominator (usually dollars) and related to each other in a bookkeeping fashion. The construction of a matrix of these flows allows the user to predict changes throughout the system of changes in any part.

The comparison of the detail in the individual input-output studies with the detail in the CITY model is biased in favor of CITY by the fact that this model uses national parameters whereas the individual studies use local data to build their matrices. Thus, the other models may be more sophisticated in that they use locally estimated data for fewer industry groups. If, however, the CITY model parameters are modified to reflect actual local interindustry relationships (as is possible), it will provide more detail than any of the input-output models shown. Table 4.2 offers a comparison of the GEM/CITY model with three input-output models.

The way one would operate one of the input-output models to

TABLE 4.2
COMPARISON OF THE CITY MODEL WITH INPUT-OUTPUT MODELS

	Input-Output Models		CITY Model
Industry Groups	CenNY	– 32	40
	SD	– 14	(12 agricultural, 11 manufacturing,
	CAL	– 29	3 retail, 5 services, etc.)
Number of Counties or States	CenNY	– 5	Variable
	SD	– 1	(the two sample areas are 14 and 6 county
	CAL	– 1	regions)

SOURCES: CenNY = Kalter (1968).
SD = Tjersland (1969).
CAL = Hansen and Tiebout (1963).

TABLE 4.3
COMPARISON OF THE CITY MODEL WITH ECONOMIC BASE MODELS

	Economic Base Models		Economic Base in the CITY Model
Number of Industries	LA	– 25	MOD – 40
	WICH	– 21	(12 agricultural, 11 manufacturing,
			3 retail, 5 services, etc.)
Number of Counties or Cities	LA	– 1	Variable
	WICH	– 1	
Measurement Variable	LA	– Employment land use, employment	
	WICH	– Employment salaries, tax base	

SOURCES: LA = Tiebout (1962).
WICH = Federal Reserve Bank of Kansas City (1952).

test impacts would differ considerably from how the model would normally be used. The conventional use of an input-output model would cause a change in the final output of one industry, a change in its input requirements and, thus, the output of all other industries because of the interrelated nature of the matrix. In the CITY model, the increase in output of one industry will not necessarily increase output of other manufacturing activities, but would cause increased sales by those local suppliers who only sell locally if they happen to have excess capacity. Thus, it will not automatically adjust supply and demand. If supply remains constant and demand increases, prices will rise in the CITY model. Prices are not generally dealt with in input-output models. The trade-off between labor and capital is also not considered. In the model, however, it is possible to change the capital/labor ratio by using overtime shifts of upgrading equipment.

Economic Base Models

Economic base models show in income and/or employment terms which activities are export-oriented (i.e., produce goods and services for export to markets outside of the local system) and which activities are service-oriented (i.e., produce goods or services for sale in local markets or used by local businessmen).

Economic base models are used to gain an understanding of current sources of income and/or employment in an area; to identify the importance of a single industry; as a government device, to identify expenditure needs and expected revenues; to forecast the impact from changes in the export sector; and in conjunction with other studies. In general, they tend to deal with fewer activities than contained in the CITY model.

Base models deal only with the demand side of a local economy, whereas the CITY model deals with both the demand and supply side. In CITY, labor shortages, depletion of resources, high local costs of land or other factor inputs, local financing, and available government supplied facilities are taken into account. These supply issues cannot be dealt with by a base model, which explains why the base model is most often used as a part of a larger modeling effort. Table 4.3 is a comparison of terms of three elements of the CITY model with two Economic Base Models.

In many ways it is not particularly helpful to compare the scope of models. The previous analysis of transportation and land use models compared to the CITY model merely illustrates the relative richness of the models in terms of the number of variables covered, but does little to indicate model form. The previous models were all either built to simulate a particular area or a particular problem. Usually the method of the designers of these models was to start with certain data and extrapolate them into the future. The models generally did not take into consideration all of the behavioral attributes of a system which caused a series of events to happen but were more concerned with the magnitude and direction of a particular growth trend as related to the data under study.

There are numerous other ways to relate the GEM model (or, to be more specific, its current version, CITY) to other modeling techniques. One of the best known typologies developed for model comparison was done by Britton Harris (1966). Harris prepared six dichotomous states; (1) descriptive vs. analytic, (2) holistic vs. partial, (3) macro vs. micro, (4) static vs. dynamic, (5) deterministic vs. probablistic, and (6) simultaneous vs. sequential. Although it is difficult to categorize a model as large and complex as GEM into such a simplified scheme, in general GEM/CITY can be said to be analytical, holistic, macro, static, probablistic, and sequential.

A more recent clarification scheme developed by Kilbridge et al. (1968) offers still another framework but possibly a more useful one as it relates twenty planning models to each other in terms of subject, function, theory and method.

As the chart in Figure 4.1 shows, the CITY model includes more subject matter than any of the twenty models surveyed by those authors. To illustrate the similarities and differences, let us take a few categories and make comparisons referring to CITY. To save time I will focus on just the main topics of subject, function, theory and method.

Land Use Models

With regard to land use, CITY model has three residential densities (single family, garden apartments, and high-rise) each of which may have a quality index that ranges from 0 to 100. Furthermore, the housing may be located on any of the 625 parcels of land, each with different locational features (distance to CBD, political jurisdiction, assessed values of land, etc.) and the infrastructure present (roads, utilities, public services in the form of schools and municipal services).

CITY model has four types of local commercial activities, three types of basic industries, and one type of construction industry land usage in the private sector, and three types of government buildings (schools, municipal services, and utilities), two types of transportation facilities (roads and terminals), and two types of park land usage (improved and unimproved) in the government sector.

Population

The CITY model deals with population in three major classes including characteristics such as educational level, number of workers, number of students, normal number of voters, and average consumption requirements. The model user inputs values for the dollar value of time and for allocation of leisure time among the options of extra work, adult education (public and/or private), recreation, and political activity.

The population units in the local system pass through several major operating programs of the model in order that their individual status may be determined. For example, the population units by class have characteristics and preferences that affect how they are handled by the migration, housing, employment, transportation, commercial, school allocation, and time allocation processes.

Transportation

CITY model deals in greatest detail with the peak hour work transportation issue. The model contains a sophisticated combined modal split and routing submodel that allocates workers to auto, bus, or rapid rail modes and specific routes based upon transport capacities, dollar costs, time costs, and personal preference.

Transportation is also an influencing factor in the commercial process and terminal use process. In other words, the assignment of personal consumption and business consumption of goods and services to specific locations is influenced by road capacities, alignments, and terminal locations.

Economic Activity

Employment is dealt with in some precision by CITY model inasmuch as population units by class, location, and education level are employed at specific employment locations (manufacturing, retail, and services) and at generalized locations (schools, municipal

FIGURE 4.1

CLASSIFICATION OF TWENTY-ONE URBAN PLANNING MODELS[5]

SOURCE: Kilbridge et al. (1968).

	MODEL NAME	AUTHOR(S)	CITY	APPROX. DATE	LAND USE
1.	New Accessibility Shapes Land Use	Hansen	(Hypothetical)	1959	
2.	Activities Allocation Model	Seidman	Philadelphia	1964	
3.	Chicago Area Transportation Model	C.A.T.S. Group	Chicago	1960	
4.	Connecticut Land Use Model	Voorhees	State of Conn.	1966	
5.	Econometric Model of Metro. Employment and Pop. Growth	Niedercorn	(Hypothetical)	1963	
6.	EMPIRIC Land Use Model	Brand,Barber,Jacobn	Boston	1966	
7.	Land Use Plan Design Model	Schlager	S.E. Wisconsin	1965	
8.	Model of Metropolis	Lowry	Pittsburgh	1964	
9.	A Model for Predicting Traffic Patterns	Bevis	Chicago	1959	
10.	Opportunity-Accessibility Model for Alloc. Reg. Growth	Lathrop	Buffalo	1965	
11.	Penn-Jersey Regional Growth Model	Herbert	Philadelphia	1960	
12.	Pittsburgh Urban Renewal Simulation Model	Steger	Pittsburgh	1964	
13.	POLIMETRIC Land Use Forecasting Model	Hill	Boston	1965	
14.	Probalistic Model for Residential Growth	Donnelly,Chapin,Weiss	Greensboro	1964	
15.	Projection of a Metropolis: New York City	Berman,Chinitz,Hoover	New York City	1960	
16.	RAND Model	RAND Corp.	(Hypothetical)	1962	
17.	Retail Market Potential Model	Lakshmanan,Hansen	Baltimore	1964	
18.	San Francisco C.R.P. Model	A.D.Little Corp.	San Francisco	1965	
19.	Simulation Model for Residential Development	Graybeal	(Hypothetical)	1966	
20.	Urban Detroit Area Model	Doxiadis	Detroit Area	1967	
21.	CITY Model	Envirometrics	(Hypothetical)	1968	

SUBJECT																			FUNCTION			THEORY								METHOD										
a. Residential	b. Industrial (MFG.)	c. Commercial	d. Govt. or Institutions	e. Roads, Streets, Alleys	f. Public Open Space	POPULATION	TRANSPORTATION	a. Interzonal Trips	b. Other Transport.	ECONOMIC ACTIVITY	a. Employment	1. Retail Trade	2. Manufacturing	3. Service	b. Trade	1. Retail	2. Other	c. Personal Income	PROJECTION	ALLOCATION	DERIVATION	BEHAVIORAL	a. Economic (Market)	b. Preference	GROWTH FORCES	a. Gravity	b. Trend	c. Growth Index	d. Input-Output	ECONOMETRIC	a. Regression	b. Input-Output	c. Markov Process	MATHEMATICAL PROGRAMMING	a. Linear Programming	b. Other Analytical Forms	SIMULATION	a. Autonomous	b. With Intervention	
●						●													●							●										●				1.
●	●	●		●		●					●		●					●		●	●			●				●			●							●		2.
●	●	●	●	●	●			●					●						●		●						●												●	3.
●						●						●	●	●				●	●		●					●		●			●							●		4.
●						●			●			●	●	●					●		●							●			●									5.
						●						●	●	●				●	●		●					●		●			●									6.
●		●	●	●	●	●														●	●		●	●											●			●	●	7.
●	●	●				●						●	●							●	●					●													●	8.
								●	●										●		●					●									●					9.
●						●		●												●	●					●												●		10.
●																			●	●	●		●												●			●		11.
●	●	●				●						●	●				●	●		●	●			●		●		●	●									●		12.
						●						●	●	●				●	●	●	●					●		●								●		●		13.
●																				●											●								●	14.
						●						●	●	●		●	●	●		●	●								●			●								15.
●						●					●									●	●		●	●														●		16.
								●								●				●	●					●		●								●				17.
●						●													●	●	●		●	●									●					●		18.
●											●								●	●	●		●	●												●		●		19.
						●		●											●	●	●					●					●					●				20.
●	●	●	●	●	●	●		●	●		●	●	●	●		●	●	●		●	●		●	●														●	●	21.

services, and transit companies) that offer salaries influenced by individual considerations. Thus is is possible to have hundreds of employment locations, each offering different salaries and having different locational advantages.

The trade section of CITY model divides local purchases into four categories (business goods and services and personal goods and services). Local consumers are assigned to these establishments based upon capacity considerations, prices charged, and transportation access.

Personal income of the local population is derived from full-time jobs, part-time jobs, and welfare payments. Personal income is calculated by land parcel and by population class. Personal consumption (fixed and variable) is made from this income and the remainder is either savings or dissavings.

Function

The CITY model is not a projection model, but trend lines do develop over a number of simulated years and these may be extrapolated by the model user at his own risk. CITY model is primarily an allocation model that matches supply and demand in the employment, transportation, commercial, time allocation, housing, and government services markets. Land use allocation is a model user function, and the user may affect the other allocations by changing locations, prices, quality of services, etc. This is presently being modified to include a land use allocation phase by machine algorithm.

Some submodels in the CITY model perform derivation functions. The land auction and land purchase program derives the market value of rural land based upon such factors as distance from the nearest terminal, the nearest residence, and the nearest employment and the presence of utilities, zoning, and road accessibility. Other derivation type programs include the calculation of federal-state aid received, social dissatisfaction, tax revenues, and utility usage.

Theory

Since the CITY model has no automatic growth process (the user inputs new activities and removes old ones) except for a slight population increase due to natural population growth, the major theoretical assumptions relate to how markets operate and how population units exert their preferences.

Method

The method used to relate inputs to outputs in the CITY model is simulation. The components of a simulation model as defined by Kilbridge et al. (status variables, exogeneous variables, functional relations, and output) conform very closely to four of the five model elements presented in this model (data base, inputs, operating programs, and output). Human intervention is also an integral part of the CITY model. It is the human intervention via director and user inputs that causes the local area to change during a cycle of the model.

Possibly more detail as to the actual method used to derive the more complex algorithms might be useful.

The Kilbridge et al. paper, when discussing the theoretical structure underlying urban models, brings up a host of concepts, only some of which are applicable to our discussion. For example, they discuss urban planning models in terms of two dichotomous classes: choice models and index models. This dichotomy is not applicable for a discussion of GEM, as the model contains both. On the other hand, delving into the Growth Forces and Behavioral Models is useful.

Growth models are said to assume statistical stability, rationality, and regularity in describing mass behavior. The basic premise of the models is the belief in a natural law which is consistent and known. Constructs of the growth model form include gravity, trend, and index models. These models are largely extrapolatory and are often used to build projection models.

The other form of model is labeled Behavioral. Kilbridge divides these into two categories. The first consists of economic models based on the concepts of rational choice, market behavior and equilibrium. The other is built around the concept of preference. These preferences are multifactor and might include such things as household budgets, activity patterns and taste norms.

This generalized dichotomy which can be recast into the areas of forecast and resource allocation models may have important ramifications in present times, particularly as the powerful techniques of modeling are brought to bear on the problems of the environment.

When the country (particularly its political and research communities) was more specifically focused on the problems of the metropolitan and urban communities, the point of view taken by its federal champions at the Department of Transportation and

Department of Housing and Urban Development was one of progression and evolved change to the system over some period of time. This helped to explain the growth of modeling methodologies which were of the forecast variety where the system under consideration was seen to be perturbed by a federal generated action and the results to the system rippling through time.

Today, the focus of these communities (and others, including those dedicated to the protection and preservation of the environment) appears to be toward the area of the immediate affect of policy changes on the system These impact models are not of the forecast type as the policy makers appear to be more concerned with the immediacy of their remedies. Possibly, the touted life and death urgency noted in the laws and promulgations fostered this. Regardless, the modeling methodology necessary to handle these types of questions generally cannot be evolved from the transportation and land use fostered models but will have to be largely of the form of resource allocation.

It is this latter technique (resource allocation) which was of most interest to us as we designed our individual algorithms.

THE CONCEPT OF BEHAVIORAL MODELING

The modeling design used in GEM rested on the idea of models based on the behavior pattern of humans and organizations as they interact on a daily basis. The concept of behavioralism is a relatively recent idea for the social sciences.

One example of its use is in a study of political power. For years traditional political science has studied power as a monolithic structure and assumed that the staff and line structures represented by the government organization chart were descriptive of the power flows also. However, in every case, there was a tacit agreement that specific people frequently had unusual sway in this process.

In the last decade or so, a number of social scientists from a variety of disciplines began to study the system using a behavioral approach to try and discover who really does govern our local communities. These studies all but ignored the formal structures of the government in favor of trying to determine who influenced the decisions on various issues which were before the government and whether these influences appeared to provide a demonstrable show of political power. The research of these scientists did indeed indicate that the expected paths of government power (staff and line) did not explain how decisions were actually arrived at in the community. This suggested that expectations of results arrived at on the basis of formal theory would often not materialize.

The discrepancy found between the actual workings of a political system and the workings of the system as described by the educator and researcher is not surprising when one understands the job of the educator. His position is to take a heterogeneous reality, which is made up of a large number of seemingly disparate features and simplify the structure into a scheme more or less readily comprehensible to his students or the users of his research.

Presently there is a question as to whether the simplified models used for pedagogical purposes should continue to be separated from the models used for policy-making. This dichotomy has persisted over the years. However, with the advent of the computer, which allows a student to experience the richness of reality without being drowned in its complexity, the dichotomy may hopefully be resolved.

THE COMPUTER AND BEHAVIORAL TECHNIQUES

The belief that the computer could indeed be powerful for memory and analytical purposes and the search for a learning/research tool led us through the path of gaming to behavioral modeling. Behavioral modeling, in its essence, is a process of matching system segments with each other on the basis of wide limits prescribed by individual characteristics. It is termed behavioral because it depends not on set optimizing or extrapolative functions, but responds heuristically to behavior patterns set by the different elements within a culture. As can be seen from the equations in the Appendix, GEM is, when viewed as a complete man-machine model, a form of mathematical programing often referred to as "satisficing."

There are two types of behavioral modeling, static and dynamic. A static behavioral model is one which relates components of a system to each other at a particular point in time. The process of relating these data to each other at the time they are loaded into a Data Base can be considered behavioral. At the same time, it is also static in that we are only interested in the interrelationship at the particular time of the data gathering.

With the second form of behavioral modeling, dynamic, we are not only interested in the relationships between the data bases as they are entered into the computer, but also in the process which allows these data bases to grow from one period to the next. These functional relationships and parameter values are of utmost concern to people building forecasting or predictive models.

The behavioral model differs from other models in that a large number of the multiplier type functions present in predictive models are loaded whereas in GEM they are actually derived from the running of the model itself. For example, in Origin and Destination Models, so familiar to the transportation economist, the basic trip data would not be loaded into the model at the beginning with the Data Base. Rather, the characteristics of employers would be noted by industry type and be matched by industry type with the characteristics of the workers. Further, all of the residences and industries would be located as would the various forms of transportation levels and the other relevant data. The actual origins and destinations would be found as a result of the model's attempt to match employers to employees.

In GEM, because the results of decisions are derived from the workings of the model and are not prespecified as part of the model design, this form of modeling has a great deal of potential for the researcher and the policy maker. For example, let us say he wishes to change a major form of transportation in a city; i.e., insertion of a rapid transit system Rather than having to perform the hypothetical analysis of the population and land use distribution resulting from the building of a mass transit system he would insert the mass transit system into the model and, because the preferences of the employer/employees are already loaded, would be able to have the model assert a modal choice for a total transportation network.

BASIC PREMISE OF A BEHAVIORAL ALGORITHM

One of the most common problems facing a researcher in science is that of defining his study population. The world and its parts are very complex and are presently not able to be analyzed as a total entity; at least not in any detail. The question of problem definition becomes still more acute when the researcher takes into consideration the fact that the various portions of this world, both its people and its environment, are not perceived in exactly the same fashion by all people, in all situations, for all time. For example, a book is a source of pleasure, information, income, escape; it is also a work of art, a classic, a collector's item, decoration; a certain size, shape, color, number of pages; printed or written on particular quality paper, with certain typescript, and has (or has not) pictures or illustrations, and so forth. Obviously, a book can be all of these things, but it would be a very rare situation should all of these facets be included or discussed in any one book. Rather, the many different people or institutions connected with a particular book would tend to only look at the descriptions of a book which particularly serve their purpose. The descriptors would have to be ones which the parties discussing the book could agree on.

The researcher, as he begins a project, must therefore take the time to define his problem so that the audience reading the work understands his assumptions. So that he does not have to completely set all of the limits of his research, he writes his work under the aegis of a particular specialty or in a given professional field. This latter set of descriptors which are agreed upon by those belonging to the discipline are being constantly defined and redefined. The constant revision of these descriptors, plus the reinforcement of the fields through professional meetings and conventions, help provide a comprehensive shorthand which makes research communications possible.

In essence, the various professional disciplines have decided only to look at certain portions of the world and from very specialized points of view. The resulting myopic picture of reality simplifies the situation so that meaningful research can be carried out within the limits of intellectual and technological capability.

This practice of limiting the scope of a problem is very important as a precedent for building behavioral models. It is a basic premise of behavioral modeling that, although every item in the total system requires a very large number of descriptors if one were to attempt to explain it fully in all of its facets, each of the parts of the system can alternatively be described in a few of these descriptors, if one is only interested in a portion of the total attributes and if the parties involved agree on the shorthand used.

The precepts followed in the building of a behavioral algorithm would be much like the psychological concept of compartmentalization. Compartmentalization is used to explain how a man can do various things which appear to be contradictory without serious damage to his ego. That is, a man could steal in his business by falsifying records or ruthlessly put a competitor out of business and still be a deacon of his church or a good husband to his wife without being emotionally destroyed by the apparent contradiction of his activity patterns. This construct is used to explain that the concept of human is very complex and different facets of a personality are combined to perform the different functions of businessman, deacon, or husband. The fact that they are all one man could be considered irrelevant unless the feedbacks from one stereotype fed into another.

The same can be said of almost any basic building block used in the model. The feature of multiple descriptors for a unit of analysis, such as people (P1's), buildings, roads, businesses, etc., are carried throughout the behavioral process and each of these is described differently for each of the matching processes in which they interact.

The Process

Our task was to derive a procedure for building a general, holistic model of the environment. The task, if we had to describe the world in all its detail, would be impossible. However, if we carefully divide the total environment more and more into its component parts and only describe these parts in terms of the descriptors needed to relate one part to another, the task, although still complex, becomes feasible. Let us then describe such a procedure for analyzing a social system in a behavioral and holistic fashion.

(1) The environment (including people) would be segmented into categories which would be consistent with the problems one hoped to use the model to investigate. Largely, this is a question of deciding upon the level of aggregation: a single individual, a family, a neighborhood, city, nation, and so on. (This process was described in some detail in the section devoted to the Sector Theory and the process utilized in the latter portion of the book to describe the CITY model.)

(2) Although the whole system is interrelated, it is usually not actively interacting all the parts with each other. Consequently, paths of interaction have to be identified and the descriptors associated with these interactions have to be noted. It may be that the model builder will be forced to only make explicit those paths which are most likely to occur and ignore others. The choice of these interaction paths (as with the system segmentation) is defined by the scope of the model, its potential use, and the skill of the model designers.

(3) The delineation of the system segments and identification of paths of interaction are common to many forms of model-building. The next stage is to define the descriptors of each of the model segments as they force each other along their respective interactive paths. Each segment is therefore handled separately and is analyzed for each and every interaction expected. Consequently, the concept of say, a school plant, might be described differently for interaction with a builder, a teacher, a parent, a student, the government, and so forth. During the process of this analysis two main features will become evident.

(a) The same individual descriptor may be used as a feature of many different perceptions of potential interaction. In the example of a school plant, all of the above potential interactions would be concerned with the plant location but not all of them would be interested in the building composition or its structural materials. Thanks to the computer we are able to store all of these descriptors, determined as necessary for the model only once and can call on these individual components to make an index or composite to be used by a particular path of interaction.

(b) The interaction of two or more system segments is not always the simple case of one sector (described by a certain set of characteristics) relating to another (defined by another set). The paths of interaction, therefore, have to be carefully defined. The descriptors of a system's sector are determined by the sector itself, by the segment interacting with it, and they are usually not using the same frame of reference. Therefore, the system sector needs to be described as a four way rather than a two way matrix. In other words, a particular relationship between two entities can be seen as a supply and demand problem where the supplier has a conception of his worth and of the demander's, and the demander has a similar self viewpoint and also a perception of the supplier's worth. For example, in the case of an employer-employee relationship, the employer has need of a particular kind of worker to fill a position he has available. He advertises the opening and offers a certain salary and set of benefits to prospective employees. The worker he seeks will be one of many he sees and will be the one he decides is best qualified to fill the position. The employee, on the other hand, looks at the place of work, both its physical and nonphysical attributes and considers the offering in terms of his other choices. His own potential is set by his age, sex, training, experience, and so forth. In both cases, the potential employer and employee set ranges within which they would be satisfied to make a contract, both being to test the market.

(4) The concept of behavioral modeling is perhaps best illustrated by this last step. The fields of economics (with such concepts as consumer and producer surplus, supply and demand, and so forth) and political science (with brinkmanship, individual decision-making and have suggested that deterministic solutions of choices of social interactions are not realistic. Instead, human interaction (directly or through institutions) is more or less random within some fairly elastic tolerance limits. The boundaries set by the system segments, as they potentially interact with each other, are set as limits rather than points and allow such intercourse.

In modeling such a system the designer might begin by dividing the system segments into discrete categories which allow some basic differentiation between individual segment categories. In the case of the employer-employee example, the employees might be divided by, say socio-economic class and the employment possibilities by SIC code. These secondary classifications might be considered bounds within which choices can be made and allow greater specificity in relating system segments to each other. Therefore, people with no skills or training in the medical areas would not seek work in that field and those looking for purveyors of these skills would not look for any people but those trained in the medical field.

(5) The delineation and definition of the system segments and their paths of interaction leaves only the method of getting the sectors together. The method of accomplishing this is done in behavioral modeling by matching goods and services with the people, institutions or things in search of such items. These matches are made by linking the various system segments which are searching for a link with each other, so that the demands of the supplier of a good or service fall within the range of the desired quality he has set, and the goods or service offered in exchange fall within the supplier's limits. This solution need not be (and often is not) the optimum choice that the sector segments could have made, but they do satisfy their requirements.

Suppose we take a simplified example to illustrate this methodology. Let us consider the problem of matching students to school plants. The students are divided by age and sex cohorts and the schools by educational level and location. The students' descriptors include socio-economic class, years of schooling, quality of performance, living location, race, religion, and, of course, age and sex.

The school plant might include size, condition, number and quality of teachers, the school as an institution, affiliations (public, private, religious), cost, and, of course, location. Before the model is used, the importance of each of these descriptors must be noted so that the particulars of cultural backgrounds can be accounted for. In a perfectly dynamic model, all of the possible permutations and combinations of the descriptors would be accounted for. However, for most purposes, each of the descriptors could be defined as being part of a particular range. The quality of student or school might be revealed by quartiles or deciles. Other descriptors could be binary in nature (yes or no). Still others could yield an absolute value from a predetermined list (e.g., religious affiliation).

These descriptors are then listed in groupings so that they can be tested against some standard set of bounds prescribed by the seeker of the service, in this case a school. Therefore, one particular plant might only handle boys from the ages 6 to 14, cost $1,000 a student per year, have a student-teacher ratio of 1 to 10, have 10,000 square feet of classroom space, have been built 2 years ago, and rank eighth in the state as a private institution. The rest of the plants could also be so classified.

The student population would be divided among socio-economic class, age, and sex. Each class would be given a set of criteria for school loading. The age and sex of the highest socio-economic class, for instance, would provide a first pass split of the population. In general, the better each of the indices for each of the school descriptors, the more likely people are to use the plant. Each specific student is also flagged if he has certain limiting needs; i.e., must go to a religious affiliated school. For our simple example, the higher socio-economic class requires at least a student-teacher ratio of 1 to 13, 10 feet of classroom space per student, be less than 5 years old, or maintained in that condition, and rank tenth or better in the state.

When such a model begins to scan for student-school matches, such factors as age, sex, location (assuming school district boundaries), cost of school and religious requirement would be automatic sorters for the populace. The process of loading the schools sets some of the other limits, such as student-teacher ratio and floor space per child. Consequently, the model matches the seekers of the service with education facilities which offer at least the service they require. In no case is there an attempt to match the best students with the best schools, unless the basic sorting criteria of the institution sets scholarship limits. In the latter case, the result would be a tendency for good students to go to this plant, but there is no requirement for hierarchical matching.

In short the students are seen as requiring certain qualities to be able to go to a particular school plant (school viewpoint) and requiring certain educational quality or skills (student view). The schools are of a particular quality, given all schools (school view) and provide a certain quality of service, given crowding and teachers (student's view). The match between students and schools takes place as each finds people or plan that falls within the standards they have set.

This modeling form has a great deal of promise, both in the short run for interrelating the information systems and data bases available in a large number of cities, and in the long run for taking these large scale sophisticated data bases and projecting them into the future.

OVERVIEW

Each of the models (indeed all models) and methodologies discussed are better as the data gets better. The results are more valid and useful as the data becomes more readily available and accurate. On the other hand, it is quite possible for a perfectly valid model to be loaded with poor data and, because it yields ludicrous results, to be thought of as a poor model. We will discuss this in more detail in a moment.

To return to the model forms presented here and the CITY model, let us first note that a model designed like CITY can be made to respond to and yield other types of models as well. This would appear to be a waste, though, since CITY is not designed to be a detailed extrapolatory device. It is structured to replicate a large number of features of the urban environment so that all of the significant features of the system are able to interact and relate to each other in such a way that the model can iterate from one time period to the next.

The model is concerned with people as participants in the growth (or decay) of the system and differentiation among urban phenomena. When each iteration represents a single year's activity, a highly structured model can be very useful as an explanatory tool. Real-world structures usually do not change very much in five to ten years, which is the usual number of cycles of such a short-term model. As data become more readily available, many of the detailed relationships represented in the model will be refined.

One iteration of the model represents one year's activity in the simulated area. The specific model relationships do not change between time periods. In other words, the model itself does not recognize trends and modify its functional relationships in response to the conditions existing in any specific simulated urban area. Many models, including most forecast models, are loosely structured and do change in structure during successive iterations. Such models cannot represent much differentiation among urban phenomena in any detail. They deal with large aggregations of people and activities over many years of real-world time.

Our aim was to construct a model which did allow a great deal of differentiation among and consideration of many characteristics of people and activities. The model was to be highly causal, with many interrelated components. CITY was also built as a man-machine model. Those structures and relationships which we felt could not be usefully understood in static terms were put outside the model itself, in the gameroom, a research or policy office. The CITY program structure itself does not change from iteration to iteration.

Since the model is highly structured, components can be extremely interrelated and interdependent. Such a structure allows more complexity than the looser structure of forecast models. More complexity and more interrelated components lead to increasingly finer degrees of resolution and therefore traces the path of each of these people (as groups of people) as they work, shop, play, go to school, etc. Although the model has changing land use, or several forms or Origin and Destination transportation trips, these are not designed as forms of growth equations but processes as the people move about. In short, the user of the model would have to call for information contained in CITY in the same way he would call for the data in the real world; by making a study or survey. The principle difference is that the data are all available and the computer is able to make an exhaustive and rapid study of these data in a relatively short time period and for very little money.

Therefore it can be said that the format of the CITY model replicates, in a very general way, the total change of a human system from time period to time period. To make this behavioral model a predictive one requires that the computer program be told to keep track of the data in which the user is interested. The advantage of this modeling form is that the same model can be used to test different parts of the system. Further, the feeds and feedbacks inherent in every real-world social system are necessarily numerous and complex, which suggests a greater degree of accuracy can be obtained with this methodology.

Chapter 5

USING MODELS: PURPOSES AND APPLICATIONS

There is a great deal of legitimate concern over the use of models. Unquestionably, models are fun to build and the builders often appear to get so involved with them that they forget the purpose for which the models were designed. The outsider and potential user, who are not afflicted with this disease, rightly ask the question of the real utility of the resulting product.

The GEM model as described in the previous chapters is meant to be a general simulation. It is to serve educators, researchers, trainees, and policy makers. (As of yet, however, the CITY model has not been used in formal research as a policy model, but the method for such utilization is documented in this chapter.)

THE NEED FOR AN URBAN AND ENVIRONMENTAL LABORATORY

The modern urban environment desperately needs solutions to its problems, and social scientists are one of the sources from which the answers will come. At present, however, these scientists lack the comprehensive means with which to arrive at real solutions. While the natural and physical scientists have taken long strides toward examining, quantifying and analyzing the natural world, those concerned with the social milieu are still making the first steps toward understanding theirs.

The social scientist today appears to need some of the techniques of his brothers in the natural and physical areas if he is to profitably study and improve man's urban environment. Until recently, such techniques were denied him, seemingly because he studies man as a social animal; which means he not only deals with a real world that apparently defies predictable physical laws, but he also faces complex dynamic variables caused by an unpredictable, if not erratic, agent–man.

Most of the early research in urban affairs has been undertaken from a single point of view. The economist, the sociologist, the political scientist, and the public administrator each studied one or more problems, suggested solutions, or attempted explanations. The emphasis on multidisciplinary approaches is relatively new. Although social scientists are increasingly incorporating knowledge of other disciplines into their studies to attempt an interdisciplinary approach, many have failed to do so when they examine the urban environment. They still see a particular problem as primarily economic, political, or sociological in nature.

There are probably many reasons for this, but I will focus on three. First, tradition or conservatism hinders man from changing his ways or freely embracing new ideas. Second, division of labor is as true in the social sciences as in any other marketplace; specialists profitably proffer these goods and services which they produce best. And third, social scientists today lack a generally accepted urban theory within which to incorporate multidisciplinary approaches. A comprehensive theory would allow social scientists to embrace an approach large and usable enough to handle the urban problem.

Since the metropolitan area is not exclusively a social, economic or political phenomenon, full comprehension is difficult with the tools of a traditional discipline. Multidisciplinary approaches without a mutual frame of reference and common vocabulary have usually proved frustrating. Thwarted, the specialists often retreat to their particular disciplines and resume their parochial views. An ancillary problem is that many of the subdisciplines are expanding their usual purviews to areas such as urban or environmental studies so that their traditional boundaries are becoming imprecise. This condition tends to duplicate the tendency toward segmentation.

OPERATIONAL SIMULATION

It might appear that just when the social sciences are being challenged to surmount the pervasive national urban and environmental problems, they are without a complex tool kit with which to complete the job.

This challenge was the basis of our earlier research for an educational tool and has been carried; forward in formulating an impact model for research and policy-making applications. Operational simulation offers the social scientist a laboratory tool similar to that of the natural or physical scientist for testing the results of his ideas on an urban environment. It is infinitely more sensible than the experimentation that goes on with real cities. It is prohibitively expensive to try out new schemes on an existing city and illogical to begin programs that cannot be completed. It is wasteful to disrupt cities with unproven methods and inhuman to use segments of the urban population as guinea pigs.

In designing a simulation, however, the builders require a deep understanding of the urban system They have to think through the dynamics and interrelationships among the system components so that the simulation will act like the real urban area. Thus, in using a simulation, planners, administrators and students will be able to experience the interrelationships and dynamics among the system components.

A simulation also gives those concerned about the urban area a common language, so that they can exchange experiences, knowledge and information. It begins to hurdle the jargon problem, enabling model builders and social scientists to talk to and work with each other.

Finally, fully realized simulations can be used to help formulate policy. As a laboratory, a simulation can let a policy-maker pretest his ideas and consider possible alternatives and their consequences before ground is broken.

The actual realization of this ambitious goal, a simulation with educational, research, and policy-making applications, has been the research focus of the evaluation. The uses of the model have been varied so a brief synopsis of some of these may be helpful.

EXAMPLES OF THE USES OF GEM-CITY

Educational Uses

There is often a feeling that a device that can be used to train adults is too sophisticated or advanced for youth. Our experience does not bear this out. Admittedly, the several runs of the model which were part of a high school curriculum did not engender the sophisticated, technical vocabulary of the training sessions involving professionals. On the other hand, the amount of experimentation which took place was often greater because the students were not imbued with conventional wisdom as to what could or could not be accomplished.

Three runs of the model (most ran for several weeks as part of the normal course work) are an indication of the experiences that students have had with GEM-CITY.

One run, with a local center-city high school was sufficiently successful that the school has made CITY I part of its curriculum. The students were very aware of the detailed day-to-day problems of a center-city resident and the probable future for people growing up in such an environment, but they had no awareness of the city as an interrelated whole. The model was therefore presented as an opportunity to add their ideas or remedies for urban ills, rather than as a device to be used to tell them what happens in a city.

The students experienced a high and sustained level of interest, not only for the model itself but for the technology associated with it. Few students missed any of the sessions with the laboratory and there was never a problem with their conduct. Further, one of the students who was cutting all the rest of his classes did not miss any of our labs, and a student who had formerly been dismissed from the school continued to show up at the lab and then disappeared once the session was over.

A second run was by a group of students from a Virginia boarding school. They structured a hypothetical city for several weeks, loaded it into the model, and then brought it to their classrooms. Not only did they gather the normal training usually associated with the application of the model but gained some of the theorist's insight into the numerous components of the social system.

A third run was with a high school in Montgomery County, Maryland which used the model as part of a course. After running the model for several simulation years, the students received the school's permission to invite their parents to run the model. Their avowed reason was that youth traditionally had to take charge of a city that their elders had structured. They wanted to reverse the process and see what would happen if their parents ran a city they had set up. The reports received were very favorable and both students and parents learned more than just urban theory.

The other formal educational use of the model is in undergraduate and graduate facilities of colleges and universities. The most significant response we received was that the student involvement increased with the educational process. One class convinced their dean to grant course credits for the laboratory. The stipulation placed on the course was that the students submit to a verbal final exam that would be administered by various members of the liberal arts and planning faculty. The students took to the exercise with great vigor and spent numerous hours in the library and in conference with professors in many disciplines as they delved into various sectors of the model. Even granting the possible Hawthorne-type effects of such use, the students and faculty felt that the experiment was a success.

A study conducted under the auspices of the National Science Foundation tells the story of the GEM-CITY model as a social science laboratory for college and university use. The initial grant was given to test the premise that a model could be used as an urban laboratory. The schools chosen were Dartmouth, Cornell, American University, Mankato State, Georgetown, and Memphis State. The class sizes ranged from seven to over fifty students and consisted of both graduates and undergraduates. The subjects included in the test were geography, planning, sociology, economics, real estate and political science. The final report (House and Patterson, 1972) showed that a holistic model was beneficial for teaching a variety of disciplines and that a multi-disciplines model could also be beneficial as an addition to a traditional course structure of individual disciplines. The only major impediment to mar the project was the difficulty of not having computer availability on each campus. The schools had to mail the inputs to us to get computer service. Furthermore, all of the participants reported that they had to spend a considerable amount of time learning to use the model. Students also stated that if they knew what an expenditure it would have been early in the modeling period, it was likely they would not have begun. After having used it, however, they felt that the time required had been worth the effort.

A final example is the case of a number of people from the Washington area who cooperated in loading the actual data base for Washington, D.C. Metropolitan Area into the model. The resulting City model will be used as a teaching device by local colleges for theoretical studies as well as local case studies.

SUMMARY

In summary, holistic models, as the result of their interdisciplinary approach, are used in a number of college and graduate courses and in university and non-university seminars to teach participants about the complexities of urban and regional systems by allowing them to become decision-makers in a realistic and dynamic environmental system. Much like a laboratory, the model can be used by the teacher (as director) to simulate certain initial system conditions (unemployment, traffic congestion, fiscal deficiencies, and/or others) and outside influences (natural disasters, new federal programs, changing national business conditions, etc). Thus, the teacher is able to confront the students with situations that put the students in charge of evaluating the situations and setting policy for economic, social and government interests in a local system.

The following two case studies are related in some detail to acquaint those readers with two other uses of GEM. The first is a report of the model's use as an education-training device. The second, as a research-policy tool.

USING THE MODEL FOR TRAINING

In March of 1970, the Landscape Architecture Department of the University of Wisconsin (Madison Campus) conducted an experiment using CITY.

The class which participated in the experiment was enrolled in an undergraduate Landscape Architecture course. Fourteen students, predominantly male, participated regularly in the gaming sessions. Their average age was about 24. None had previously played an urban game.

Background

In order to broaden the perspective of design students beyond the traditional views of urban planning, the class assumed "real world" decision-making roles in each of two formats. The first format involved identifying the major decision-makers who are responsible for the management of financing, construction, and public response to urban development schemes.

The second format consisted of the functions in the GEM-CITY. These functions included only those pertaining to business (the economic sector). During the gaming sessions, the participants were encouraged to incorporate positions and strategies representative of their housing design process roles into the conduct of their GEM-CITY economic decision-maker functions. Research exercises and analyses of the elements of GEM and some of its underlying assumptions were also included to complement the role-playing activity.

Conduct of the Course

All of the students were assigned to decision-making roles in the economic sector of the model. Decisions in the other two sectors, government and social, were made by the game director. There were no social sector decisions made during the course of the play, and government decisions were made only in response to demands from the economic sector for additional public services.

There were seven economic teams, six of which controlled residential, commercial and industrial economic activities and several square mile parcels of undeveloped land. The seventh economic team was designated the Public Housing Authority. This team was responsible for residence and an eight-square-mile undeveloped area in the northwest corner of the city earmarked for low-rent housing.

Specific Economic Functions

Several decision-making roles can be derived from the GEM-CITY model economic sector which have real-world counterparts. The following list includes those counterparts to which the students could relate.

Realtor	In this decision-making role a player can: purchase and sell land; bid on outside owned land; work in caucus for equitable assessment and property taxes; and perform other land-owning functions as described in the developer role.

Landlord	As a landlord, a player: specifies maintenance levels[13] and rents; encourages government to provide good municipal services and schools for each residential location; attempts to get lowest prices on personal goods and services (for maintenance) and minimize transportation costs to those establishments; works in caucus with other decision-makers to determine equitable assessments and property taxes.
Housing Developer	This function includes: the purchase of land from a realtor; the determination of the type of housing (single family, multiple-family, high-rise); desire for a particular square-mile site on the part of the developer; the determination of the level of intensity of development (1-8 levels possible, each level requires 12 percent of a square mile of land, etc.); obtaining necessary zoning and utilities; arranging financing; and determination of the quality index (40-100) at which the residence will be developed.
Personal Commercial Operator	Two types of commercial establishments (PG and PS) sell their products to the resident population units and to landlords for maintenance of their residential properties. Managers at existing concerns make maintenance and pricing decisions as well as setting the wage level for each type of population unit (PL, PM, and PH) they employ. Thus, both the commodity market and the labor market must be analyzed by these managers in order to most efficiently operate their businesses. Housing development decisions must be planned since an expanded housing market generates increased consumption demand and a greater supply of labor. Transportation networks are also an issue for these managers.

The final two areas of economic decision-making (Industrial and Business Commercial Operation) were not emphasized to the players because these concerns are peripheral to the housing question. But, as will be seen in the write-up of the actual play, they became central to the planning and redevelopment process as conducted by the class.

Industrial Establishment Operator	These activities (HI, LI, NS) sell their output to the Outside System at an outside determined price. Players determine the maintenance level and salaries. Major concerns are the transportation system (closeby terminals are necessary), supply and price of goods and services, and property taxes. When local conditions (such as availability of labor) permit, new levels of these plants may be constructed following the typical development procedure; utilities, zoning, financing, site location, land purchase, construction. Each new level provides a substantial number of employment opportunities.
Business Commercial Operator	Managers of BG and BS establishments sell most of their output to LI, HI, and NS. Consequently, they are located in the vicinity of industrial land uses. Decision-makers set prices, wage levels, and maintenance level. As with personal commercial establishments, managers of BG and BS have two market considerations. New levels of each type are feasible only if there is a growth of industry in the system.

Dunbeath Urban Housing Scenario (Given to Students)

Dunbeath is a medium-sized city of 290,000 population encompassing a developed area of 42 square miles. There is a large amount of privately owned undeveloped land within the core area as well as on the fringe.

The industrial and commercial area is centered within a two to three mile radius of an export terminal, which is a focal point in the city. The low-income residential section of Dunbeath extends into the northeast which contains apartment complexes which constitute most of the slums in the city. The remaining low-income housing is of mediocre quality and generally overcrowded. The public facilities serving the northeast section of town are all inferior to those in the other parts of town. The school in the northeast is overcrowded, with a poor student-teacher ratio of 25-1 and a low value ratio of 65, compared to student-teacher ratios in the other schools. The municipal services department is uniformly bad throughout the city as police and fire stations and hiring policies have continually lagged behind Dunbeath's recent rapid growth. Likewise, the road system in the northeast has been allowed to deteriorate significantly. In addition, the bus service that exists does not serve the low-income people of northeast. Finally, the planning and zoning department has failed to provide any parkland at all in the northeast residential area, while providing abundant parkland in the south and northwest.

The southwest section of Dunbeath is a high-income residential area where all public services, except municipal services, are plentiful and of high quality. The northwest neighborhoods and a few residential developments in the southeast are largely middle income with some higher-income people.

The growth pattern of Dunbeath has been a mad rush of land speculation and almost unrestricted development since the municipal planning agency is nothing more than a tool of the economic interests and has been granting all zoning changes which have been requested. For this reason new developments have leapfrogged large tracts of undeveloped land in order to build housing on cheaper land which is farther from the center city. This has resulted in a very uneconomic land use pattern with large, totally vacant areas in and near the center of the city, particularly in the northern half.

The government has responded to the urban sprawl of low density housing by placing single-family-type housing under special assessment restrictions. Moreover, the outgoing lameduck mayor called for and received a complete zoning freeze to allow the incoming administration some margin of control over future development. A block of land in the northwest, originally purchased by the city under public domain for renewal purposes, has been razed and presently lies formant and vacant.

The possibility that the Public Housing Authority (acting as Team F) will increase its capacity to offer low-rent housing is strong. This is based upon the expectation that Dunbeath will have an influx of low- and middle-income residents within the next two years.

As decision-makers in Dunbeath, you will assume roles of economic decision-makers. As such, you will concentrate your efforts and decisions on housing and business activities and government activities affecting housing. Thus, you will be the builders, developers, and landlords in the simulated city.

Other roles normally played in the City simulation will be assumed by the Landscape Department staff and Envirometrics staff. They will respond to your essential development requests for government approval and services, and will generate citizen response to housing conditions.

As part of these simulation exercises, you will be expected to have a thorough understanding of housing and other conditions in this city. You will be responsible for developing a series of indicators to measure the quality of housing which you own and develop. These indicators will later form the basis for measuring your performance in the role you are assuming.

Round One

Several modifications were made to the starting Round One output with which the students began their play. As is outlined in the scenario presented to them in the introductory session, several ownership, zoning, assessment and financial accounting data were changed. For example, cash balances were reduced to small positive amounts which would enable construction of two levels of multiple-family residences; e.g., townhouses, in the absence of other financial arrangements.

During the next class meeting, players were briefed on their roles and suggested activities based on the scenario. After the students analyzed the scenario, examined the Round One output and completed the introductory phase, they were invited to make sample housing decisions based on the Round One output. Among the decisions attempted, were upgrades of residences (increasing the intensity of development on a particular parcel), rent changes, and adjustments of maintenance levels.

Round Two

There was a planned four-week lag between the introductory play and the next gaming session. During this period, the students were directed to research their class roles as well as identify some of the GEM concepts pertinent to the housing development problem. A means through which to enhance this research was the Master Plan design process. The task was reshaping Dunbeath as it existed in Round Two to a city which satisfied the varied desires of each type of decision-maker. Obviously, tradeoffs would have to be negotiated. The goals of developers and contractors might be counter to the goals of federal government, social workers, and citizen groups.

The land use Master Plan was diagrammed and mailed to Envirometrics. Contrary to the original intention, it was not based on the supposition of transition from Round Two. Instead, the class designed a Master Plan for a hypothetical urban area. Nevertheless, a basic analysis was drawn up in order to demonstrate the massive investment necessary to complete redevelopment. This Master Plan and the cost figures were used as examples of extreme redevelopment and budget requirements to guide the decision-makers for the remainder of the play.

The first stages of the Master Plan were implemented onto the

Round Two output. In addition to rezoning the entire board, five demolitions were implemented. All of the demolitions involved housing in the northern part of the city. A large-scale highway project was begun, according to the Master Plan. First of all, four segments of the east-west superhighway were torn down in order to focus redevelopment on the central and north-south corridor of the city. Next, the road improvements to the southwest fringe of the city were input in preparation for the intensive industrial park outlined in the Master Plan. Finally, utilities were installed and municipal services districts were rearranged so that the new proposed development could be completed and not be at a disadvantage to existing developments in terms of housing indicators.

Round Three

At the start of the next gaming session, the players were presented the implications of the Master Plan along with the updated output (Round Three). This marked the beginning of the most instructive sequence of play.

Immediately, the students reacted somewhat harshly to the stark impracticability of their Master Plan, which provided an excellent graphic of how an unplanned city can both differ greatly from an ideal concept and cost a considerable amount of money to correct.

The tactic then employed was to examine the possibility of maintaining the spirit of their plan within the scope of their financial resources. They concentrated on two major areas of redevelopment:

(1) Renovation and/or demolition of all substandard housing (all located in the northeast quadrant of the city).

(2) Relocation of the old industrial center situated in the heart of the city.

This latter effort was directed as an ecological and aesthetic improvement to the area. It was desired that Heavy and Light Industry be located on the fringe of the populated centers and border a greenbelt area, rather than in the center of the residential complex.

In order to facilitate the government's rulings and subsequent decision-making, proposed zoning and utility changes were posted on a blackboard visible to all. The chart provided an approval check on the part of the teams. Consequently, all the players knew what type of developments were likely to appear during the following rounds.

Round Four

Three new participants joined the Monday evening session (at which time decisions were made based on Round Four output). These persons, affiliated with the Landscape Architecture Department, added some degree of imagination to the play by demolishing all the slums on one square mile parcel and developing public institutional land in its place. While some of the other players decried this as somewhat frivolous, the move did serve to highlight the flexibility and variability of approaches that are possible in the model.

To stress the necessity of eliminating the old industries from the center of the city, a special assessment zone was input. In this zone, encompassing nine square miles, an assessment ratio of 90 percent on all Light and Heavy Industry was applied. This meant that the developments had to be assessed at 90 percent of their market value. Since the normal ratio was 50 percent, the effect of the input was to almost double the property taxes.

Rounds Five, Six, and Seven

Play continued in the next class session. By this time the students were quite familiar with their roles and had established personal objectives. These sessions were well-organized and productive.

Debriefing

In the debriefing several points were stressed. First, the use of gaming and simulation as a methodology is a technique which can and should be employed in all situations where a systematic approach to a problem or condition is possible. Several examples were readily given. Two of the examples, which were particularly appropriate to the Landscape Architecture Department, were ecology and the urban planning/development process.

Gaming, they found, is potentially a good training and educational tool. And of particular benefit is the capability of reconfiguration and redesigning of the model. To reload and restructure the model required full comprehension of the problems, parameters, etc. of an urban system.

A second area of discussion was the appropriateness of the GEM-CITY model and, in particular, the Dunbeath configuration. All were in favor of a somewhat smaller aggregation.[14] However, they did recognize that in order to do that, the perspective and focus of the model would have to be narrowed. Moreover, several students desired to play the Social Sector in addition to the Economic Sector roles. The main reason was to obviate some of the conflicts and opposition which occur during stages of redevelopment. Several suggestions were made regarding the conduct of playing the model. These are discussed in the section on evaluation of recommendations.

The following section summarizes the physical changes made in Dunbeath over the seven rounds of play.

Results of the Seven Rounds of Play (See Figures 5.1 through 5.3).

The changes in the socio-economic composition of Dunbeath in the seven rounds played by the architecture students are reflected in eight tables and four figures. Although none of the statistics is discussed in depth, the significant features and trends in the data are noted. The following discussion pertains to the data contained in tables, each of which is analyzed in the order of its appearance.

Table No. 1: Population (total for each income class)—Total population expanded at an extraordinary rate from Round Four to Round Seven. The primary reason for this growth was the rise in available housing. Note that high-income population units moved into the city at an even rate throughout the play. Both of the other classes, on the other hand, experienced one year of population decline. This was caused by the housing redevelopment which demolished slum housing and replaced it with housing suitable for high-income. (See Figure 5.1.)

Table No. 2: Population per Residential and Developed Square Mile—The stability of total developments is easily inferred by comparing the lower graph in Table No. 2 with the total population graph in Table No. 1. Both slopes are remarkably similar. After a peak in year four, the students made a strong effort to alleviate the housing density. Applying the above information on total development, business land uses were being displaced by residential land uses. Expansion stopped in year seven. The growth in population was not matched by new housing. (See Figure 5.1.)

Table No. 3: Average Dissatisfaction of All Population—This information has only minor relevancy to the play in that the government and social sectors were not active sectors. Notwithstanding, several housing indicators, such as rent and quality index, contribute to this index. Consequently, the level suggests that after initial strong improvement in housing quality, rises in rent and declines in public services overrode altruistic ambitions. (See Figure 5.1.)

Table No. 4: Total Housing Units by Type—This table illustrates both the students' preference in housing types and the expansion of housing. By the end of Round Four, all redevelopment demolition had been completed. From that point, ten units of RB, nineteen units of RA, and one unit of RC were successfully constructed. In order to understand the actual supply of units this equals, two relationships must be known. (See Figure 5.2.)

First, a dwelling unit is defined as that occupied by a low-income population unit (PL1). An RA has a capacity of two dwelling units; an RB, twelve, an RC, fifty. Each middle-income population unit (PM1) occupies one and one third dwelling units and each high-income population unit (PH1) occupies two dwelling units. Thus, if housing is constructed specifically for high-income, its capacity in terms of total population units able to occupy the housing is half that of similar housing developed for low-income units. A reasonable rule-of-thumb is to assume that each level of RA housing provides space for 1.3 population units; each RC, thirty-three population units.

Table No. 5: Systemwide Vacancy Rate—Throughout the play, the housing market was extraordinarily tight. As entrepreneurs, the players could not miss by developing housing. Of course, social conditions were worse because of the crowding. Some gains were made after the early demolitions eliminated almost all vacant residences. However, by Round Seven nearly all space was again filled. (See Figure 5.2.)

Table No. 6: Residential Descriptors: Total Number of Parcels Devoted to Residential Land Use; Number of Overcrowded Parcels (those occupied at over 100 percent of capacity); Slums (those residences with Quality Indexes less than forty)—Line A illustrates that housing construction was in fact a redevelopment project in the city. Either by relocation or by razing and rebuilding, the total number of residential parcels only increased by one. Thus, the

FIGURE 5.1
RESULTS OF THE SEVEN ROUNDS OF PLAY

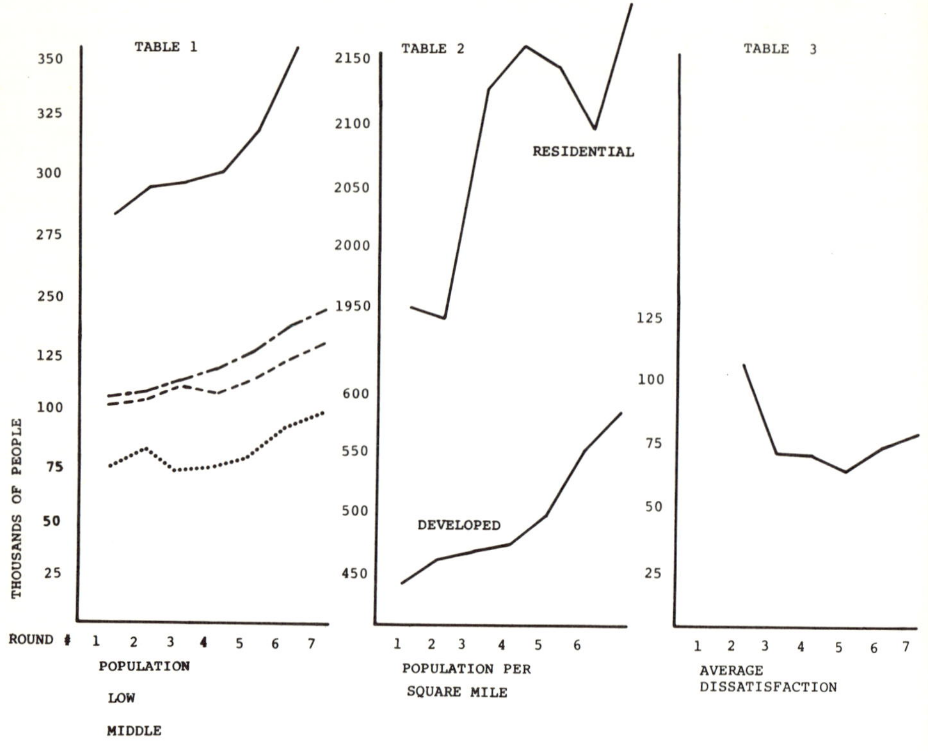

increase in total units was accomplished by increasing the density (development level) on parcels already developed with residences.

Line B is a source of disappointment as it indicates that little or no success was met in the objective of eliminating overcrowded housing. Line C, on the other hand, points out the most clear-cut achievement of the players; by Round Five they had eliminated all slum housing. (See Figure 5.2.)

Table No. 7: Systemwide Unemployment Rate—This table is not as instructive as it is in most CITY plays. Here it indicates the large economic impact a Heavy Industry has on the system. Note that Heavy Industry employs sixty population units. In Round Three, one Heavy Industry was demolished in accordance with the Central City redevelopment. In Round Four it was relocated. In Round Six, another Heavy Industry was razed. In this instance, however, it was not replaced. (See Figure 5.3.)

Table No. 8: Tax Base: Assessed Values of Land (lower line) and Developments—Again, the large economic impact of industries is apparent. In addition to the HI caused fluctuations in Rounds Three, Four and Six, an upward revaluation in Round Five of all industries in the central city pushed the tax bases up.

The model, then, can be seen as a useful training tool with sufficient flexibility to handle a special prupose group. By no means does the previous example exhaust the model possibilities nor is it meant to be a guideline for use. However, the example does serve to highlight not only the things that the directors thought were important but how the problems that the participants were interested in were handled. (See Figure 5.3.)

THE SIMULATED CITY: USING THE MODEL AS A RESEARCH AND POLICY TOOL

To demonstrate the use of a behavioral model for research and policy-making, we used the latest version of the GEM-CITY model and ran it as a man-machine simulation. This use of the model has several constraints. Among these are the specific forms of the functions in the model itself, the parameter values chosen, and the rationality of the decisions made for the four years. The first two of these general objections are well taken. To guard against continuation of a problem of poor relationships or parameter values, the

FIGURE 5.2
RESULTS OF THE SEVEN ROUNDS OF PLAY

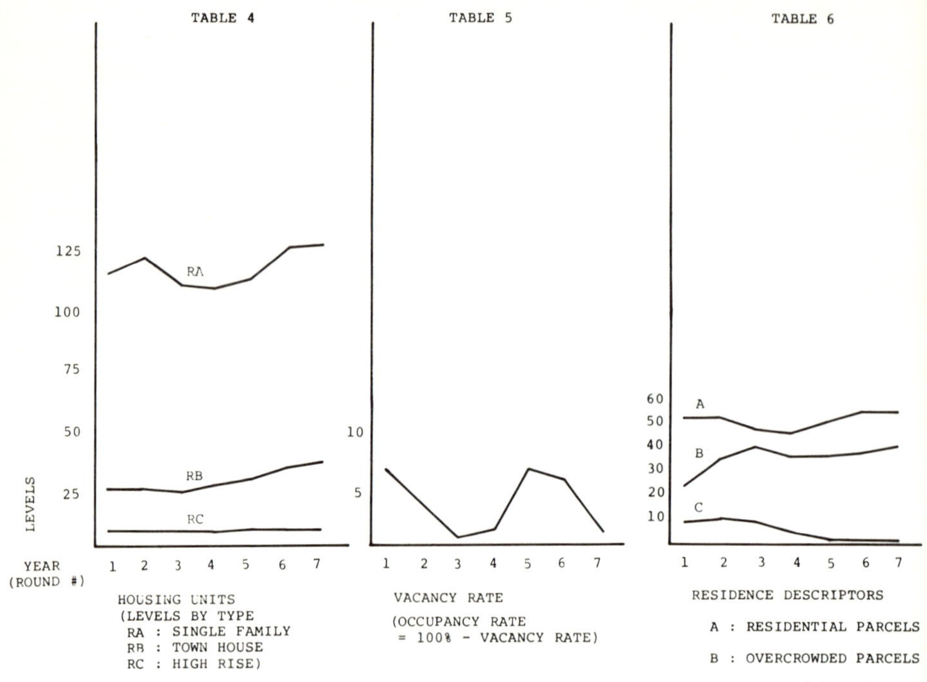

FIGURE 5.3
RESULTS OF THE SEVEN ROUNDS OF PLAY

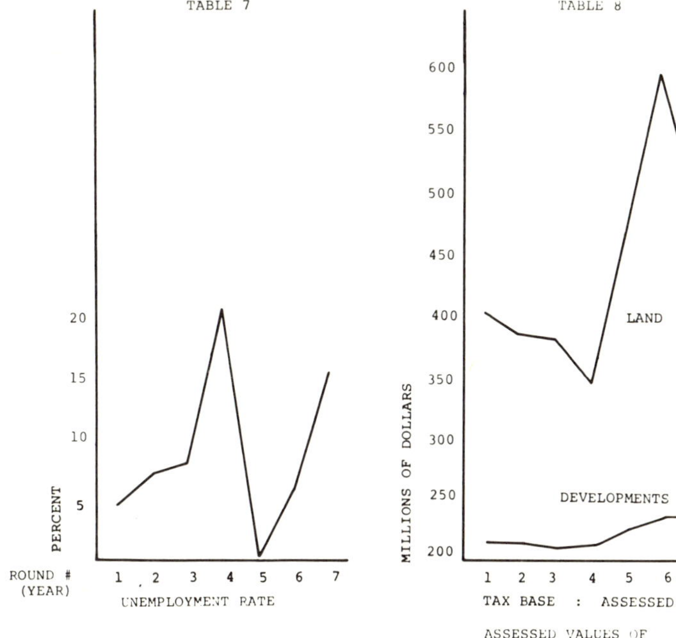

model was designed in a modular fashion to allow simplified adjustment when simulating specific geographical areas. The latter comment as to the rationality of our choices is all but impossible to defend or even discuss as rational or not, as are almost all policies of the various portions or sectors in the real world.

The purpose of this exercise is to determine the possible effects of making automobile travel more expensive, by doubling the base costs for use of the automobile in order to reduce pollution from automotive emissions.

Technique

The technique employed to accomplish this task has been to use the model as a man-machine simulation for four time periods.[15] The model was run and at the end of each year decisions were made based on conditions prevailing within Simulated City at that point in time. Decisions were made according to several criteria.

(1) In the Social Sector decisions were made in order to accomplish two ends: to minimize dissatisfaction and to maximize personal income.

(2) In the Economic Sector, decisions were made with an eye toward maximizing profit and maintaining a rate of return higher than the current interest rate.

(3) In the Government Sector, decisions were made by each department and were based on the department's specific criteria.

The School Department made decisions in order to (1) maximize the percentage of students attending schools within the public school system of Simulated City, (2) to maintain adequate facilities in terms of value ratio, (3) to prevent overcrowding of facilities and maintain use indices at or below 100.

The Municipal Services Department made decisions designed to (1) maintain use indices for each municipal service at or below 100 and (2) to maintain adequate facilities and physical plants. The Highway Department decisions were based on a desire to maintain uncongested and well maintained roads, and to provide road access to newly developed or developing parcels.

The Utility Department decisions were made in order to provide adequate utility service to all parcels affected and to maximize income. Bus company decisions were made with an eye to maximizing revenue and providing adequate bus service within Simulated City.

The Zoning Department of Simulated City was very passive and granted any zoning requested by private concern. Within the Economic Sector decisions were made which provided for new construction at a number of locations, primarily expansion of existing residences and industry, plus the addition of a second Business Services in the upper northwest.

In summary, the actual construction completed was as follows:

The School Department construction consisted of the upgrading of a single school in District 2 and sufficient maintenance in order to raise or maintain the proportion of students attending school within the public school system.

Highway construction within the four periods consisted of new roads within the center of town and in the southeast in anticipation of future development in the area.

Municipal Services construction consisted of upgrading two municipal services facilities in order to provide expanded service and capability to the residents of Simulated City.

Simulated City–Period 1 (See Figure 5.4.)

One of the problems encountered when dealing with as complex an entity as a city is that it is frequently difficult or impossible to determine directly cause and effect stemming from a given decision. Part of the problem of determining causality is that each decision has both direct and indirect effects on a number of facets of the city. In the case of this experiment (doubling of auto cost) the direct effects are primarily concentrated on the population and any changes in the governmental or economic sectors result from differences in the composition of the population and not directly from the doubling of auto costs. Consequently our focus in this discussion will be on those aspects of the city which were most strongly affected.

Government Sector–Like many governments everywhere, the government of Simulated City found itself extremely hard pressed to provide all of the necessary services and facilities which constitute the difference between mere existence and comfortable living for its citizens. The discrepancy between revenues from taxes and expenditures and appropriations, forced the city government to float short-term bonds annually in amounts of $6 to $9 million.

The current period showed little promise of reversing the trend of continual government indebtedness. Revenues from the property and local sales taxes amounted to only $50 million while appropriations to the various departments and agencies of the city government totaled $59 million. The deficit had to be covered with short-term municipal bonds which, in the past, had borne an interest rate of 3 percent.

FIGURE 5.4
SIMULATED CITY LAND USE MAP

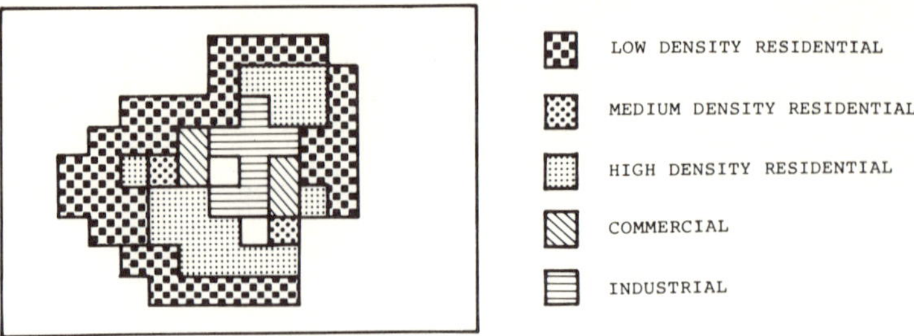

FIGURE 5.5
SIMULATED CITY STREET MAP

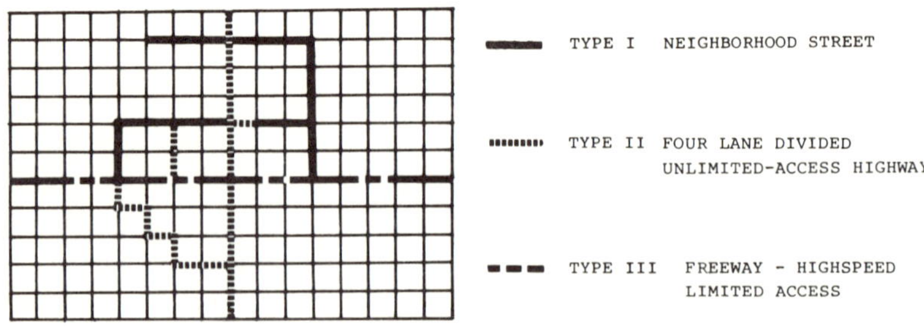

TABLE 5.1
SCHOOL ENROLLMENT IN SIMULATED CITY

School	Number of Students	Number of Teachers	Student/Teacher Ratio	Use Index
1	18,700	1,140	15:1	72
2	14,600	600	24:1	192
3	15,000	1,100	11:1	52
4	9,000	800	9:1	48
Total	57,300	3,640	16:1	94

Ideally, to full understand conditions in Simulated City it would be necessary to examine in detail each of the governmental departments and agencies. However, in most instances the response of governmental agencies to doubling of auto costs is both marginal and indirect in the time period viewed. We will, therefore, examine the three government departments which reacted most strongly to the doubling of auto costs–Schools, Highways, and Bus.

School Department–There are approximately 68,000 school age children in Simulated City. Of these, 57,000 attend public schools and approximately 11,000 attend private schools. Students attend private schools for one of two reasons: (1) the school in whose district they reside is grossly over capacity, or (2) the quality of education to be received in that school is below expected standards for the socio-economic class to which the student belongs. The first reason applies primarily to low- and middle-income students; the second, to high-income students.

The quality of public education in Simulated City is uneven, with students in high- and middle-income neighborhoods receiving better quality schooling than those in lower-income areas. Student-teacher ratios range from 9-1 to 24-1, and use indices vary from 48 percent to 192 percent of capacity. Table 5.1 provides a detailed comparison of the City's schools.

The School Department is also charged with providing Adult Education in Simulated City. The current capacity of the School Department for Adult Education is 3,000 students. There are currently 2,997 students enrolled and a waiting list of 5,145.

Highway Department–The Highway Department is charged with the construction and maintenance of all streets and roads within Simulated City. Roads are, on the whole, adequately maintained and 73 of the 86 miles of streets within the city have depreciations of less than 20 percent. Congestion of traffic is not a major problem and is, in most cases, only slight or moderate in nature. Streets in the central part of Simulated City, however, are quite heavily traveled with congestions up to 184 percent of designed capacity. (Figure 5.5 shows the road network of Simulated City.)

Bus Company–The Bus Company of Simulated City maintains 6 routes covering 25 miles of bus service. Currently 12,280 persons use the bus annually. Fares are $.15 base cost plus $.02 per mile traveled.

The average trip length for bus riders is 2.8 miles. The Bus Company has been operating at a loss for some years with fares covering only about two-thirds of operating expenses.

Economic Sector—The Economic Sector of Simulated City includes all those activities of a private, entrepreneurial nature, such as industry, wholesale and retail establishments (including both goods-oriented and service-oriented businesses).

In discussing the economic life of the city we must be concerned with employment. With respect to employment, there is a substantial proportion of the low-income population unemployed and an excess of employment opportunities for high-income workers. While there is unemployment among middle-income workers there is also a surplus of middle-income jobs as well as middle-income persons employed in low-income occupations. The current unemployment rate is 3.7 percent of the labor force, or 3,160 workers. The vast majority of the unemployed, 3,000, are low-income workers for whom the unemployment rate is in excess of 10 percent. The remaining 160 unemployed workers are middle income, for whom the rate of unemployment is one-half of 1 percent (0.5 percent).

On the whole, the economy of Simulated Sity is sound, with most businesses returning about 7 percent profit on the initial investment. There are, however, several firms which have shown losses. These losses are due primarily to an excessive depreciation of the physical plants which has cut productive capacity by as much as 40 percent.

Social Sector—Simulated City is situated on flat ground at the intersection of two major highways. The center of town is occupied by commercial and industrial interests and the population is distributed within this area in five distinct neighborhoods. (The five neighborhoods are located on Figure 5.6.)

Neighborhood 1 is located to the northeast of the center of town and is occupied by the low-income population of Simulated City. There are a few old-line middle-class-income families scattered about the area. Neighborhood 1 covers 13 census tracts and has a population of 81,000. Housing is predominantly garden apartments.

Neighborhood 2 is located on the northeast of the town center and is an exclusively middle-income area. Five of the six census tracts in this neighborhood are devoted to single-family homes, with a single garden apartment project on the sixth square mile. The population of Neighborhood 2 is 20,500.

Neighborhood 3 is the second exclusively middle-income area; it covers four census tracts and is located east of the center of Simulated City and south of Neighborhood 1. It is comprised predominantly of single-family detached dwellings and has a population of 17,500.

Neighborhood 4 is a thoroughly mixed neighborhood of middle- and high-income families. It is a crescent-shaped area extending from the west side of town southeast, with its easternmost end due south of the downtown area. Covering 12 census tracts, it is an area of mainly townhouses with a few high-rise apartments and single-family homes. Its population is 116,000.

Neighborhood 5 swings in the same arc as Neighborhood 4 and is just outside, in terms of distance, from the downtown section. Its area is the largest of the five neighborhoods, covering 15 square miles. The population of 35,000 is exclusively high-income families living in single-family homes. (See Table 5.2 for summary.)

Simulated City–Period 4–Normal Auto Cost

The changes which the city demonstrates from Pd. 1 to Pd. 4 are the result of natural ecological processes at work in the city. Among the processes at work are the movement of new residents into the city, the movement within the city of persons who have become dissatisfied with their housing, jobs, or the quality of public services in their neighborhood. The movement out of the city by these same people occurs when their attempt to find a better location fails.

Government Sector–In the intervening time, the provision of necessary public services to the community has forced the government of Simulated City to go deeply in debt and by the end of Pd. 4 the amount of governmental debt is serious. Bond payments on a two-year bond of $18 million are in excess of $9.5 million and bond payments on two loans, each of $9.87 million, are in excess of $10.3 million. Bond payments in Pd. 4 represent approximately 12 percent of governmental expenditures.

In order to finance as much of city operations as possible from local sources, the government has instituted a local income tax of 2 percent. The income tax was instituted because of rising city costs and a relatively stable property tax base.

School Department–The education offered by the public schools in

Simulated City is still uneven and suffers now from an increased school age population. Of the total school age population (79,390), 67,040 attend public schools. The remaining 12,350 attend private schools. (See Table 5.3.)

Adult Education services 10,000 night students. There is a slight unmet demand of 1,210 students.

Highway Department—By Pd. 4, the Simulated City Highway Department has constructed several miles of roads, with the net effect that, for the most part, road congestion in Pd. 4 is less than in Pd. 1. However, the streets in the center of town still have congestions ranging from 102 percent of designed capacity of 161 percent of designed capacity.

Bus Company—In Pd. 4, as in previous years, the bus company has consistently lost money. Total ridership on the bus system is 31,800 passengers and there are still seven bus routes for a total of 25 miles. Bus fares have been changed to $.16 base cost plus $.01 per mile traveled.

Fares received from passengers amounted to just over $1.5 million. Fare income just covered payments on previous loans and the entire cost of operating the bus system, $1.77 million, had to be borrowed.

Economic Sector—The overall unemployment rate for Simulated City in Pd. 4 is 5.49 percent. However, this is concentrated entirely in the low-income classes for whom the unemployment rate is in excess of 16 percent. There were a few high- and middle-income job openings available and 13 middle-income population units were employed in low income occupations. (See Figure 5.7.)

The general state of the economy of Simulated City improved to the point where there are only two businesses (out of four) Pd. 1 showing losses. Both businesses are Business Services establishments. The loss is due to the introduction of the second establishment into a situation which did not warrant competition.

Rates of return on investment averaged about 7.5 percent for all business.

Social Sector—The distribution of population in Simulated City changed greatly over the four periods under study. Neighborhood 1 exhibits the least change of all five neighborhoods. There is some infusion of middle-income persons into the area; however, the basic

FIGURE 5.6
SOCIO-ECONOMIC DISTRIBUTION, PERIOD 1

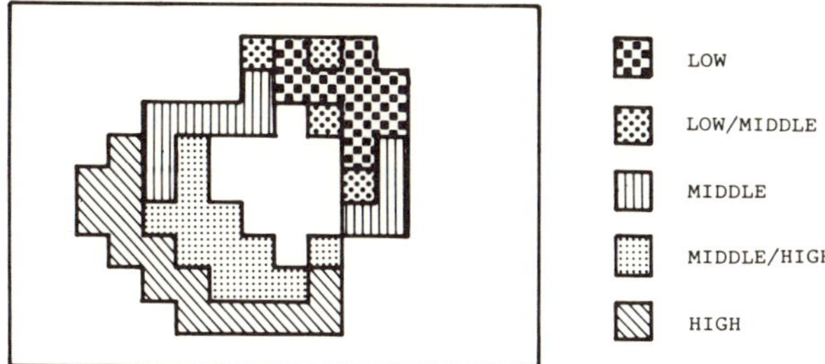

TABLE 5.2
SUMMARY OF DEMOGRAPHIC CHARACTERISTICS

Neighborhood	Class	Area	Population	Density
1	L/M	13	81,000	6,231
2	M	6	20,500	3,417
3	M	4	17,500	4,375
4	M/H	12	116,000	9,667
5	H	15	35,000	2,333
Total		50	27,000	5,400

TABLE 5.3
SCHOOL ENROLLMENT—PERIOD 4—NORMAL

School	Number of Students	Number of Teachers	Student/Teacher Ratio	Use Index
1	21,950	1,220	18:1	88
2[a]	16,540	1,040	16:1	72
3	17,870	1,280	14:1	72
4	10,680	1,040	10:1	72
Total	67,040	4,580	14:1	77

a. School 2 has been upgraded from a level 1 school to a level 2 school; i.e., it has had its capacity doubled.

character of Neighborhood 1 remains the same: an area of low-income families with some older middle-class groups. The population of Neighborhood 1 has become 85,000.

The characters of Neighborhoods 2 and 3 completely change. No longer exclusively middle class, they are now a thorough mixture of middle- and low-income families, with low-income families being 22.4 percent of the 24,500 population of Neighborhood 2 and 26.8 percent of the Neighborhood 3 population of 28,000. In addition, Neighborhood 3 has seen the largest growth in population, with a 60 percent increase for the four periods.

Neighborhood 4 displays only minor changes in the distribution of socio-economic classes within it and still represents a thorough mixture of middle- and high-income groups. The population of Neighborhood 4 has increased to 139,500 persons.

Neighborhood 5 displays a change from an exclusively high-income area to an area which, while still predominantly high income, has had a slight movement of middle-income families into the area. The population of Neighborhood 5 has grown to 39,000 of which 10.2 percent are middle-income persons. (See Table 5.4 for summary.)

Causes of Change—Period 4—With Normal Auto Costs

The movement of people into new areas within Simulated City is caused by several factors, the most important of which is the attempt to reduce overall transportation cost and distance to work.

The low-income population of Simulated City, in a successful attempt to reduce the length of their trip to work has moved into the middle-income areas: Neighborhoods 2 and 3 immediately adjoining the urban core. This movement reduces the average low income trip to work from 3.1 miles in Pd. 1 to 2.6 miles in Pd. 4. In addition, the four periods see a drastic shift in the mode of travel used by low-income workers, from a reliance on the automobile (55 percent in Pd. 1, 34 percent in Pd. 4) to increased dependence on the bus system (26.5 percent in Pd. 1, 46.8 percent in Pd. 4). During this same period of time, the low-income population of Simulated City has increased 14 percent from 73,500 to 84,000. The movement of low-income families in Neighborhoods 2 and 3 has caused some of the middle-income families living there to move into Neighborhoods 4 and 5, with a net result that the average trip length of middle-income workers has increased slightly from 1.4 miles in Pd. 1 to 1.6 miles in Pd. 4.

The middle-income population has increased approximately 14.5 percent, in the period under study, from 99,000 to 113,500. The effects of the movement of middle-income groups away from the central city can be seen in the utilization of the various modes of transportation. In Pd. 1, the predominant mode of transportation was walking; i.e., much of the population lived in residences sufficiently close to their jobs so as not to require transportation. The walkers comprised 48.8 percent of the middle-income population in Pd. 1 versus 42.1 percent driving, and only 9.1 percent riding the bus. In Pd. 4, slightly more than half the middle-income population drives to work, 50.2 percent; 11.9 percent take the bus; and walking is used by only 37.9 percent.

The movement of middle-income persons into the areas previously occupied by the high-income residents of Simulated City has caused high-income residents to move out slightly from their previous locations. The result is that the average trip length to work for high-income residents has slightly increased, from 2.6 miles in Pd. 1 to 2.9 miles in Pd. 4. Even more interesting than this, however, has been the reduction of trip length, from 3.0 miles in Pd. 3 to the 2.9 miles in Pd. 4, representing a slight reintegration of middle- and high-income groups in the portions of Neighborhoods 4 and 5 located closer to the urban core of Simulated City. The high-income population of the city has increased approximately 21 percent from 98,000 to 118,500. This increase has resulted from the construction of several new businesses which offer an abundance of high-income jobs.

The distribution of population by mode of transportation has changed only slightly. Table 5.8 gives a complete summary of trip lengths by class and mode for Pd. 4. Figure 5.8 shows the distribution of socio-economic classes in Pd. 4.

Simulated City—Period 4—Double Auto Costs

The single change which occurs between the computer runs has been the institution of a double base cost for automobiles. This double cost was introduced in an attempt by the governing body of Simulated City to reduce use of the automobile and, consequently, reduce pollution of the atmosphere from automotive emissions. The net result has been to force low-income residents to seek housing even closer to their jobs in order to minimize the cost to work for all modes of transportation. This results in some changes of a substantial nature from the conditions which existed in Pd. 1.

FIGURE 5.7
SOCIO-ECONOMIC DISTRIBUTION, PERIOD 4
(Normal Auto Costs)

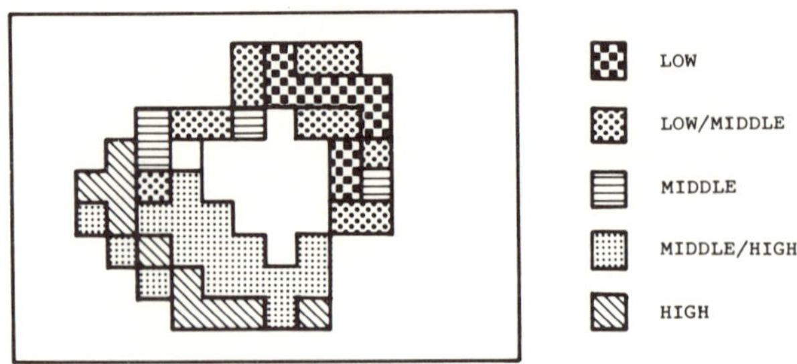

FIGURE 5.8
SOCIO-ECONOMIC DISTRIBUTION, PERIOD 4
(Doubled Auto Costs)

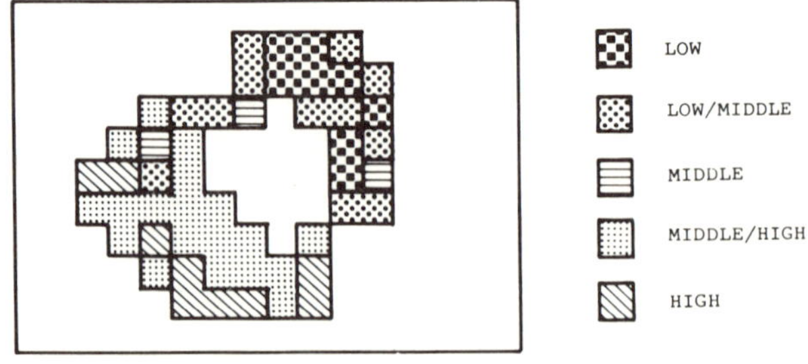

TABLE 5.4
SUMMARY OF DEMOGRAPHIC CHARACTERISTICS—PERIOD 4—NORMAL

Neighborhood	Class	Area	Population	Density
1	L/M	13	85,000	6,538
2	L/M	6	24,500	4,083
3	L/M	4	28,000	7,000
4	M/H	12	139,500	11,625
5	M/H	15	39,000	2,600
Total		50	316,000	6,320

Government Sector—The decision to double the cost of automobile transportation within Simulated City has had profound effects on the financial situation of the government. In Pd. 4 doubled revenues from taxes amounted to only $69 million, while appropriations were $78.1 million. In order to meet this deficit and pay off outstanding bonds, $18.5 million in new bonding had to be raised.

School Department—School age population in Simulated City in Period 4 under doubled auto cost conditions is 78,560 students. Of these, 66,730 attend local schools and 11,830 attend private schools. Educational quality is still quite varied within the town, with lower-income students receiving poorer quality schooling than high- and middle-income students. (See Table 5.5.)

Highway Department—The effect of the decision to double base auto costs has significantly reduced congestions citywide and most dramatically within the area of the center of the city, where congestion now runs from 101 percent to 129 percent of designed capacity (compared to nearly 184 percent in Pd. 1).

Bus Company—The doubling of auto costs within Simualted City has increased bus ridership to 23,640 persons for the entire 25 miles of bus routes. However, the Bus Company continues to lose money at the rate of approximately $1.5 million per annum, which is largely a loss from preceeding short-term bonds which covered earlier operating losses.

Economic Sector—The overall unemployment rate in Simulated City in Pd. 4 under conditions of doubled auto costs is 6.94 percent. However, this is concentrated entirely in the lower socio-economic strata for whom the unemployment rate is 19.88 percent (as compared to 10 percent in Pd. 1). Industrial and commercial activities remain profitable, with an average return of 7.5 percent on the investment. The only segment of the economy in which establishments are not profitable is in Business Services.

Social Sector—In Neighborhood 1 the population of the area remains constant and a slight rearrangement of the middle-income population in terms of residential location occurs. In Neighborhoods 2 and 3 a change which occurs is that these neighborhoods are no longer exclusively middle income and are thoroughly mixed areas of middle-

and low-income population. Neighborhood 2 has become the only area in Simulated City in which all three socio-economic classes reside. The population of Neighborhood 2 has increased from 20,500 to 23,000 and the population of Neighborhood 3 increased from 17,500 to 28,500. Neighborhood 4, the area of middle- and high-income population south of the urban core, shows a slight increase in the relative proportion of middle-income population residing there. Middle-income families constituted 46 percent of the population of Neighborhood 4 in Pd. 1 and 49 percent of the population in Pd. 4. Additionally, the population in Neighborhood 4 increases from 116,500 to 141,500. In Neighborhood 5 there has been a movement of middle-income people into the formerly high-income neighborhood and population has increased to 39,000, of whom 9 percent are middle-income families. (See Table 5.6 for summary.)

Causes of Change, Four Periods, with Doubled Base Automobile Costs

The net effect of doubling of auto costs during the four periods has been to spur population growth in the low- and middle-income classes and to retard population growth in the high-income class; bus ridership has increased, walking as a mode of transportation has decreased and, surprisingly, the average use of the automobile has increased.

The institution of a doubled base auto cost in Simulated City, in order to reduce atmospheric pollution from automobile emissions, has forced the low-income population to seek residence locations and jobs in such a manner that the trip length to work will be minimized. The infusion of low-income population into Neighborhoods 2 and 3 is a result of low-income populations of Neighborhood 1 attempting to get closer to the urban core and to places of work. This has had the effect of reducing overall trip length of low-income residents from 3.1 miles in Pd. 1 to 1.9 miles in Pd. 4. Additionally, the use of automobiles has declined substantially by approximately 60 percent. Ridership on buses has doubled that of Pd. 1 and the proportion of persons walking to work doubled from Pd. 1 to Pd. 4. In the same period the low-income population increased 16.3 percent to a total of 85,500 persons.

The movement in substantial numbers of low-income people into Neighborhoods 2 and 3 has forced middle-income residents of these areas to seek housing even further from the urban core, with the net result that the average trip length to work for middle-income residents of Simulated City has risen from 1 mile, in Pd. 1, to nearly 2 miles, in Pd. 4. This has also had the effect of reducing substantially the proportion of walkers among middle-income residents. The movement out from the urban core has also forced the middle-income population to rely more heavily on the automobile as the major mode of transportation. The use of the automobile has increased from 37 percent of the population in Pd. 1 to 45 percent of the population in Pd. 4. Bus ridership has increased from 12.2 percent of the population to 16.9 percent of the population, and walking has decreased from 50.2 percent of the population to 38.1 percent. In this same period of time, however, the middle-income population of Simulated City has increased 17.3 percent, and the new population is 115,500.

The movement of middle-income people into formerly high-income areas has again caused high-income population to shift residence locations with the effect of raising the average trip length. This movement has taken the population even further from existing bus routes and residence locations from which walking is feasible, with the result of raising the proportion of the population relying on the automobile from 55.6 percent in Pd. 1 to 71.4 percent in Pd. 4. Again we see a peak trip length in Pd. 2 of 2.9 miles and a reduction of that average trip length in Pd. 4 to 2.8 miles which, again, represents a slight reintegration of middle- and high-income population in areas of Neighborhoods 4 and 5 that are closer to the urban core. In the four periods, high-income populations of Simulated City increased 14.3 percent, to a total of 112,000 people.

Comparison of Period 4—Normal and Period 4—Double

The doubling of base auto costs had a number of interesting effects in the Government Sector as well as in the Social Sector of Simulated City.

In the Government Sector, the patterns of school attendance were significantly changed as a result of the different composition of the population with the doubling of auto costs. Table 5.7 shows the enrollment for each school under normal and doubled auto cost conditions.

Doubling of auto costs had the desired effect of lowering overall highway congestion within the city. However, due to inadequacies in the bus system these reductions were not as substantial as expected.

TABLE 5.5
SCHOOL ENROLLMENT–PERIOD 4–DOUBLED AUTO COST

School	Number of Students	Number of Teachers	Student/Teacher Ratio	Use Index
1	22,020	1,240	18:1	88
2	15,460	1,040	15:1	72
3	18,210	1,240	15:1	72
4	11,040	1,040	11:1	48
Total	66,730	4,560	15:1	73

TABLE 5.6
SUMMARY OF DEMOGRAPHIC CHARACTERISTICS

Neighborhood	Class	Area	Population	Density
1	L/M	13	81,000	6,231
2	L/M/H	6	23,000	3,834
3	L/M	4	28,500	7,125
4	M/H	12	141,500	11,792
5	M/H	15	39,000	2,600
Total		50	313,000	6,260

TABLE 5.7
ENROLLMENT IN PERIOD 4–NORMAL AND PERIOD 4– DOUBLE

School	Enrollment Pd. 4 Normal	Enrollment Pd. 4 Double
1	21,950	22,020
2	16,540	15,460
3	17,870	18,210
4	10,680	11,040
Total	67,040	66,730

The bus company, which should have been the major beneficiary of the decision to double auto costs, was only marginally affected. Although ridership did increase, the increase was not as significant as it could have been owing to the poor location of bus routes.

Differences in the Social Sector between Pd. 4 Normal and Pd. 4 Double are, on the whole, considerably different from what would have been expected. The doubling of base auto costs forced low-income residents, for whom use of an automobile represents a larger proportion of income, to move and seek work at locations which greatly minimized their trip length and cost to work. This movement of low-income population into areas immediately surrounding the urban core provoked a movement of middle-income population into areas more distant from the urban center, with a result of greater trip length and increased dependence on the automobile due to an inadequacy of bus transportation in areas to which the middle-income people were forced to move.

The difference in the rate of population growth from Pd.1 to Pd.4 Normal and from Pd.1 to Pd.4 Double is reflected in the fact that movement of low- and middle-income persons within the urban area had effectively denied housing, in many cases, to potential high-income migrants. The net result was that increased automobile cost made the city less desirable for high-income persons who, on the whole, are biased toward use of the automobile. (See Figure 5.9.)

The movement of low-income population into areas closer to the urban core and the selection of new jobs in order to minimize total transportation costs are reflected in the reduction of the average low-income trip length from 2.6 miles (normal auto cost) to 1.9 miles (double auto cost). These factors are also reflected in the reduction of the percentage of the population relying on the automobile in both Pd.4 Normal and Pd.4 Double. The significant factor, however, is the fact that the proportion of low-income persons relying on walking as a mode of transportation is approximately twice in Pd.4 double auto cost compared to the proportion in Pd.4 under normal auto costs.

A noticeable effect on low-income population is the greater rate of increase of the low-income population under the conditions of double auto cost than under conditions of normal auto cost. The increase in low-income population from Pd.1 to Pd.4 doubled, is 16.3 percent. The increase from Pd.1 to Pd.4 under normal auto cost conditions is 14.3 percent. Consequently, one can surmise that doubling auto costs forces low-income residents to seek housing

FIGURE 5.9
POPULATION GROWTH UNDER NORMAL AND DOUBLE AUTO COSTS

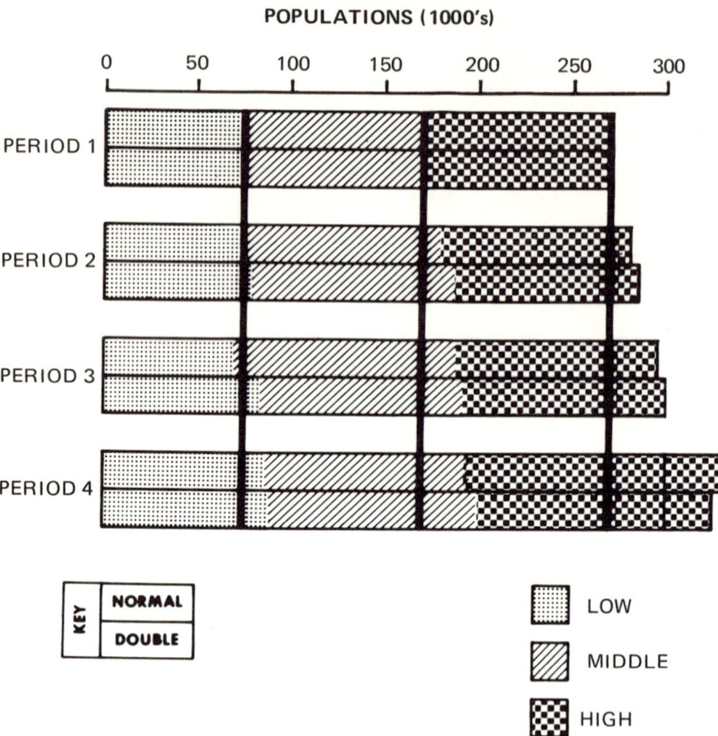

closer to their place of employment, thereby improving the desirability of the city as an area in which low-income persons would locate.

Doubling of the auto cost had immediate and profound implications for middle-income residents of Simulated City. In Pd.1, under conditions of double auto cost, it was possible for middle-income persons to seek jobs which, while not offering the highest initial salary, still produced a maximum net income due to significantly reduced transportation costs; this made the average trip length—under conditions of double auto costs—1 mile for middle-income residents. However, in the period from Pd.1 to Pd.4 Double, the movement of low-income persons into areas previously occupied by middle-income population groups forced the middle-income residents to move out from the center of the city. As a result the average trip length for middle-income persons increased from 1 mile to 1.9 miles under conditions of the doubled auto cost. Under conditions of normal auto costs the average trip length only increased from 1.4 miles to 1.6 miles.

It is easy to see that middle-income residents moved out further from the center of the city because of the greater infusion of low-income persons into previously middle-class areas. In addition, the movement of middle-income people out from the center of the city forced a greater reliance on the bus system. The proportion of the population using the bus in Pd.4 is approximately 50 percent greater under conditions of a doubled auto cost than under conditions of a normal auto cost. The decline in importance of the automobile as a means of transportation is attributable to the fact that, in spite of increased trip lengths, middle-income persons tended to relocate in areas which either were closer to their place of employment, thus allowing them to walk to work, or more distant from the urban core which were situated on adequate bus lines. Neither the fact that middle-income people have a greater trip length under doubled auto cost conditions than under normal auto cost conditions nor the fact that the absolute increase in trip length is greater under doubled as opposed to normal auto cost conditions meant that the city was less desirable as a place for middle-income persons to live. On the contrary, it is a more desirable residence location, as witnessed by the fact that the increase in middle-income population is 17.3 percent with the doubled auto cost as opposed to 14.6 percent with normal auto costs.

The effects on high income residence locations and on the average trip length of high-income populations served to increase the initial trip length under conditions of doubled auto cost. With doubling of auto costs, average high income trip length rose from 2.6 miles (Pd.1 Normal) to 2.7 miles (Pd.1 Double). While this difference in average trip length is hardly significant, it does point up the fact that in order to compensate for increased automobile costs, high-income workers were forced to seek jobs slightly further from their residences in order to maximize income. In Pd.4, however, the average high-income trip length is only 2.8 miles with doubled auto costs as opposed to 2.9 miles without. This modest decrease in average trip length is due less to movement of high-income persons to residences closer to the urban core in Pd.4 doubled than it is to the fact that the increase in high-income population in Simulated City was only 14.3 percent under doubled auto cost conditions, as opposed to 20.9 percent under normal conditions. Consequently, we can assume that the reduction in average trip length by the doubling of auto costs is due primarily to the fact that fewer high-income persons moved into the city and, as a result, increased settlement in the fringe areas did not occur. (See Tables 5.8A and 5.9B for analysis.)

Summary

In summary, we note several significant differences in the distribution of socio-economic classes within Simulated City as a result of increasing the expense of automobile usage: population increases and average trip length. Increased cost for automobile usage had the net effect of speeding the process of demographic succession.

(1) The movement of low-income populations into formerly middle-income areas is hastened due to the necessity of low-income people to drastically reduce the transportation cost and trip length.

(2) The desirability of the city increases in the perception of low- and middle-income populations and decreases in the perception of high-income populations. These changes in desirability are reflected by the increased population growth for low- and middle-income populations and the decreased rate of population growth for high-income populations. The additional influx of low-income populations creates a situation which forces certain locations to be denied to high-income population groups with a consequent reduction in the number of high-income migrants. It is a case not so much of high-income populations leaving, but more simply, a reluctance on the part of high-income populations external to Simulated City to move into the metropolitan area.

TABLE 5.8A

TRIP LENGTH ANALYSIS

	Period 1–4 Normal Auto Cost Pd. 1	Pd. 2	Pd. 3	Pd. 4
Low Income				
Average trip length	3.1	2.8	2.7	2.6
Auto passengers	73 (55.3)	78 (55.3)	46 (43.4)	48 (34.0)
Bus passengers	35 (26.5)	36 (25.5)	52 (49.1)	66 (46.8)
Walk	24 (18.2)	27 (19.2)	8 (7.5)	27 (19.2)
Total workers	132	141	106	141
Unemployed	15	10	37	27
% pop. increase		2.7	–2.7	14.29
Middle Income				
Average trip length	1.4	2.4	1.5	1.6
Auto passengers	83 (42.1)	108 (52.4)	105 (47.3)	114 (50.2)
Bus passengers	18 (9.1)	16 (7.8)	24 (10.8)	27 (11.9)
Walk	96 (48.8)	82 (39.8)	93 (41.9)	86 (37.9)
Total workers	197	206	222	227
Unemployed	1	1	1	0
% pop. increase		4.6	12.6	14.6
High Income				
Average trip length	2.6	2.7	3.0	2.9
Auto passengers	151 (77.0)	152 (72.7)	172 (77.5)	175 (73.8)
Bus passengers	0	0	0	4 (1.7)
Walk	45 (23.0)	57 (27.3)	50 (22.5)	58 (24.5)
Total workers	196	209	222	237
Unemployed	0	0	0	0
% pop. increase		6.6	13.3	20.9

TABLE 5.8B
TRIP LENGTH ANALYSIS

	Period 1–4 Doubled Auto Cost Pd. 1	Pd. 2	Pd. 3	Pd. 4
Low Income				
Average trip length	3.1	2.7	2.4	1.9
Auto passengers	83 (62.9)	56 (40.6)	45 (35.2)	35 (25.6)
Bus passengers	25 (18.9)	40 (29.0)	50 (39.1)	53 (38.7)
Walk	24 (18.2)	42 (30.4)	33 (25.7)	49 (35.7)
Total workers	132	138	128	137
Unemployed	15	15	33	34
% pop. increase		4.1	9.5	16.3
Middle Income				
Average trip length	1.0	2.4	1.9	1.9
Auto passengers	74 (37.6)	109 (52.2)	112 (53.6)	104 (45.0)
Bus passengers	24 (12.2)	16 (7.7)	24 (11.5)	39 (16.9)
Walk	99 (50.2)	84 (40.1)	73 (34.9)	88 (38.1)
Total workers	197	209	209	231
Unemployed	1	0	0	0
% pop. increase		5.6	5.6	17.3
High Income				
Average trip length	2.7	3.3	2.9	2.8
Auto passengers	109 (55.6)	147 (70.7)	160 (72.1)	160 (71.4)
Bus passengers	20 (10.2)	3 (1.4)	4 (1.8)	5 (2.2)
Walk	67 (34.2)	59 (27.9)	58 (26.1)	59 (26.4)
Total workers	196	208	222	224
Unemployed	0	0		
% pop. increase		6.1	13.3	14.3

(3) Increased automobile costs force low- income populations to drastically reduce their average trip length and transportation cost simply because transportation represents a larger proportion of their income than it does for middle- and high-income residents. Again, this causes a movement of low-income population groups into areas formerly occupied by middle-income populations, forcing middle-income residents into areas primarily available to high-income migrants. This population movement increases the density and occupancy rate of these locations and therefore discourages the movement of high-income migrants into these areas.

The fact that average trip lengths for middle- and high-income populations increased in terms of a comparison between Pd.4 Normal and Pd.4 Doubled, reflects the fact that middle- and high-income populations have been forced to move out to locations at ever-increasing distances from the center of the city. The reduction of average high-income trip length from Pd.3 to Pd.4 both under conditions of a normal auto cost and doubled auto costs, reflects the fact that there has occurred in both instances a slight reintegration of middle- and high-income populations at locations closer to the urban core.

It cannot be emphasized too strongly that the results presented here are illustrative and not predictive. Current research suggests that travel and travel cost relations are highly inelastic and that the magnitude of shifts suggested here are grossly exaggerated; this is particularly so given any reasonable time period. On the other hand, the distortion as presented did serve its true purpose, that of displaying the potential richness of a GEM-type model for policy and research purposes; particularly in the ability of the model to point out potential effects beyond the direct.

The next chapter will deal with our experiences in building models and in the light of this, the very difficult questions of model data needs and predictability.

Chapter 6

MODELING EXPERIENCE

The decision to build a general model should be considered carefully. Since our own preparations were far from painstakingly conceived, it is by no means suggested that others follow this path. In our case, a high degree of staff dedication, public and private interest and inordinate good fortune often made up for a lack of planning. To summarize briefly:

DESIGN RESOURCES

As with every product, the resources necessary can be parsed into time and money. In building models, of course, space and computers must also be included.

The concept of model cost was meaningless in our early days of model development. To begin with, an enormous price had to be paid for public relations and advertising. Further, the principal accounting procedure followed by many of us during the four years of model development consisted of substituting time for money.

DESIGN TEAM

The best method we derived for the design process includes the following:

(1) A small multidisciplined team who makes up an overall design plan and has the last word on what goes into a model.

(2) This design team should be supported by a second level group who, with the designers, is concerned with how to present the system in model terms so that the routines can be efficiently programmed.

(3) There should be someone on the team who has the group confidence as a synthesizer and another member who is responsible for making sure that the algorithms which are arrived at include what the design group desires.

(4) The research should be made easier by encouraging many design meetings. In this way everyone is building the same model and each design stage benefits from all viewpoints.

(5) If the group is small, the model relatively simple, and time and money of non-prime importance, then models can be built using "group awareness." CITY I and II were built in this way, with no formal plan. The design staff met constantly and the models evolved out of these encounters. It seems doubtful, however, that more complex models could be built so informally. A design plan or overall theory becomes necessary as the size of the model and group increases.

(6) The design and programming staffs should be separated during the formative stages of the model. Interaction between the two groups should only occur when programming actually begins, making certain it is the design staff which specifies the model and not the programmers.

MODELING PROCESS

There are numerous rules-of-thumb we have used in building our models. A few changed with time, some have remained constant. For example:

(1) In the early days of our models, REGION I, II, and CITY I, we were not concerned with the accuracy of model relationships, at least not in the way that those who build policy models usually are. In fact, the models were designed so that they enabled game players to make decisions which were not always valid but would give more realistic results within the constraints of the model.

(2) Fortunately we chose a type of gaming called "systemic" as our early modeling technique. What we interpreted this to mean was that as many decisions as possible were to be made during the game and the

problems which arose were to be a product of the model itself rather than of an "umpire" or the result of a preconceived scenario. Our prejudice to use the systemic approach was fortunate in that the model does not depend upon contrived happenings, and a strict adherence to this objective led to a closer simulation of reality. Further, during the designing of our model, the discussions of each portion of the system were so structured that all inputs and outputs of the model sector would be a function of things which happened in the gameroom or as part of the pure machine portion of the model.

(3) We never accepted another researcher's findings for inclusion in our model unless it also fit the experience of the design team.

(4) The various parts of the model were added, subtracted, or modified, on the basis of suggestions made by a large number of players and numerous colleagues and an almost maniacal concern for model balance. By balanced we usually meant that the population was looked at in numbers which related to, say, the land unit or money unit size.

Further, the resources available to the players and decision makers were of constant concern. There was an attempt to balance the amount of resources available to the various gameroom participants.

This section suggests that one break almost all of the commandments previously held by the modeling community. We used the models to discover relationships rather than using an accepted theory. Our exploration therefore resulted in an evolved theory rather than a planned one; we ignored defined factors or decision points and focused instead on functional processes in a system; did not worry about data availability or form, did not research the literature for algorithms, vocabulary, or support; and finally, we felt our way through such areas as model balance and aggregation.

CONCLUSIONS

The second half of this book will concern itself with more detailed documentation of the current GEM derivative, CITY IV, with the hope that it will be of use to others who choose to tread the path of large scale model building.

Obviously, after four years of experience, many more uses could be discussed. However, now that the model is free to the user and is in widespread use, it is preferable that the user become familiar with the manuals and documentation available elsewhere.

In the meantime, the reader can make his own assessment of the usefulness and validity of using the GEM form of impact models for his purposes. If he decides this form suits his needs, then the framework presented here can be the backdrop for his own research.

DATA

For the past several years, there has never been a group discussion concerning our model which did not eventually bring up the question of data availability. This preoccupation with data is often confusing. Perhaps there is great security in reams upon reams of numbers which are real and measure something. What is worrisome is that in the business community lawyers and accountants are never in control of a company unless the company is in financial trouble. Their intellectual soul-brother, the empiricist, is usually in control of the modeling community. The health of the current state-of-the-art of modeling might be questioned on this basis.

It would seem that the theoretician and the empiricist ought to be able to have an equal stance in model design. Although it is not certain that the same man would provide these two services, both of their inputs are required before a model can be used for policy purposes.

The real users of the data are the researchers, not the policy makers. The fact that there are X policemen or Y fireman per square mile is not ordinarily useful data to the people running a city unless attached to a policy question. The data to be useful to a researcher have to be conceived of as part of a general schema or theoretical structure. This suggests that the theoretician's model can be thought of as a separate entity and not dependent on data. Of course the model, if accurate, can be made more of a predictive tool with better data.

MODEL ERRORS

One of the present allegations made by a number of the model designers is that a model, even if it is not an accurate forecast device, is still a valuable tool for testing alternative policy choices. I believe that outright acceptance of such an idea would be reassuring to a model builder but potentially dangerous for users. The argument has face validity only under a very special set of circumstances.

Let us divide the factors which might cause results obtained by model use to differ from reality into two different categories. The first of these, a Type A Error, is caused by a poor model design. These types of errors might be the result of a complete lack of understanding of the system being modeled, a poor design of a single subsystem, or may be due to a failure to include all the necessary major subsystems. The second general category, the Type B Error, is a result of poor data. Type B Errors would include poorly aggregated data, wrong relationship values, missing data, or poorly estimated numbers.

Briefly, the results obtained with a model containing a Type A Error are not useful for any purpose. The second problem area, a model with Type B Errors, may or may not be useful for comparing policy alternatives but will likely be a good educational or training device. If the model appears to replicate reality in a consistent fashion (no Type A Errors) but there is insufficient data to do more than indicate the general direction of growth or change, then although it would not be a good forecast device, it may be possible to use the model as a control device or a constant against which various policies could be tested. This use of the model, although not as satisfactory as the use of the same model for both forecast and laboratory testing purposes, is a far cry from the unstructured, almost random approach taken by many decision makers today.[16] The principal caveat to be remembered with a model with a serious Type B Error is that it can be as useless for any form of policy testing (not to mention forecasting purposes) as one containing Type A Errors.

Unfortunately, the discussion of Type A and Type B Errors does not really shed much light on the use of models as policy laboratories. We have said that good forecast models are good laboratory models, but that some models which are not good forecast models may be good as laboratory models, yet in reality, there is often no way of testing which of these errors account for an invalid model.

The final frontiers of social science model-building will not be in the research for better modeling forms or even for clearer understanding of the relationships in the social system. Nor will it be in the area of the usefulness or availability of data or in its retrieval. The area of research where most work is yet to be done is that of model usage.

For example, there is a provocative argument that can be made for the inherent nonfeasibility of large-scale man-machine modeling as a predictive device for decision makers. Briefly, the thesis assumes a model which is valid and the availability of adequate data.

To use a man-machine model (say, of the GEM type) for policy purposes, let us postulate that the model is of a sort that requires the inputs (decisions) of leading policy makers from the business, social, and government communities of the modeled area. If those men were given computer print-outs of the portion of the environment over which they exercised control and interacted in real life and, if they were also able to communicate with each other and had access to the data banks, then they could act as endogenous branch points for the model's iteration. (Let us also assume that the exogenous inputs are known and automatically fed to the model.)

The session, if carried out without feedback from the model, would be expected to be a good approximation of the state of the system for the next year–assuming no large unexpected exogenous interventions.

However, the model, to be used for policy purposes, would have to have its results surveyed by its users. Unless the situation was highly fortuitous, there would likely be one to several decision makers who would be able to better their position by changing their decisions. If they are allowed to (for they certainly will in reality if they believe in the model's validity) then the second iteration will find the local resources reallocated so that relative advantages and disadvantages are shifted. After each attempt, the least well off will wish to change their decisions.

In short, the model will have to be continually recycled from the starting point with altered decisions until a mini-max solution is reached. That is, until the decision makers are convinced that no reallocation of their resources could yield them a greater return (or sustain them a smaller loss).

This equilibrium position is obviously several times more sophisticated a decision-making schema than is found in real life. Further, men who are sufficiently rational to accept the mini-max point in one sense belie the existence of race tracks, Las Vegas, card games, and the like. In fact, such rationality might be antithetical to the very entrepreneurial instincts which made many of the policy makers the leaders they are.

This example, as well as several others, highlights the many problems ahead as the social scientist wrestles with using advanced technology to create his own laboratory. The milieu of the model user will prove fruitful ground for the researcher.

VALIDITY AND PREDICTABILITY

Validity refers to replicability, how well the model represents what it purports to; and predictability, how useful it is in extrapolating in some way a current situation to a future time so that the user would have confidence in the results.

There does not appear to be any agreed-upon method for proving either validity or predictability for most complex social science models. There are ways to see if the models do not meet minimum criteria. If the problem to be modeled were one which only depended on (1) quantifiable variables for a solution, and (2) if we were able to restrict the number of variables to be considered for solving the problem, then a model could be tested against observed data and its validity and predictive capability evaluated. This would be particularly true if the phenomenon being studied was one which covered a fairly homogeneous and common event, such as the amount of traffic on a particular street during rush hour. Under such conditions the model could be run over and over again to predict an expected output. The success with which it achieved the goal of anticipating the phenomena would be a measure of its predictability. Hamilton et al. (1969: 111-113), have arrived at a similar conclusion.

> "Model validity" is a bad choice of words in that the words carry the connotation of a simple dichotomy–the model is valid or not valid. In practice, the problem is never that simple. The real issue is, "Is the model good enough to answer my questions?" Here also, the answer is almost always clouded. At present there are few objective tests that can be applied. Especially there are none that can give an answer relative to a specific use of the model. So the question becomes one of whether the builder has confidence in his model for the use to which he plans to apply it–admittedly a subjective evaluation. This being so, he cannot prove the validity to anyone else, but he can answer the question for himself.[17]

Attention to three areas can contribute to the model-builder's confidence in his model.

> (1) *Microstructure.* Is the microstructure of the model reasonable? Have the appropriate variables been included and is thir dependency on other variables sensible? Is the form of the dependency reasonable? Is the direction of cause and effect correct?
>
> (2) *Statistical fit.* Have the sensitive parameters been carefully derived from data? Have the residuals been carefully studied for signs of missing variables?

(3) *Overall model behavior.* Is the overall model behavior reasonable? Are there peculiar biases toward special modes of behavior that one would not reasonably expect? If the model is run over a period of time for which there is historical data, does it reproduce history reasonably well?

Designers generally agree that the term "model validity" is inappropriate. Since, however there are no objective tests that can be applied, the answer becomes subjective. In the end, the builder may not be able to prove the validity to anyone else, but he can use the model as a tool and aid for his own decision-making. This is somewhat analagous to a policy maker who cannot objectively discuss why he trusts his advisors, but does so anyway because he has faith in their predictions and knows how to interpret their opinion in light of a specific, current situation.

There is an important distinction that must be made between models designed for a specific purpose and general models. Social science, unlike physical science, is studied as an action-reaction phenomenon. Almost any event which takes place is the result of a large number of activities, some more or less important at a particular point in time, but all interacting to produce a particular result. This result, after its occurrence, is unique and cannot be exactly replicated by a simulation unless all the events which led up to its occurrence are exactly replicated.

For example, let us take the example of trying to simulate the game of baseball. Despite all the rules which this game has developed to handle exceptional circumstances, the overall theory of the game itself is very simple. There are nine men who play both an offensive and defensive role with nine other men of similar ability. The offensive object of the game is to hit a ball which is thrown past a single member of the offensive team by a member of the defensive team. The object of the offensive team member is to hit the ball and run around a diamond-shaped track, touching each of its points of intersection. There are a limited number of times the offensive player and the defensive player can participate in this duel. If the offensive team is successfully prevented from hitting the ball and running around the diamond within a specified number of opportunities, the teams change sides and the offensive team becomes the defensive. The defensive team is expected to prevent the offensive one from hitting the ball, or if the ball is hit, from running around the diamond.

The prevention of hitting the ball is the prime responsibility of a member of the defensive team called the pitcher and his partner, the man who receives the ball, called the catcher. Successfully throwing the ball between them a specified number of times in a specified fashion, without its being hit by the offensive player, results in the necessity of the offensive team replacing the hitter. This may only be done three times. If the ball is hit, then it becomes the responsibility of the rest of the defensive team to retrieve the ball and tag the offensive team member who hit the ball before he runs around the diamond, tagging the four intersections. If the offensive player runs around the diamond and is not tagged, he scores a run. The team which scores the most runs wins.

Obviously, we have only superficially described the game of baseball. However, it is a game which could be successfully simulated and programmed for the computer. The resulting model would be sufficiently realistic that the statistics of two teams could be loaded into the model and computer baseball games played.

Given this model, let us now load in the data of two real-world teams and replay yesterday's games and play tomorrow's games. If we had unlimited time and money at our disposal, we would be able to replay yesterday's games with a high level of exactitude but might still not be able to predict exactly the results of tomorrow's games. What does this say for our model? First, if we did not have to redesign the model to take into consideration the events of each specific game but only had to readjust the parameters, then we likely have an excellent general model. Second, it says that the model works well (is valid) and will replicate the past provided we can state definitively all of the occurrences of the past. Third, that ability to recreate the past is no guarantee of the ability to predict the future, if one requires specific results–such as the winner of a particular game. In fact, with the most valid model of all, the same teams in the same field in the same day, the first game of a double header does not necessarily presage the events in the second.

This model is, as mentioned, a relatively simple zero sum game and relates to models of the general environment only in that a number of factors are required to interact for a solution. The differences between the simple case of a baseball game and modeling the environment are obviously enormous.

As difficult as it is to discuss validity and forecasting in the case of baseball, the problem is greatly compounded when we talk about the total environment. The question, therefore, is not one of what techniques to use for validating a model, but whether validation is indeed possible in light of such seeming complexity.

Point to Point Prediction

As McLeod notes in a recent issue of his S^3, the most popular test of a model's validity is point-to-point prediction.

> Probably the most time-honored method of validating a simulation is to compare the response made by the model to various stimuli with the observed reaction of the *system modeled* (the "simuland") to similar disturbances. This method has two obvious shortcomings, as well as some not-so-obvious ones, beyond the scope of this discussion.
>
> (1) It might be impossible—or impractical—to manipulate the simuland (the real-world system) in the required manner. In this case one must resort to observing the past response of the simuland to naturally occurring disturbances, then try to simulate these disturbances to elicit meaningful responses from the model.
>
> (2) Even should the response of the model to a given stimulus be identical to that of the simuland, this does not constitute proof that the internal dynamics of the model are like those of the simuland. But if model and simuland react in the same manner to step, ramp, and sinusoidal inputs, they will almost certainly exhibit the same response to other inputs. There, if considered as a "black box" the model may serve as a valid simulation of the simuland.

The argument suggests that a model is valid and has predictive capability if you start at point A and can project to point D. However, if this test of validity is accepted, except for very simplified models, there are not sufficient data at this point in time to objectively test complex models (Figure 6-1). If one were to assume that current research efforts to gather data are successful and the parameters for the model become available, can testing them be considered useful? The premises behind testing come from the physical science community. Their models, if properly tuned, when loaded at point A will always produce identical output at point D. In other words, the models are deterministic. Unfortunately, little, if anything, in the social sciences is that simple. Solutions to problems in the social area must be thought of as probabilistic, not deterministic.

Conceiving of reality as the most perfect model and imagining the ability to conjure up instant replays, the decade 1950 to 1960 may or may not replicate itself in detail. In short, the present may be said to be a historical accident. The points 1, 2, or 3 on the hypothetical distribution (Figure 6.2) are all valid solutions to the series of iterations from A to D (reality might be thought of as any one of the three also). A social scientist can project the future in terms of probability. To derive his distribution, he must run the same model with the same starting points many times. He then must resort to sampling theory to discuss the odds of reasonableness of an event's outcome.

A general model of the environment, if well constructed, would replicate the events between two time periods and produce results in specified areas which would agree with the real world. Unfortunately, we are not apt to know whether any existing models are valid using this criterion—at least in the foreseeable future—because we simply do not have the data available to load the model. Tests which attempt to use this method must therefore be highly suspect since failure to arrive at a particular result which has historical validity in real time may not be the fault of the model but of the data.

Since the principal concern for validity is as a measure of the predictive capability of a model, the inability to prove the validity of a general model also calls to question its predictability. We should expect a model which is reputed to be useful as a predictive tool to tell us what the odds are of a particular event occurring, given a specific set of inputs. Therefore, prediction becomes a probabilistic rather than deterministic feature of a model and, as such, a more readily attainable goal.

The running of a model to test the results of some particular inputs on a specific event (remembering that there are many other possibilities not called for) now goes through successive iterations, such that the results can be studied and a probabilistic outcome defined.

The summary of this brief discourse seems quite pessimistic. We have despaired of the data availability and have suggested that standard predictability testing is not useful. We have further stated that to arrive at the necessary probabilistic solutions for complex social science model solutions, the model must be run numerous times. The latter is not only an expensive process, but suggests particular problems when multiruns are of man-machine simulations.

An Alternative

As an alternative to testing validity, we might perform a test of the following order. We have said that it is important to proceed from A (a point in the past) to D (the present), and more important to go on to E and F (the future). This test, even if it worked, would still not give us absolute confidence that say, D to F was a valid extrapo-

FIGURE 6.1
MODEL FORECASTING

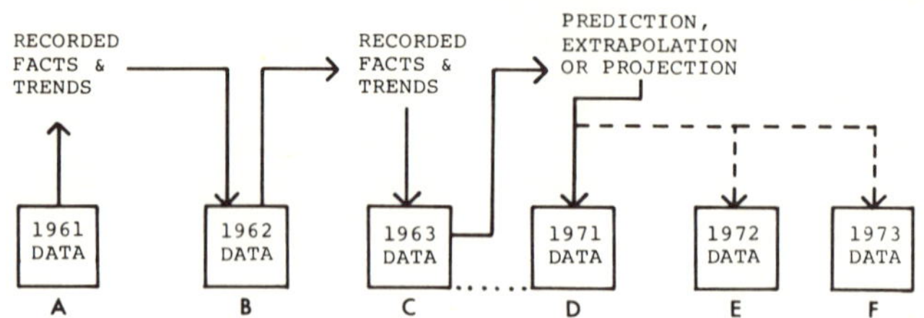

FIGURE 6.2
MODEL RUNS

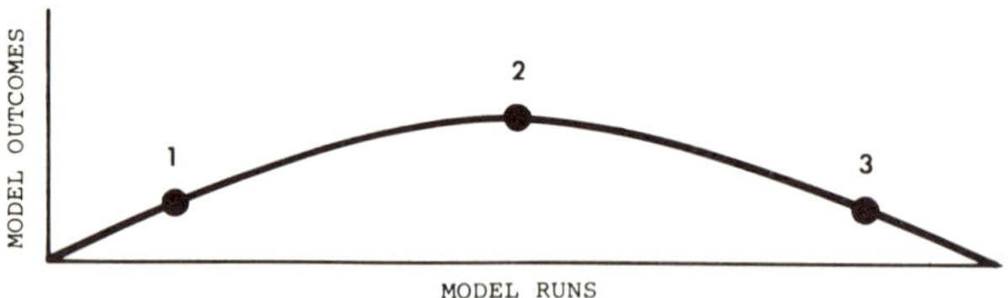

FIGURE 6.3
OUTPUT POSSIBILITIES

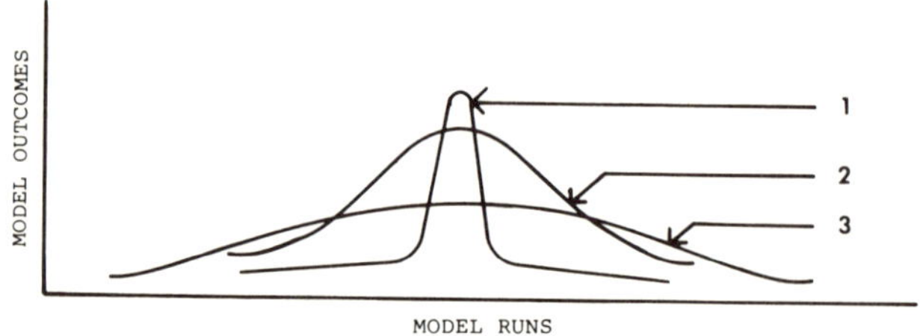

lation, even if A to D were valid. In point of fact, almost no test will satisfy this demand. What we really want to know is, will the model at least move from point A to point D (assuming data availability) if we control the intervening iterations. In other words, could one of the solutions, using the model being tested, have been the A to D result? If so, we at least have the confidence that the model is valid insofar as it would have been able to solve the A to D extrapolation. This test does not tell us, however, whether the odds of our model in solving the A to D problem are the same as the odds were in reality. Nor do we have any more than superficial confidence that the projected movement from A to F is a realistic distribution.

We do have some confidence on short run projections. The first distribution (1) might represent a situation which was almost certainty. In modeling and projection terms, if the principal variable we have under consideration is time, we can state that if we have confidence in the model's ability to go from point A to D in a realistic fashion (let us say if it passes the above prescribed test and we add some subjective validation to the reasonableness of the iterations and the projected distribution of A to D data) then the shorter the time span, point E, the greater the confidence in the model results and the tighter the distribution (2). Running the model into the distant future would result in a distribution like (3) and be almost meaningless for predictive purposes. Remember, we are discussing general purpose models. These results might not apply to highly aggregated models which focus only on a relatively few parameters. But highly aggregated models fall prey to the danger of possibly not including enough parameters to arrive at realistic results in the long run. (See Figure 6.3.)

While we await the day when we are able to definitely test a model to assure that it mirrors the future faithfully, we will have to be content with the rough and ready guidelines suggested here and depend on the subjective evaluation of usefulness. In the meantime, we can use behavioral models to study the possible parameters of the present.

Model Use as a Policy Device

As noted elsewhere, it is difficult to discuss questions of a model's usefulness for predictive purposes because the movement into the future can be fraught with unexpected happenings, many of which are often of great consequence for local areas. I suspect that the problem of prediction can be handled only for relatively short periods of time and then only with models which are rich enough to incorporate the many parameters which are apt to be pivotal for total system direction.

Rather than focus our attention here on attempting to prove the ability to forecast the future, let us instead discuss the model as a different type of policy device. First, we will load the model with the data base of a particular area. If we describe validity as the ability of a model to reflect present system reality, then demonstrating the validity of a behavioral model would be relatively simple, since the model's operation can be checked against present data. Once satisfied that the model replicates reality tolerably well (within a particular time period), the behavioral model becomes a useful tool for doing impact studies.

An impact study is probably the most familiar form of research methodology used in the social sciences. Its essence is the description of a system, in whole or part, and the insertion of a new parameter or parameter value to the system. The system is then analyzed in light of this change and the resulting changes noted.

Impact models do not take time into consideration, at least at first, but reallocate system resources in light of what would have happened both with and without a specific run input. With the GEM model one could add human decisions to the results of the impact state and judgmentally forecast the results of the new stimulus. However, this last step is not crucial to the usefulness of the technique although it helps to satisfy the incessant yearning for models with forecast ability. This ability is sorely needed by our policy makers, many of whom hope to have highly sophisticated data banks at their disposal in the near future but, as yet, have no way to relate and use the data. A behavioral model does not search for solutions such as the gravity models, which generally do not represent reality except in the grossest fashion, nor does it merely extrapolate the past as does a trend model; instead, it can give answers to policy changes which are not only realistic but yield implications of results in all areas and not just the one or so usually supplied by the analysts who are specialists in single sectors. This ability to note effects throughout the system has obvious advantages, particularly where some policies cause unanticipated stimuli in other parts of the system.

Conclusions

If we are not always sure a model is valid and consequently are not positively able to predict with it, why use such complex, sophisticated models at all? The reason is not that the problems have necessarily become more difficult to solve so that more sophisticated models are needed, but that our measures of the effects of policy decisions become more accurate with complex models. Many solutions to problems tried previously may have actually been failures but the time taken to discover this took so long that often other factors intervened to solve the original dilemma.

If, as some suggest, our country's resources are not unlimited and are in fact becoming increasingly scarce, one might legitimately ask if we should continue testing ideas in the real marketplace when an alternate policy can be tested with large-scale computer models which would likely be more successful and save precious resources.

Computer resources combined with a functional theoretical structure of the total system are a necessary bridge in dealing with environmental decisions. It will not be long before we all feel the full force of the computer revolution. This machine, once accepted as a valid resource, has provided us with an increased ability to problem solve. Present policy makers and others in decision arenas are experiencing all of the cultural lags which accompany a new invention. The youth being trained now, however, are quite conversant with this new technology. But the intellectual credence and power mostly lie with those who are not.

Holistic models with man-machine simulations can be an invaluable tool in making this transition for dealing with modern-day problems. It is our hope that we will be able to create computer software which is not only on the edge of the current state-of-the-art, but is done in such a fashion that users—regardless of training era—can benefit. If we all fail, then the results of present decisions and ongoing changes will indeed be painful; even revolution proceeds by steps.

PART TWO

Chapter 7

THE CITY MODEL: A DETAILED USE OF THE SECTOR FRAMEWORK

The previous section of the book is complete in itself and should satisfy those who are interested in the general structure of the GEM model. However, there are some who will be concerned with the details and parameters which are used in such a model, particularly those used in the research and training examples in the previous chapter. While a complete analysis of the flow charts of the model would be prohibitive and unnecessary for our purposes, we will attempt in the following pages to treat the model in a descriptive but abbreviated form so that the reader has a chance to see the general structure of the GEM-CITY model. It is important that this be done because it is one of the few instances that a very complex theoretical structure—such as the Sector Theory—has actually been implemented in an operating fashion. There are several manuals elsewhere which have as their purpose detailed descriptions of the use, application, and documentation of the CITY model. If the reader refers to other of these works he may find differences in some details. Generally, this is due to the fact that GEM is constantly evolving and each edition of the manuals presents these changes. Further, there is an almost constant mismatch, more or less serious, even in this book, between the intended design, the previous operating program, and the current version, as modules get rethought and reprogrammed on the basis of experience. As noted earlier, the purpose of this book is to wed a number of complex ideas together; detail would be distracting to the main focus and is left to other works.

In an effort to follow the Sector Concept presented in the first section, the model is discussed in terms of economic, social and governmental areas. Within each of these Sectors, there are a number of Operating Programs which interact across the Sectors. For example, employment affects the Economic, Government and Social Sectors; however, to repeat the total employment process in each of the Sectors would not only be repetitive, but tiring. Therefore, it is mentioned in those areas in which it first occurs, or where it has the greatest effect. This means that the Economic Sector is overburdened with definitions of Operational Programs at the expense of the Government and Social Sectors. Nonetheless, on the whole, the reader should be able to find sufficient information to enable him to comprehend the examples of model use in the following material.

OUTSIDE SYSTEM OF GEM-CITY

Most systems lack some degree of closure. A decision usually needs to be made by the analysts, therefore, on how to handle those portions of the environment that are not part of the immediate model. The designer decides (usually based upon the purpose for which the model was constructed) which portions of the universe are likely to affect the parameters of his model. Having made this determination, he then proceeds to represent these feeds in his simulation. On the other hand, the modeler can choose to hold other things equal and, like the scientist working in a controlled laboratory experiment, run his simulation without taking into account the effects of parameters outside his immediate concern. Both solutions are less than perfect, but by choosing to limit the things the model will ignore, a greater degree of confidence in the results can be allowed.

Defining the actual simulations in either of the above approaches would, of course, depend upon the level of generality being simulated. The principal constraint to their construction is that it is not considered possible to simulate all of the necessary levels of generality above and below the one being used. For the GEM model, the outside system is represented with general simulators which give gross application of inputs instead of with the hundreds of smaller ones that would be required if the whole system were completely modeled (Figure 7.1).

The outside system influences on the local system represented in GEM can also be divided along Sector lines: economic, social, and governmental. The economic influences are those generated by the national money market (interest rate and funds available), the national business cycle (prices paid for goods by SIC category, cost of goods and services by SIC, and rates of return on investments), national business mobility (nationally owned businesses moving to or from the local system in response to economic conditions), tourism (the attraction of outside the system consumers to local recreational resources), outside construction industries (costs and time needed to complete construction of new structures), and taxes paid to and funds received from higher level governments.

Some of the influences on the Social Sector that are interrelated with the outside system are those from migration (movement of population units in response to jobs, housing and amenities) and taxes paid to and personal payments received from higher level governments and outside institutions.

Influences on the Government Sector include those that are created by the outside system from intergovernmental aid (capital and current, regular and special) and from regulation by higher level governments.

National Markets

The computer simulates a national market mechanism that recreates a national business cycle, changes the prices paid for goods and services in the national market, and sets interest rates for various types of loans and bonds. The national business cycle is based upon historical trends and varies by major types of goods and services. The conditions generated by the set of national cycles, such as the prices and loan rates, feed to other national market mechanisms.

Business Cycle

The business cycle routine generates an index number by year for each of the following items:

(1) Overall national business conditions
(2) Prices paid

FIGURE 7.1
OUTSIDE SYSTEM

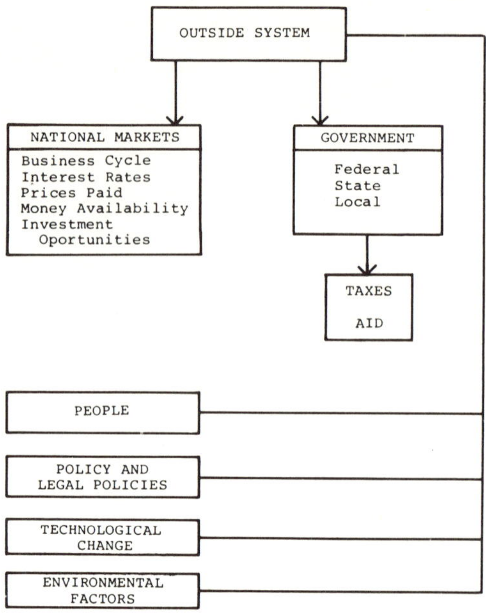

(3) National interest rate
(4) National bond rate
(5) Return on conservative investments[18]
(6) Return on speculative investments[19]

The variation in HI (Heavy Industry) average prices is greater than that for LI (Light Industry) which is, in turn, higher than that for NS (National Services). The price received per unit of output for any basic industry in the local system is calculated by multiplying the normal price per unit for that type of basic industry times the business cycle index for that industry.

The outside system model decides the price to be paid for goods and services sold at national markets. The model also generates the interest and bond rate which is determined by the system average and the price of borrowing money, based upon national conditions the model determined the type of loan and the financial status of the borrower. Finally, depending on local system profitability conditions, the outside system controls the number of levels of each business activity that will move to the local region.

Federal-State Relations

The major federal-state decisions considered in this model relate to: (1) conventional and innovative financial aid programs to local governments and private organizations, (2) regulations, (3) taxing and (4) physical structures built; i.e., military bases, state offices, parks, universities, etc. Financial aid is available for specified current and capital programs when appropriate grand conditions are met (e.g., matching, minimum standards, etc.).

The local region is very much affected by the taxing policies of state and federal authorities. Federal income and excise taxes and state sales and income taxes are largely outside the control of local system decision makers. Yet the Social and Economic Sectors are directly affected by rate levels and the local governments are, in a sense, in competition with the higher governments in their quest for revenue from taxes.

Federal, personal, and business income taxes are paid by local system population units and businesses. State sales taxes are paid by all private purchasers of goods and services whether the selling establishment is in the local or outside system.

FIGURE 7.2
ECONOMIC SECTOR

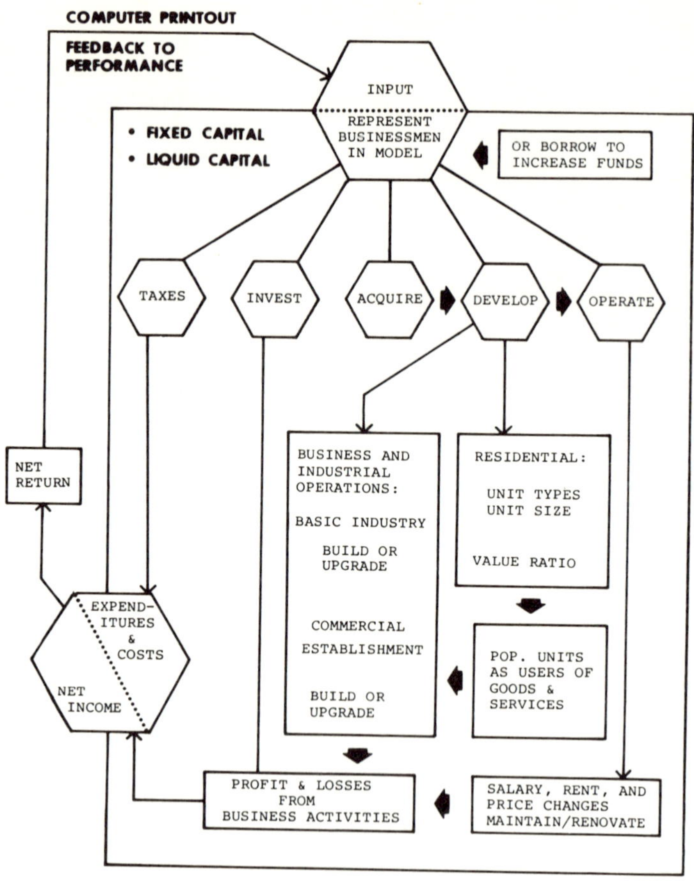

ECONOMIC SECTOR

The Economic Sector of GEM deals with all non-government physical structures, all business activities, and all locally controlled financial and real estate institutions (Figure 7.2). More specifically, Economic Sector activities involve building construction operations; the business operations associated with agriculture, mining, construction services, manufacturing, retail trade and services; and the activities associated with banking (transfer of cash, borrowing, lending, and investing) and with real estate (transfer land, renting housing, and renting office space; Figure 7.3).

The Economic Sector is in constant interaction with the other two sectors (Social and Governmental). Furthermore, the Economic Sector has an impact on the physical dimensions of the local environment by the land it consumes, the buildings it constructs, the transportation links that it uses, and the pollution it creates. Conversely, the physical characteristics of the local geographical area such as available space and the topography have an impact on decisions within the Economic Sector.

The Social Sector acts as a supplier of labor and a demander of goods and services with respect to the Economic Sector. Interest groups represent the Social Sector in a formal manner and affect the supply of labor through unions and the purchase of goods and services through consumer organizations. The Economic Sector may influence decision-making of the interest groups through the instrument of dues and donations.

The Government Sector provides many of the services and grants some of the privileges that are required by economic activities. The Economic Sector pays for these services through taxes and charges.

Functional Classifications in the Economic Sector

A number of different considerations were involved in the determination of the business activities to be employed in the model. The Standard Industrial Classification (SIC) codes, prepared by the Office of Statistical Standards of the U.S. Bureau of the Budget, served as the basic building blocks for the non-farming business activities.

Since we wanted the various types of business activities in GEM to interact realistically with one another, we used the interindustry relationships contained in the 1958 Input-Output Study (most of the

FIGURE 7.3
AGGREGATE INTERACTIONS BETWEEN THE ECONMIC SECTOR AND OTHER SECTORS

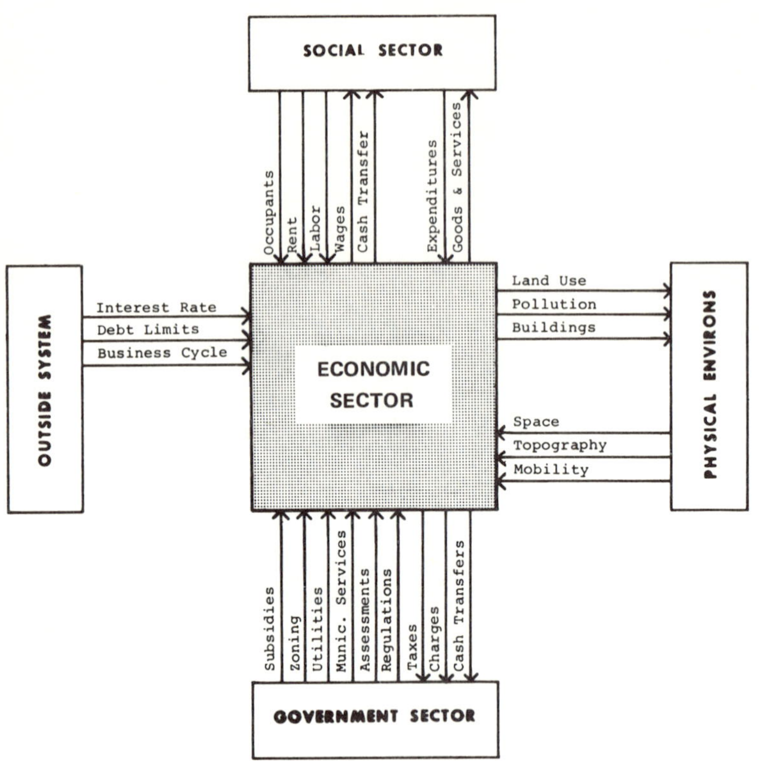

other model data bases used the 1960 Census, or data available as close to that date as possible). Through the use of these relationships, it was possible to derive an aggregated and average number of standardized units of intermediate products that would be required to produce a standardized unit of final product for any business activity. We converted the dollar figures contained in the input-output table to standardized units of output (tons of hypothetical units) so that the effect of changing prices could be represented when the model is run in a dynamic fashion.

There are eleven general types of economic land uses in GEM. These land uses are divided among basic, industrial, commercial establishments and residents.[20] They include:

Basic Industry[21]

HI	Heavy Industry: steel, petroleum, etc.
LI	Light Industry: electronics, pharmaceutical, etc.
NS	National Services: insurance, consulting, etc.

Commercial Establishments

BG	Business Goods: intermediate products, raw materials, etc.
BS	Business Services: computer, accounting, legal, etc.
PG	Personal Goods: food, drugs, appliances, etc.
PS	Personal Services: banking, restaurants, etc.

Residences

RA	Single family housing
RB	Townhouses, garden apartments
RC	High-rise apartment buildings

Taxes—All economic decision makers pay local and federal-state taxes.

The local taxes include property and sales taxes. Property taxes are applied to all privately owned land as well as to developments. Sales taxes are applied to all purchases of goods (from BG and PG) and all purchases of services (from BS and PS) by a particular development. All local tax rates are variable. Federal-state taxes are set for business income and sales. The rates for these taxes are summarized below:

Business Income (State)	5 percent of (gross income minus deductions)
Business Income (Federal)	22 percent of first $25,000 of (gross income minus deductions)
	plus 48 percent of rest (minus the same deductions)

Sales Tax (State)	3 percent of the total purchase from BG and BS or PG and PS establishments

Basic Industry (See Table 7.1 for Level One Characteristics.)

Income—Each of the three types of basic industry in the model (HI, LI, NS) sells its output to the outside system. The income to the local system for these sales is primary input for local economic activity. In model terms, the maximum output for an industry at level 1 is 1000 units. The average price per unit of output is determined by the outside system, although they usually range around $190,000 per unit for HI, $115,000 for LI, and $110,000 for NS. The price paid for HI output is the most variable and the price paid for NS output is the least variable in the business cycle (Figure 7.4).

Expenditures—Expenditures for basic industry are for maintenance and normal operations, utilities, salaries, transportation and taxes. Transportation costs are incurred by industry when acquiring the goods and services from BG and necessary for maintenance and normal operation, and (except for NS) for shipping finished goods to terminals from which they are distributed to the outside system. These costs vary according to type of road, user, and destination.

Production Process—Production of units of output or capacity by a particular business is dependent upon the level of business activity, the quality and quantity of labor hired, and plant and equipment used. Thus, inputs feed into the production process directly (desired business levels, building levels, and equipment units) and into the production process indirectly (maintenance on building and equipment, salaries offered, and overtime). Both the Depreciation-Obsolescence Process and Employment Process must operate before the Production Process is begun. (Both of these processes are described in detail later.)

The Employment Process yields the number of workers hired by class and the educational level of these workers. Both the quantity and quality of the hired workers are functions of the salaries offered. Overtime requests also affect the number of workers hired if sufficient labor is available. If certain minimum numbers of workers are not hired, then the levels of business activity are automatically reduced. In some cases, a shortage of workers (because of low wages,

TABLE 7.1

INDUSTRIAL ESTABLISHMENTS (Level One Characteristics)

	FL	SG	MP	MF	NL	EL	TE	FO	TA	PA	CR	NS
Location Requirements												
1. Percent of parcel	28	40	48	20	15	12	12	20	6	16	28	12
(maximum possible levels)	(3)	(2)	(2)	(5)	(6)	(8)	(8)	(5)	(16)	(6)	(3)	(8)
2. Zoning required	—	—	—	—	—	—	—	—	—	—	—	—
	00	00	00	00	00	00	00	00	00	00	00	00
	10	10	10	10	10	10	10	10	10	10	10	10
	20	20	20	20	20	20	20	20	20	20	20	30
	21	21	21	21	21	21	21	22	22	22	22	31
3. Minimum level of utility service	1	1	7	1	1	2	2	3	1	3	4	1
4. Annual utility units consumed	50	100	700	100	100	200	200	300	100	300	400	76
5. **Construction Costs** (millions of dollars)	300	240	240	320	150	140	180	230	120	250	250	50
Depreciation												
6. Annual percentage (due to aging)	3.0	2.0	4.0	3.5	3.0	4.0	5.0	2.0	1.5	1.5	3.0	3.0
7. MS Effect (maximum percentage)	3.0	2.0	4.0	3.0	3.0	4.0	5.0	2.0	2.0	2.0	3.0	3.0
8. Fire (maximum percentage)	3.0	2.0	4.0	3.5	3.0	4.0	5.0	2.0	1.5	1.5	3.0	3.0
9. Flood	Depends upon amount input by director and location in flood plain											
Flood multiplier	.6	.6	.6	.6	.6	.6	.6	.5	.5	.5	.5	
10. Water quality (maximum)	1.0	NA	1.0	NA	NA	NA	NA	1.0	1.0	1.0	1.0	
Water Characteristics												
11. Surface water user	x		x					x	x	x	x	
12. Consumption (MGD)	61	10	225	9	12	5	8	49	17	333	31	.18
13. Days in operation per year	260	260	260	260	260	260	260	260	260	260	260	260
14. Consumption (MGY)	15860	2600	58500	2340	3120	1300	2080	12740	4420	86580	8060	46.8
15. Recycling cost per MG	200	NA	200	NA	NA	NA	NA	200	200	200	200	NA
Maximum percentage of water able to be recycled	100	NA	100	NA	NA	NA	NA	100	100	100	100	NA

TABLE 7.1 (Continued)

	FL	SG	MP	MF	NL	EL	TE	FO	TA	PA	CR	NS
16. Effluent treatment construction cost per level (millions of dollars)												
CL	.5	NA	.8	NA	NA	NA	NA	.45	.2	1	.3	NA
PT	5	NA	8	NA	NA	NA	NA	4.5	2	10	3	NA
ST	15	NA	24	NA	NA	NA	NA	13.5	6	30	9	NA
TT	45	NA	72	NA	NA	NA	NA	40.5	18	90	27	NA
Employees												
17. Full time population units (P1's)												
PH	8	14	19	24	21	30	25	15	15	23	24	23
PM	8	18	18	18	20	18	22	19	10	17	24	9
PL	35	23	18	17	18	17	15	24	30	20	14	9
18. Part time (leisure time units)												
PH	0	80	80	80	80	80	80	0	0	80	80	80
PM	80	160	160	160	80	80	80	80	0	0	80	0
PL	240	160	320	160	160	80	80	80	240	160	80	0
Capacity Measures												
19. Maximum employment effect	1000	1000	1000	1000	1000	1000	1000	1000	1000	1000	1000	1000
20. Maximum units produced	1000	1000	1000	1000	1000	1000	1000	1000	1000	1000	1000	1000
Income Factors												
21. Normal price per unit sold (thousands of dollars)	196	155	176	232	147	200	184	148	100	183	185	110
22. Typical income from sales (millions of dollars)	196	155	176	232	147	200	184	148	100	183	185	110
Expenditures												
23. Business goods (units)	400	200	140	300	100	400	200	30	20	100	150	60
24. Business services (units)	120	40	35	180	54	246	174	10	10	44	50	23

TABLE 7.1 (Continued)

	FL	SG	MP	MF	NL	EL	TE	FO	TA	PA	CR	NS
25. Purchases per 1% maintenance												
BG units	10	8	10	8	8	6	10	5	4	4	4	1
BS units	2	1	4	4	4	4	6	2	2	2	5	4
26. Typical utilities costs (millions of dollars)	.5	1.0	7.0	1.0	1.0	2.0	2.0	3.0	1.0	3.0	4.0	.76
27. Water (millions of dollars)												
Recycling (assuming 100% recycled)	3.17	NA	11.70	NA	NA	NA	NA	2.55	.88	17.32	1.61	NA
Intake process (assuming water quality of 4)	1.59	NA	5.85	NA	NA	NA	NA	1.27	.44	8.66	.81	NA
Outflow treatment (operating costs)												
CL ($1000)	397	NA	1463	NA	NA	NA	NA	319	111	2165	302	NA
PT	1588	NA	5852	NA	NA	NA	NA	1276	444	8660	808	NA
ST	3176	NA	11704	NA	NA	NA	NA	2552	888	17320	1616	NA
TT	4764	NA	17556	NA	NA	NA	NA	3828	1332	25980	2424	NA
Municipal supply (assuming water costs of $450 per MG; millions of dollars)	NA	1.17	NA	1.05	1.40	.59	.94	NA	NA	NA	NA	.02
28. Transportation (Per unit of output on type 3 road)												
To BG	2500	6000	7000	2700	7000	1000	2500	1000	5000	2000	2000	1250
To BS	1500	1500	1500	1500	1500	1500	1500	1500	1500	1500	1500	1250
To terminal	2500	2000	2000	1500	1000	500	1500	1000	500	1500	1000	NA
Terminal units	1000	10000	6000	2000	1000	1000	2000	3000	1000	3000	3000	NA
29. Salaries (full employment)	Depends upon salary levels offered.											
30. Taxes												
Property	Local rate times assessed value											
Sales	Fixed state sales tax times purchases of goods and services											
Income	Federal-state tax plus local tax, if any											
31. Rate of return	Net income divided by sum of business value and land value											

TABLE 7.1 (Continued)

	FL	SG	MP	MF	NL	EL	TE	FO	TA	PA	CR	NS
32. Units of pollution per MG												
BOD (Lbs/MG)	600	500	1000	500	400	800	500	6000	6000	3000	2000	100
Chlorides (Lbs/MG)	100	100	170	150	150	200	180	400	130	380	600	0
Nutrients (Lbs/MG)	1000	1000	500	700	100	200	100	10000	4000	3000	800	0
Coliform (parts/MG)	20	10	20	30	20	20	30	300	20	150	50	20
Temperature deviation	9	0	6	0	0	0	0	9	18	16	4	0
Oil & floating solids	1	0	1	1	0	0	0	1	1	1	1	0
High level wastes	0	0	0	0	0	0	0	0	1	1	1	0
33. Intake treatment costs per MG (dollars)												
Quality of water												
1	10	NA	20	NA	NA	NA	NA	50	20	20	30	NA
2	60	NA	60	NA	NA	NA	NA	60	60	60	60	NA
3	80	NA	80	NA	NA	NA	NA	80	80	80	80	NA
4	100	NA	100	NA	NA	NA	NA	100	100	100	100	NA
5	180	NA	180	NA	NA	NA	NA	180	180	180	180	NA
6	300	NA	300	NA	NA	NA	NA	300	300	300	300	NA
7	450	NA	450	NA	NA	NA	NA	450	450	450	450	NA
8	600	NA	600	NA	NA	NA	NA	600	600	600	600	NA
9	Cannot be used.											

FIGURE 7.4

ANNUAL OPERATION OF A BUSINESS

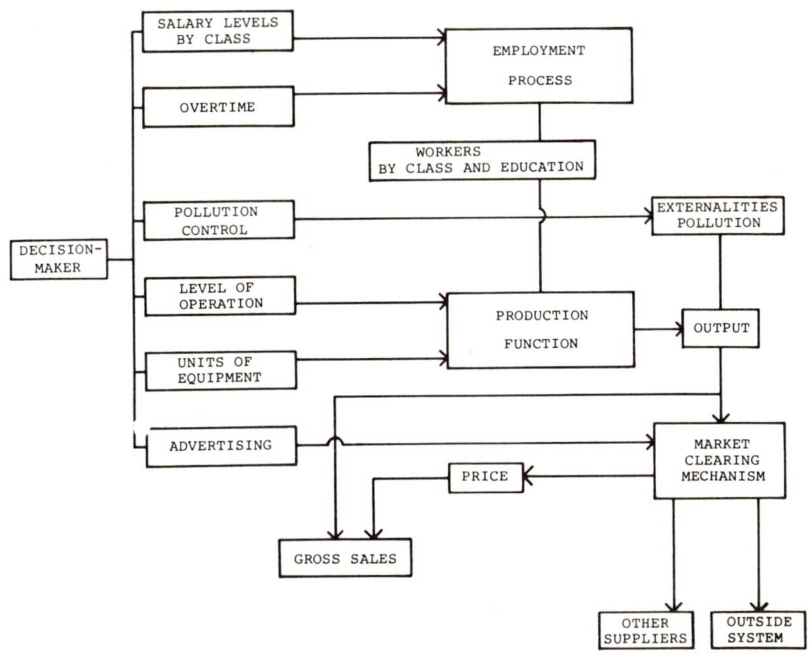

FIGURE 7.5
THE PRODUCTION PROCESS

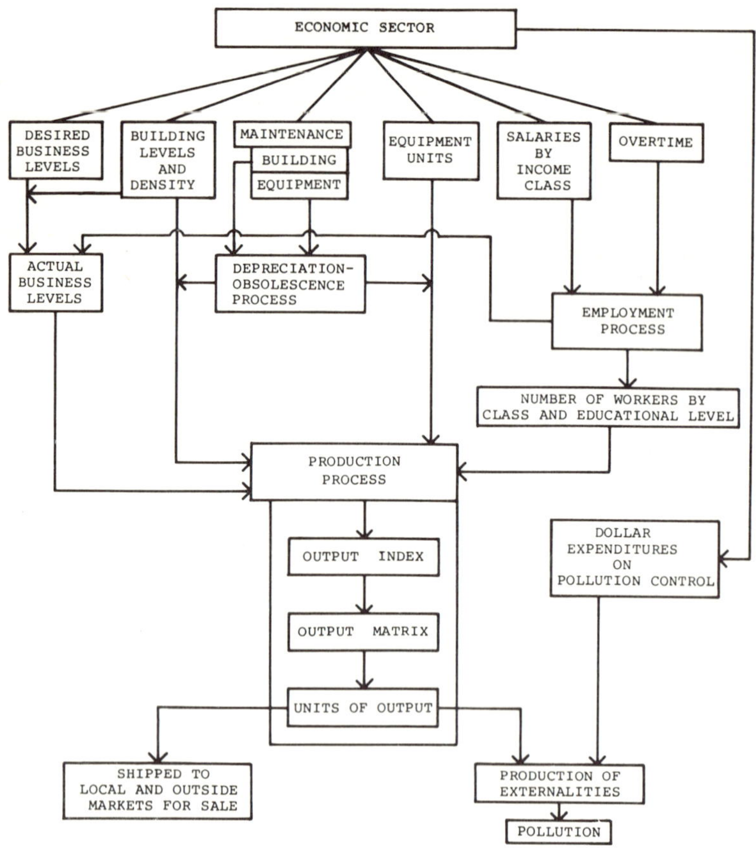

bad location, or labor deficiencies) may cause a business to automatically suspend operations altogether.

The productivity of plant and equipment is reduced as the result of annual obsolescence and may be reduced as the result of depreciation unless ofsetting maintenance expenditures are made. The decision to make these maintenance expenditures on plant and equipment is controlled through the setting of maintenance levels for each of these factors of production.

The quantity and quality measures of labor, plant, and equipment are combined in the production function to yield an output index.

Figure 7.5 illustrates the decision flow and interrelationships in the production process.

Commercial Establishments—The commercial land uses in GEM (BG, BS, PG, PS) trade with each other, with other establishments in the Economic Sector and with the Government and Social Sectors. The buyer-seller relationship with commercial establishments is best summarized in the following:

	Buyers		
Sellers	Economic Sector	Governmental Sector	Social Sector
BG	HI, LI, NS, PG, PS	SC, MS	
BS	HI, LI, NS, PG, PS	SC, MS	
PG	RA, RB, RC		PH, PM, PL
PS	RA, RB, RC		PH, PM, PL

Each iteration the commercial allocation process assigns buyers to sellers, each buyer being assigned to shop where he can obtain his goods or services most cheaply. The cost which a buyer perceives at each of his options for a shopping location is a function of the transportation cost to get to the location, the crowding at that location, the seller's price, and a model bias for shopping at the establishment where he shopped the previous round. (See Figure 7.6.)

The allocation process is iterative. Each buyer selects the shopping location which is cheapest for him, and after all buyers have selected shopping locations, all re-evaluate their selections in light of the crowding created by the previous selection process. Crowding, or overusage, at a commercial establishment can be viewed as a cost to

FIGURE 7.6
PROCESS TO ATTRACT OUTSIDE INDUSTRIES

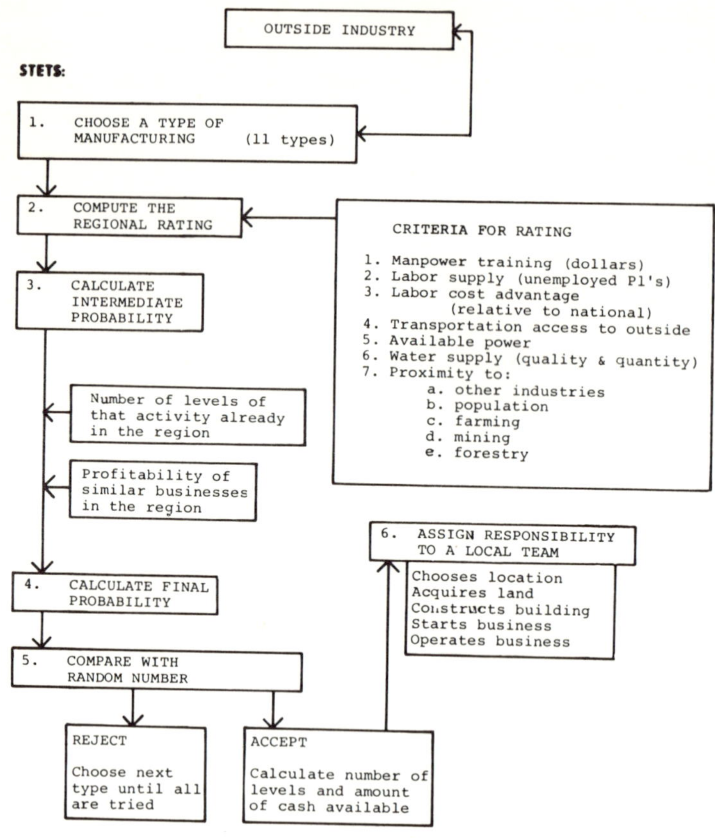

the buyer in terms of annoyance, poor or inadequate service, or length of time waiting for an appointment. The entire selection process is repeated until between two successive evaluations no buyers decide to change their selections from the previous iteration. Every buyer evaluates all possible shopping locations each iteration.

The allocation process employed by the model assigns all buyers to sellers simultaneously. Each commercial establishment's usage as seen by a prospective customer is affected by the establishment's usage after the previous iteration, or in the case of the first iteration in a round, affected by the establishment's usage after the final iteration in the previous round.

The shadow cost for a buyer to shop at a commercial establishment is a function of: (1) its base perceived usage; (2) the added usage which would result if the buyer were to shop there but did not shop there on the previous iteration; (3) the establishment's effective capacity; (4) its price; (5) the buyer's least transportation cost to travel to the location; and (6) the buyer's bias toward shopping where he shopped last round. The result of this function if the shadow cost to a buyer to shop at each commercial establishment. Each buyer selects the commercial establishment with the least shadow cost to him. If the least shadow cost is the Outside System, the buyer does not use a local establishment (Figure 7.7).

A buyer's actual expenditure is the real transportation cost and actual price charged at the commercial establishment which he selects on the final iteration. (See Figure 7.8.)

Table 7.2 for commercial developments shows profitability (typical rates of return and break even points) for the various land uses. The rate of return is the percent of development cost that is earned each year by a development (net income) assuming certain conditions. The break even point is the capacity at which a commercial development must operate in order to cover the fixed and variable costs of staying in business. These rates represent a sort of "typical average maximum rate of return." That is, it is a rate of return a businessman could expect if all prices were at their typical values, the business cycle was at its average value, and all other variables were at their typical, average, or normal value. (See Figure 7.9.)

Residences—There are three types of residences (RA, RB, RC) in the model. As with commercial establishments, residences earn income by charging prices (i.e., rents). The number of population units which can live in a given residence depends on its type and its level of

FIGURE 7.7
COMMERCIAL PROCESS

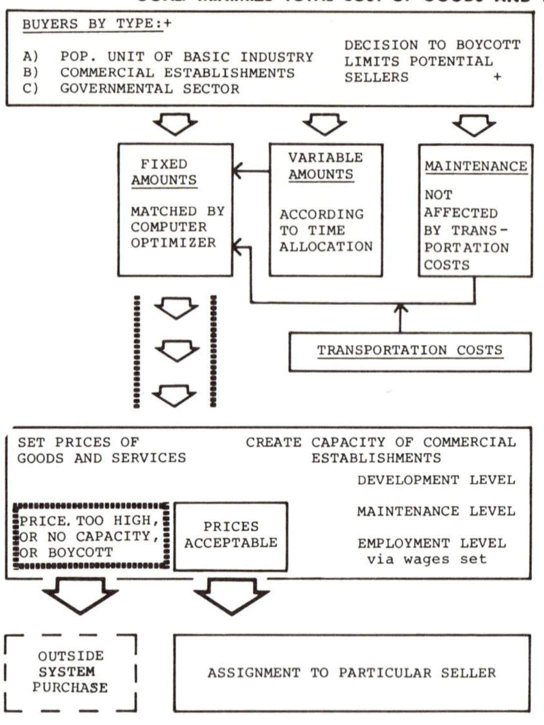
GOAL: MINIMIZE TOTAL COST OF GOODS AND SERVICES
BUYERS BY TYPE:+
A) POP. UNIT OF BASIC INDUSTRY
B) COMMERCIAL ESTABLISHMENTS
C) GOVERNMENTAL SECTOR
DECISION TO BOYCOTT LIMITS POTENTIAL SELLERS +
FIXED AMOUNTS
MATCHED BY COMPUTER OPTIMIZER
VARIABLE AMOUNTS
ACCORDING TO TIME ALLOCATION
MAINTENANCE
NOT AFFECTED BY TRANS-PORTATION COSTS
TRANSPORTATION COSTS
SET PRICES OF GOODS AND SERVICES
CREATE CAPACITY OF COMMERCIAL ESTABLISHMENTS
DEVELOPMENT LEVEL
MAINTENANCE LEVEL
EMPLOYMENT LEVEL via wages set
PRICE, TOO HIGH, OR NO CAPACITY, OR BOYCOTT
PRICES ACCEPTABLE
OUTSIDE SYSTEM PURCHASE
ASSIGNMENT TO PARTICULAR SELLER

TABLE 7.2

COMMERCIAL ESTABLISHMENTS (Level One Characteristics)

	BG	BS	PG	PS
Location Requirements				
1. Percent of a parcel consumed	12	10	12	12
(Maximum possible levels)	(8)	(10)	(8)	(8)
2. Zoning Required	—	—	—	—
	00	00	00	00
	10	10	10	10
	30	30	30	30
	32	33	34	35
3. Minimum level of utility service	2	1	1	1
(Annual utility units consumed)	112	71	99	77
4. **Construction Cost** (millions of dollars)	25	10	30	10
Depreciation				
5. Annual percentage (due to aging)	1.5	2.0	1.6	2.2
6. MS effect (maximum percentage)	2.5	3.0	2.6	3.2
7. Fire (maximum percentage)				
8. Flood (maximum percentage) Flood multiplier	1.5	1.4	1.3	1.2
9. Use (percentage at 100% use)	1.5	2.0	1.6	2.2
Water Consumption				
10. Millions of gallons per day (MGD)	.13	.17	.23	.18
11. Days water is used per year	310	310	310	310
12. Millions of gallons per year (MGY)	41	53	72	56
Employees				
13. Full time population units (P1's)				
PH	14	20	8	6
PM	7	9	13	11
PL	8	9	23	16
14. Part time (leisure time units)				
PH	80	80	0	0
PM	0	0	80	80
PL	0	0	160	160
Capacity Measures				
15. Maximum employment effect	5000	1500	16000	8000
16. Maximum effective capacity	5000	1500	16000	8000
17. **Normal Price per Capacity Unit Sold** (Thousands of dollars)	100	100	10	10
18. **Typical Income From Sales** (Millions of dollars)	500	150	160	80
Expenditures				
19. Business goods (units)	NA	NA	.037/CU	.03/CU
20. Business services (units)	NA	NA	.017/CU	.01/CU
Outside service charges (thousands of dollars)	83/CU	58/CU	NA	NA
21. Purchases per 1% maintenance				
BG units	NA	NA	2	.75
BS units	NA	NA	1	.25
Outside service charges (thousands of dollars)	250	100	NA	NA

TABLE 7.2 (Continued)

	BG	BS	PG	PS
22. Typical utilities costs (millions of dollars)	1.12	.71	.99	.77
23. Water (assuming water costs = $450)	18135	23715	32085	25110
24. Transportation (per unit of capacity on HY3)				
To BG	NA	NA	.0425	.0375
To BS	NA	NA	.02	.0125
To terminal	1	NA	NA	NA
25. Salaries (full employment)	Depends upon salary levels offered			
26. Taxes				
Property	Local rate times assessed value.			
Sales	Fixed state sales tax times purchases of goods and services.			
Income	Federal-state tax plus local tax, if any.			
27. Rate of return	Net income divided by sum of building value and land value.			

FIGURE 7.8
CONSUMPTION FUNCTION PROCESS

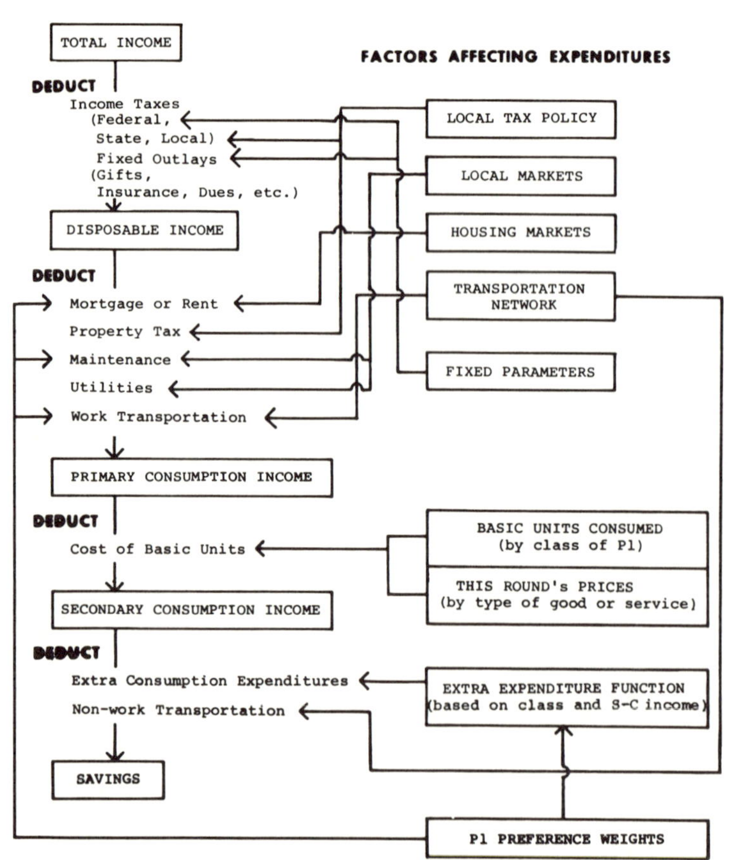

FIGURE 7.9
PERSONAL COMMERCIAL ALLOCATOR

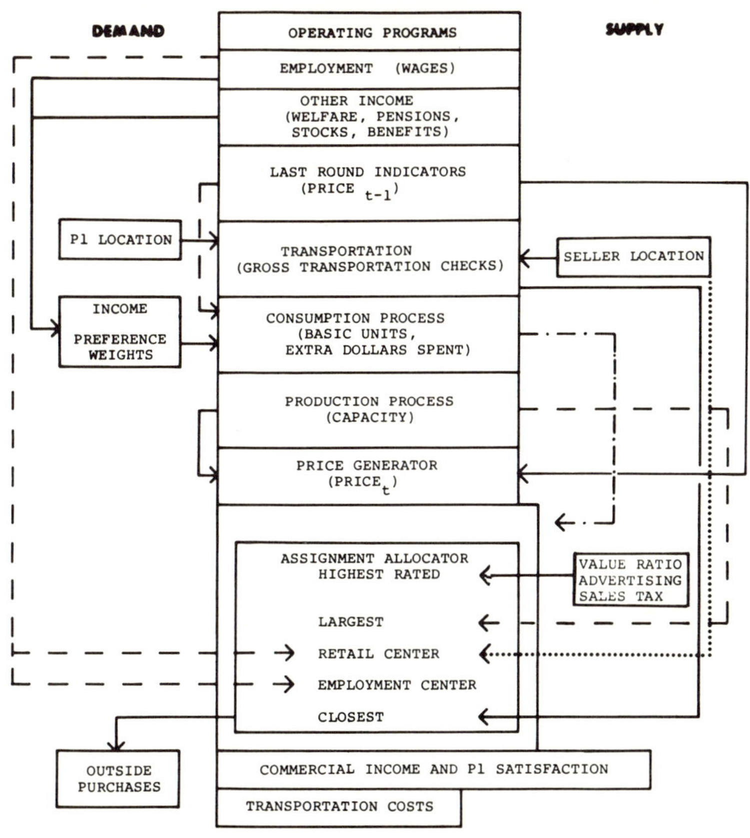

FIGURE 7.10

OPERATION OF HOUSING FOR SALE OR FOR RENT

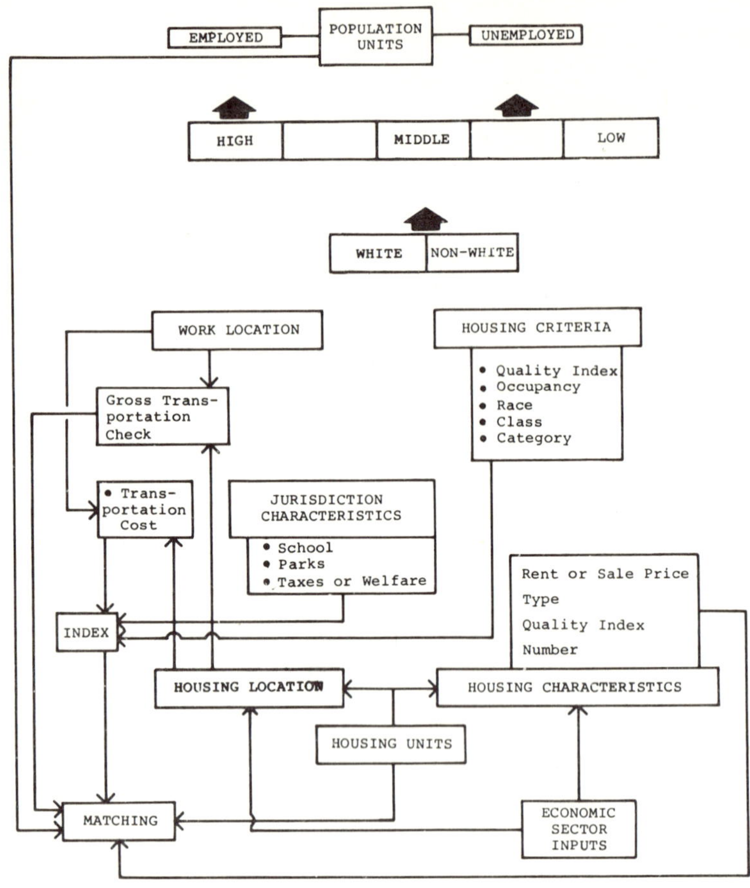

development. The quality index (QI) for residences indicates the physical conditions of the housing; the higher the QI (0-100), the better the conditions. Further, the QI and the amount of overcrowding will determine whether or not a particular socio-economic class will move into a given residence.

Income and Expenditures—Middle-income renters pay 1.33 times as much and high-income renters pay two times as much as low-income. The principal criteria for determining rents is the quality index. The typical rents that can be charged to tenants of each class are $330,000 per PH, $200,000 per PM, and $140,000 per PL regardless of residence type.

Total income from operating a residence is, therefore, determined by multiplying the number of occupants from each class times the rent charged to each class.

Operation of Housing for Rent or Sale—There is no place where the Economic Sector comes in closer contact with the Social Sector than in the sale and rental of housing. The computer matching process takes into account direct economic and social inputs as well as indirect government inputs in achieving a match between population units and living quarters (as expressed in housing units; Figure 7.10).

As the upper portion of the flowchart shows, population units are differentiated by category, class, and employment status in their pursuit of housing. If a population unit is employed, the work location provides a locus of parcel locations within which housing will meet the gross transportation check. Each type of population unit has different housing criteria that must be satisfied. In addition to this, the Social Sector places measures of importance on such factors as quality index of housing, transportation costs to work, quality of schools, availability of parks, jurisdiction taxes or welfare payments, and neighborhood composition. All these factors are combined to yield a preference index that feeds directly into the matching process.

The Economic Sector inputs that set the housing characteristics (rent or sale price, type of housing, quality of housing, and amount of housing) are also fed directly to the matching process. (Table 7.3 illustrates the activities involved in housing operation.)

Vacancy Rates—Since building space is a separate entity from business activities that occupy building space, there may be times when excess building space exists in the local system. To the extent that there are sizable amounts of unoccupied space, a misallocation of resources is implied and unfavorable rates of return for the owners of the buildings will result. This has some favorable effects by giving more options to the migrating population units and keeping the rents at a lower level than when demand is nearly equal to total supply.

The many aspects of level change in government (schools, police, fire, etc.) are carried out by a more automatic process while the construction of transportation units and links use only parts of the Build Process; see Figure 7.13).

Value Ratio (VR) and Quality Index (QI)—Value ratio is a measurement of the physical condition of a building. It ranges from a high of 100 (a newly constructed or restored building) to a low of 0 (a completely deteriorated structure). VR is defined as the ratio of the present value of a development to its original value.[22] Value ratio affects the output or capacity of a business; i.e., a value ratio of 50 means that output or capacity is 50 percent of what it would be otherwise.

The VR applies to all buildings except residences. The physical condition of residences is measured by a quality index (QI). Like VR it also ranges from 0-100, but new residences may be built at one of seven different QI's (40, 50, 60, 70, 80, 90, 100).

Resources

The classical factors of production—land, labor, capital, and entrepreneurship—along with financial assets such as cash and investments are the resources of the Economic Sector.

Land—Land has the characteristics of location (the parcel on which it is located), size (the number of acres), quality (indicated by the land code which encompasses slope, soil type, and presence of water or bedrock), status (whether developed or undeveloped), and zoning (the uses to which the land may be put, as determined by a government agency). Land can be put to agricultural or forestry use or it may be developed and then used for manufacturing, commercial, or residential purposes. Construction feasibility and cost are a function of the quality of the land. Taxes paid on land may vary dependent upon the status and use of the land.

Land Requirements—All economic establishments occupy a given amount of land on a parcel. The amount of land required for a particular establishment varies by its type and level of development. (Figure 7.11 illustrates decision flow and interaction during land acquisition.)

Water—Bodies of water are also considered a resource. The water represents a basic ingredient for all industrial, commercial and residential land uses in the model. On the other hand, the carrying out of these chores often results in pollution of the water supply.

Three types of surface water can be represented: rivers (flowing bodies of water), small lakes and large lakes. Large lakes are full parcels or combinations of full parcels of water. Large lakes have an unlimited volume of water and a loaded water quality level that does not change during the course of a run of the model.

Small lakes are fractions of a parcel of land. They are defined as having a specified water volume and percent of parcel consumed. Their water quality level is calculated in the same manner as for rivers.

Rivers are loaded as being on a particular parcel, having a specific volume, flowing at a specific rate, and emptying into a designated adjacent parcel. Rivers may or may not consume a significant (1 percent or more) portion of land or parcel. In other words, the land area consumed by a river may not be large enough to take into account.

All volumes are expressed in parcels of gallons per day (MGD), and rates of flow are expressed in parcels of land traversed in a day by a particle of water in the river. The following summarizes:

Types of Surface Water	Volume	Water Quality Level	Rate of Flow
Rivers	Specified	Calculated	Specified
Small Lakes	Specified	Calculated	Not Applicable
Large Lakes	Unlimited	Specified	Not Applicable

Labor—Labor is hired by the Economic Sector through a competitive labor market process. Employees are essential to the functioning of all non-residential land uses (HI, LI, NS, BG, BS, PG, PS) in the model. These employees are hired from the population units (1 population unit—500 persons) which inhabit the simulated area. The number of workers in a given population unit is related to the

TABLE 7.3

RESIDENCES (Level One Characteristics)

	RA	RB	RC
Location Requirements			
1. Percent of parcel consumed	2	2	2
2. (Maximum possible levels of development)	(50)	(50)	(50)
3. Zoning required	—	—	—
	00	00	00
	40	40	40
	41	42	43
4. Minimum level of utility service required	1	1	2
5. (Annual utility units consumed)	(4)	(26)	(117)
Construction Factors			
6. Cost (millions of dollars)	1	6	25
7. Quality index (when new, equal to or greater than)	40	40	40
Depreciation			
8. Annual (due to aging)	2.0	3.0	4.0
9. MS effect (maximum)	2.0	3.0	3.0
10. Fire (maximum)	2.0	2.0	2.0
11. Flood (maximum depends upon damage set by director and location on flood plain)			
12. (Flood multiplier)	(1.1)	(1.0)	(.9)
Water Consumption (Depends upon occupants)			
13. MGY per PH	29	25	22
14. MGY per PM	25	18	11
15. MGY per PL	11	11	7
16. Number of days during year water is used	360	360	360
17. MGD per PH	.08	.07	.06
18. MGD per PM	.07	.05	.03
19. MGD per PL	.03	.03	.02
Occupants			
20. Space units provided	2	12	50
21. Space units demanded:			
PH	2	2	2
PM	1.5	1.5	1.5
PL	1	1	1
Rent Per Space Unit (Thousands of dollars)			
22. Maximum	210	210	210
23. Normals for various classes			
PH	165	165	165
PM	150	150	150
PL	140	140	140
Income (Assuming 100% occupancy; thousands of dollars)			
24. At maximum rent	420	2520	10500
25. At rent of $150,000 per space unit			
PH occupants	300	1800	7500
PM occupants	300	1800	7500
PL occupants	300	1800	7500

TABLE 7.3 (Continued)

Expenditures			
26. Maintenance			
PG units per 1% maintenance	.7	4	17
PS units per 1% maintenance	.3	2	8
Normal total costs per 1% maintenance	10	60	250
27. Normal utilities charges (thousands of dollars)	40	260	1170
28. Taxes			
Property	(local rate times assessed value)		
Income	(federal-state tax plus local tax)		
Sales	(local rate times purchases for maintenance)		
Net Income	income from rent minus expenditures		
Rate of Return	net income divided by sum of residence value and land value		
Environmental Indexes	comprised of pollution index plus residence quality, rent, MS and school use indexes, and taxes or welfare		

FIGURE 7.11
ACQUISITION OF LAND

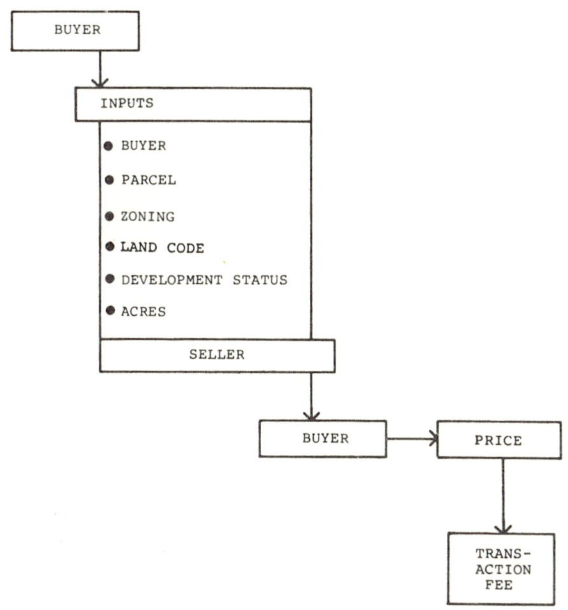

population unit's class. Socio-economic class also determines the salary range which is paid to a worker.

Each commercial and industrial land use has a different employment requirement which describes the number and socio-economic mix of full-time and part-time employees necessary to ensure maximum gross income. The individual employers try to hire the best-educated workers within each population class. At the same time, the workers try to work for the employers who offer the best working conditions. The salary offered is weighted very heavily by the prospective employees in their evaluation of working conditions. The educational level of the local labor force is an index that might more appropriately be called the productivity index, since it is assumed to have a direct effect on the production generated per worker.

Employment Allocator—The number of people looking for jobs at any one particular time is comprised of those who are new in-migrants, the unemployed, those fired because of cutbacks, workers dissatisfied with their present job, and a small percent of all other workers.

The jobs available are comprised of those that result from workers quitting, increased business level activity (old and new businesses), automatic employment growth, new local government hiring, and changes in the external number of jobs.

Each income class is considered separately, highest first. There are two major sections to the employment process: choosing a job and selecting the best mode of transportation to work. The former section will be discussed in detail first.

This operation occurs during the processing of each year's decisions. In this process, all jobs are considered open and are examined each round for possible new employment by qualified workers. However, workers do not always change jobs each round.

Another overall consideration is that in the first sort, in which workers of all classes decide to retain their present job or change to a possible new one, and in all subsequent matching, the process is performed in order of class with high-income class processed first. This process is always top down, meaning that in a job shortage high income workers can take middle-income jobs but never the reverse. Where workers of the same class are competing for the same job opening, the ones with the higher education level win.

There are occasions when some high-income workers will be

unemployed while all middle-income workers will have jobs. This situation occurs when a high-income worker cannot afford to either remain in his present job or take a new one (because his costs are too high, or because both job openings do not pay enough).

Note here that the emphasis is on what workers will or can afford to accept and not so much on what is available. This relationship is conditioned by several things, among them the supply and demand curve, what economic decision makers decide to pay, how the Government Sector is providing transportation and general Social Sector dissatisfaction.

In order to choose a job, a Pl's estimated transportation cost to each job (using last year's conditions) must be calculated. The best route is the cheapest; this is derived from the amount of usage of the transportation network last round and the dollar value of time spent traveling. Although the time cost is not paid by a worker in dollars, it is a significant factor in the selection of routes and models of travel.

Generally, the transportation cost (weighted by time and money) is subtracted from the salary offered by each employment location, yielding the direct net income a worker would receive there. To reflect job stability the direct net income from a possible new job must exceed that of the last year's job by at least 10 percent before a worker will consider changing.

All high-income P1's on a parcel have the same educational level. The best educated groups of P1's try for jobs with the greatest direct net income. If there are not enough job openings for all high-income living on the parcel at their best employment location, as many as possible are assigned jobs there. The rest look for their next best job, again comparing the artificially inflated income of their present job with the direct income of a possible job (the repeat of the process mentioned above). The process is repeated until all of these workers on the parcel have jobs or until both the artificial and direct incomes are negative. Then the next best-educated group is considered for jobs. If workers living on two or more parcels have the same educational level, the order of consideration is random. The least educated group is considered for jobs last (Figure 7.12).

When all workers in each socio-economic class have tried for jobs, the part-time employment process occurs. The entire employment process runs each time for the next lower class, plus those of the previous class still without full-time jobs who are put at the top of the list because of their higher educational levels.

When employment has been run for all classes, the new traffic

FIGURE 7.12
EMPLOYMENT PROCESS

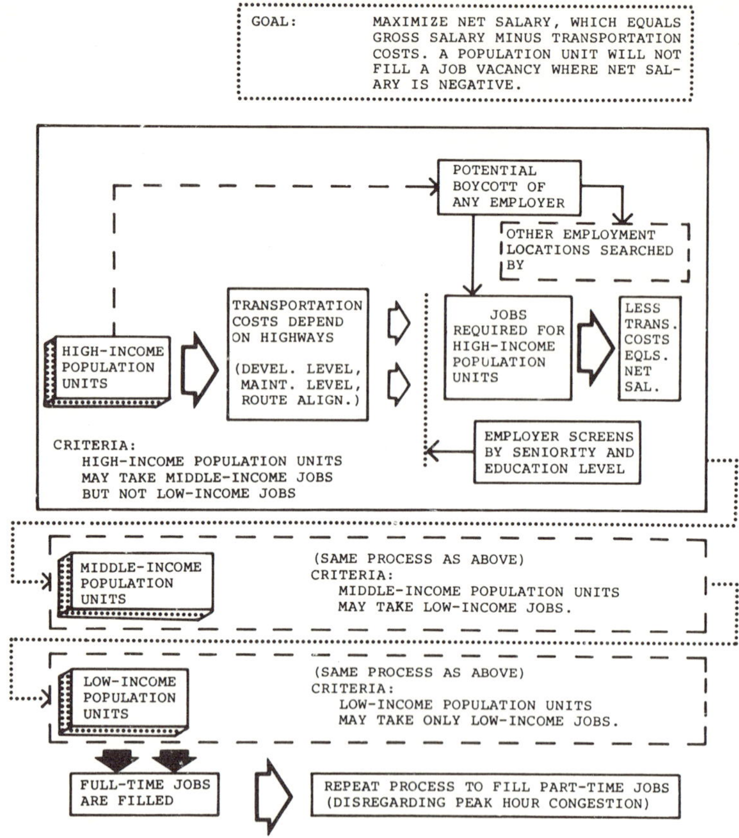
GOAL: MAXIMIZE NET SALARY, WHICH EQUALS GROSS SALARY MINUS TRANSPORTATION COSTS. A POPULATION UNIT WILL NOT FILL A JOB VACANCY WHERE NET SALARY IS NEGATIVE.
POTENTIAL BOYCOTT OF ANY EMPLOYER
OTHER EMPLOYMENT LOCATIONS SEARCHED BY
HIGH-INCOME POPULATION UNITS
TRANSPORTATION COSTS DEPEND ON HIGHWAYS
(DEVEL. LEVEL, MAINT. LEVEL, ROUTE ALIGN.)
JOBS REQUIRED FOR HIGH-INCOME POPULATION UNITS
LESS TRANS. COSTS EQLS. NET SAL.
EMPLOYER SCREENS BY SENIORITY AND EDUCATION LEVEL
CRITERIA:
HIGH-INCOME POPULATION UNITS MAY TAKE MIDDLE-INCOME JOBS BUT NOT LOW-INCOME JOBS
MIDDLE-INCOME POPULATION UNITS
(SAME PROCESS AS ABOVE)
CRITERIA:
MIDDLE-INCOME POPULATION UNITS MAY TAKE LOW-INCOME JOBS.
LOW-INCOME POPULATION UNITS
(SAME PROCESS AS ABOVE)
CRITERIA:
LOW-INCOME POPULATION UNITS MAY TAKE ONLY LOW-INCOME JOBS.
FULL-TIME JOBS ARE FILLED
REPEAT PROCESS TO FILL PART-TIME JOBS (DISREGARDING PEAK HOUR CONGESTION)

congestion and actual transportation to work costs and modal choices are calculated. In other words, the origins and destinations of work trips are now known and the routing and modal choice must be determined. The new and old congestions are compared. If the new congestion exceeds the old on any road segment, or bus, or rail route by more than the percent population increase plus 10%, the best route to work is recalculated for everyone based on the new congestion. Jobs are not sought anew–only routes to work. Of course if a road or route is not overcrowded, the percentage increase in congestion is ignored in determining whether to recompute routes. The routing and congestion comparison process is repeated up to three times or until the change in congestion does not exceed the percentages given above. The final routes to work and their usage, my mode, become the congestion factor considered in the next year's employment process.

In the case of government employment, no specific place of employment (i.e., no parcel) is designated. Rather, fixed transportation costs and travel times are used for each population class in round one. The dollar and time cost to travel to government full-time employment (SC, MS, BUS, RAIL) in subsequent rounds is the average for all other working population units. A single average time cost is calculated for all three population classes, but the average dollar cost is calculated separately for each class.

Part-Time Employment Allocation–As with the full-time employment allocation process, the P1's educational level is the most important factor in the assignment of part-time work units to extra time allocation.

The supply of part-time work units, eighty of which are equivalent to one full-time job, is primarily determined by the levels of business activity in the system. A variable supply of part-time work is also available from schools and is allocated by jurisdiction. The school department provides public adult education according to the number of middle- and high-income part-time work units it hires. This specification obviously can fluctuate considerably year to year.

Two lists of part-time work units are created for each population class: one supply of and the other demand for part-time work. The suppliers of part-time work units are ordered by salary offered (proportional to full-time wage offered), with the highest salary placed first. This demand is ordered on the basis of average education level with the highest levels first.

FIGURE 7.13
THE BUILD PROCESS

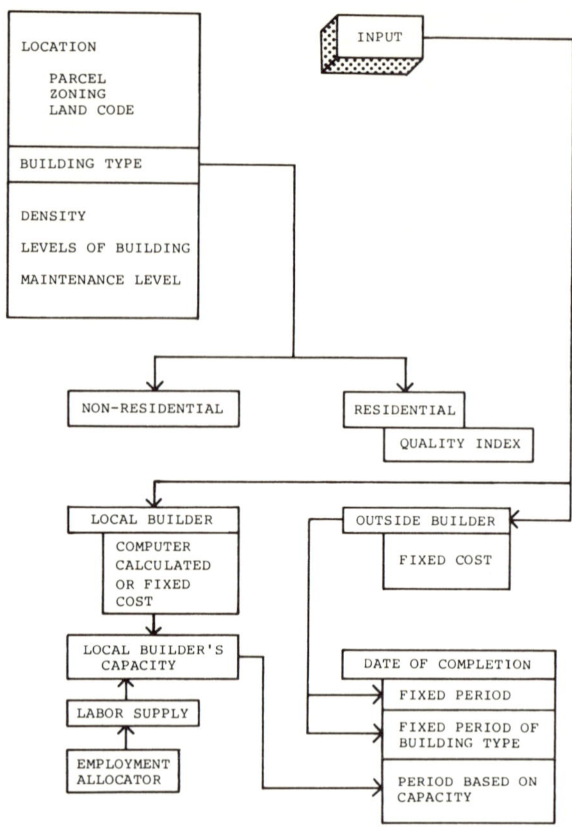

For each complete pass through the list of residence groups, the part-time work allocation process attempts to assign, by class, ten units of extra work to each population unit which has an unfilled extra work allocation. The process continues until either all requests (unfilled allocations) are filled or until the supply of part-time work units is exhausted.

Capital

Capital is divided into plant and equipment. Both the quantity (in standard units) and quality (as measured by the value ratio which reflects the results of both use and age) of plant and equipment has an effect on the production function of the economic activities. Depending upon local conditions as to the cost of labor and equipment, the economic decision makers are able to make some tradeoffs between labor and capital.

Build Process—Build is an operational program which will process inputs for the construction of concretions (buildings and links). The Build Process is designed principally for the construction of concretions for use in the Economic Sector. Buildings are constructed by either local or national construction firms. Both hire local workers and purchase local goods and services (Figure 7.13).

Depreciation-Obsolescence Process—Every building and unit of equipment in the model is subject to annual depreciation and obsolescence. Depreciation is the wear and tear on physical items that can be offset through maintenance expenditures. Obsolescence is the decline in the relative productivity of plant and equipment that occurs with time. (Figure 7.14 illustrates the relationships in the Depreciation-Obsolescence Process.)

The value of all economic developments decreases during each iteration. The rate at which a development depreciates is determined by (a) an annual depreciation rate (i.e., time), plus (b) the amount of depreciation caused by the quality of municipal services[23] serving the parcel on which the development is located, and (c) for commercial establishments only, the depreciation caused by use (Figure 7.14).

Maintenance and Normal Operation—Developments depreciate at a rate which is specified as a percent of their original value. Their value

FIGURE 7.14
THE DEPRECIATION-OBSOLESCENCE PROCESS

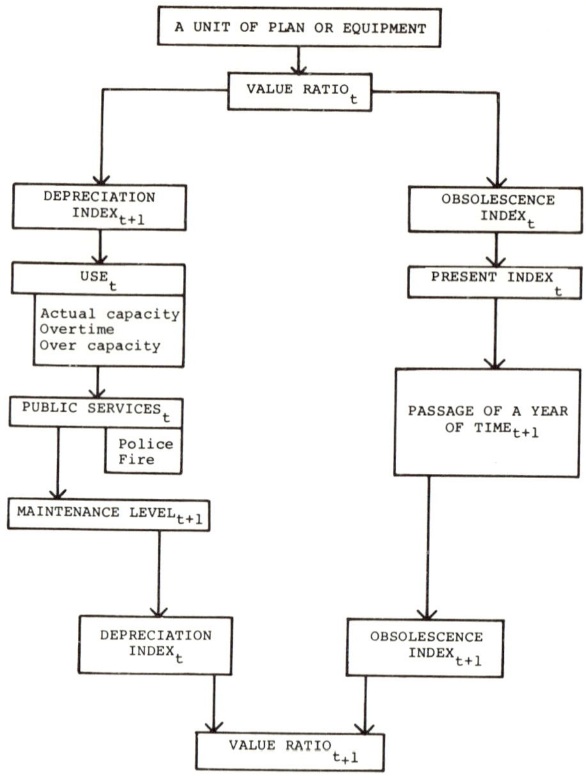

ratio may be maintained at a specified value ratio (or quality index) by specifying the maintenance level (0-100) at which one wants the development to remain. The costs of maintaining the value ratio at a specified level are automatically deducted. The costs of maintenance of a development involve purchases of goods and services and are allocated throughout the system.

Summary

The Economic Sector deals with capital and allocates these resources in a number of different ways: investing, purchasing goods and services or employing people. These decisions are meshed with those of other sectors and yield a new data base. (See Tables 7.4 and 7.5.)

The next section will discuss the Government Sector and its resource allocation.

GOVERNMENT SECTOR

Functional Characteristics

The Government Sector is designed to allow model users as many options as possible for experimenting with government structures and policies. There is practically no limit on the number of jurisdictions, special districts, and departments allowed, and no restriction for their organization. Model users are therefore able to experiment with a wide variety of regulatory, taxation, and federal/state aid policies for whatever purpose they desire.

The Government Sector includes most functions normally performed by state and local governments and certain functions performed by the federal government. The government is mainly concerned with allocating funds among departments, providing adequate services in a general sense, raising sufficient revenues, and competing for economic development, investments and federal and state government expenditures in their areas (Figure 7.15).

Many of the procedures followed for the Government Sector are identical to those followed in the Economic Sector.[24] For example, government physical plants and equipment will depreciate according to the same formula (with different parameters, however) as used for business facilities. Likewise, with a few modifications, government will employ workers in the same fashion as businesses,

TABLE 7.4
ECONOMIC SECTOR

Limitations on Debts	
Maximum amount of debt	80% of net worth
Normal range of outside interest rates	4.3% to 6.2%
Normal Range of Rates of Return on	
Speculative stock	–1 to 10%
Conservative stocks	5 to 7%
Normal Range of Price Relatives	
Heavy industries	.90 to 1.12
Light industries	.93 to 1.10
National services	.95 to 1.06

Developments (level one)	Range for Construction Costs (Millions of Dollars)	Range for Land Requirement (Percent of a Parcel)
Heavy industry		
Surface water users	240-300	28-48
Municipal water users	140-320	12-40
Light industry		
Surface water user	120-250	6-28
National services	50	12
Local commercial	20-45	10-12
Residences (100 quality index)	1-25	2

Economic Boycotts[a]

Possible Boycotting Activities	Activities that Can Be Boycotted
FL, SG, MP, MF, NL, EL, TE, FO, TA, PA, CR	
NS, PG, PS	BG, BS
RA, RB, RC	PB, PS

a. This does not include any social boycotts that might be directed against economic teams. For example, population units may boycott working at any economic employment location or shopping at any PG or PS establishment.

TABLE 7.5
ECONOMIC (Level One Characteristics)

Activity	Percentage of a Parcel	(Maximum Possible Levels)	Minimum Level of Utility Service	Annual Utility Units Consumed	Construction Costs (Market Value)	Full Time Employees PH	PM	PL	Terminal Units	MS Drain (MS Capacity Units)
FL	28	(3)	1	50	300	8	8	35	1000	150
SG	40	(2)	1	100	240	14	18	23	10000	50
MP	48	(2)	7	700	240	19	18	18	6000	200
MF	20	(5)	1	100	320	24	18	17	2000	150
NL	15	(6)	1	100	150	21	20	18	1000	100
EL	12	(8)	2	200	140	30	18	17	1000	150
TE	12	(8)	2	200	180	25	22	15	2000	200
FO	20	(5)	3	300	230	15	19	24	3000	250
TA	6	(16)	1	100	120	15	10	30	1000	150
PA	16	(6)	3	300	250	23	17	20	3000	200
CR	28	(3)	4	400	250	24	24	14	3000	300
NS	12	(8)	1	76	50	23	9	9	NA	50
BG	12	(8)	2	112	25	14	7	8	One per CU sold	25
BS	10	(10)	1	71	10	20	9	9	NA	10
PG	12	(8)	1	99	30	8	13	23	NA	30
PS	12	(8)	1	77	10	6	11	16	NA	10
RA	2	(50)	1	4	1	NA	NA	NA	NA	10
RB	2	(50)	1	26	6	NA	NA	NA	NA	60
RC	2	(50)	2	117	25	NA	NA	NA	NA	250

FIGURE 7.15
GOVERNMENT SECTOR

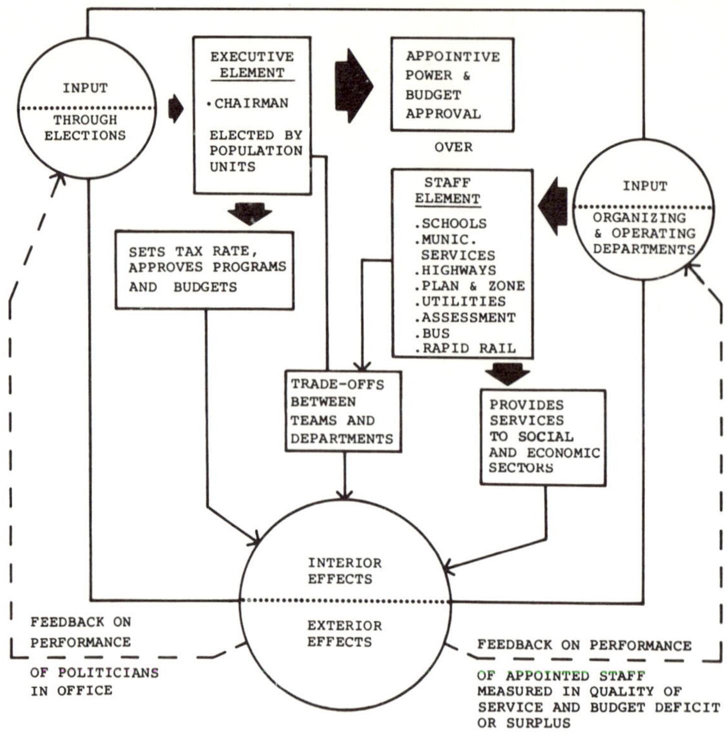

including overtime and part-time employment. (Government purchases of goods and services also employ the same procedure as Economic Sector purchases.)

The computer serves the same functions for government as it does for the other sectors, with one addition. Whereas the computer keeps the accounts for all sectors, allocates demand and supply, and represents the Outside System (this includes federal-state aid in the case of government), it serves in some cases as an enforcer of government policy. If a government institutes a tax, the computer collects that tax according to the criteria set by the government decision maker. If a planning and zoning department zones parcels, the computer allows no private use in violation of zoning.

The government authorities specifically provided for in the model are:

GEM		CITY
Highways		Highways
Education		Education
Public Welfare		Municipal Services
Hospitals	Municipal Services	Parks and Recreation
Health		Planning and Zoning
Police		Assessment
Fire		Utilities
Parks and Recreation		General Administration
Planning and Zoning	Planning and Zoning	
Housing and Renewal		
Assessment		
Utilities		
General Administration		

Those government functions not specifically included in the model (such as libraries) are subsumed under the general administration department expenditures. These fixed expenditures are part of the data base loaded for a particular simulated area. Because the model is intended to be able to represent any combination of governments, a very general structure has been designed for the sector.

Each government authority is comprised of specific functions at a specific decision level. For example, a school department constructs and operates schools, hires people, maintains its facilities, and receives and allocates revenue.

Different decision levels make different types of decisions. They may also differ in the scope of their resources and in their areas of authority. By specifying the geographic area of authority for each

FIGURE 7.16
AGGREGATE INTERACTIONS BETWEEN GOVERNMENT SECTOR AND OTHER SECTORS

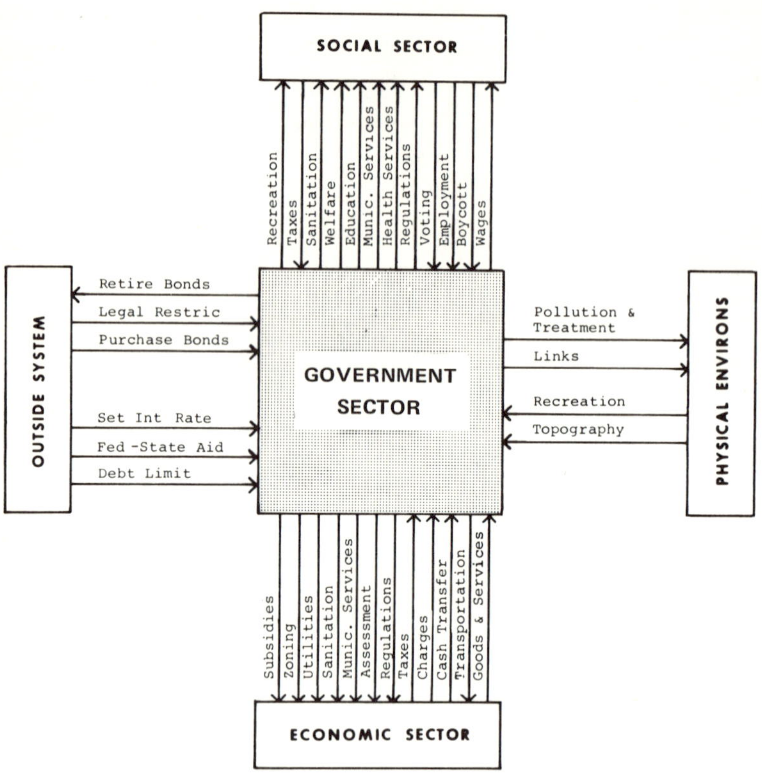

department, we allow for as many special districts, levels of government and departments as may be desired. For example, a county department might have authority over one-third of the area and a town highway department might have half the county. Each could make highway decisions only in its area and each road would be labeled (with the department ID) as to which of the departments were responsible for it. Likewise, a school operated by the county but located in the town would have the label of whatever county department was running the school.

Decision Entities in the Government Sector

Conceptually, decision entities in the Government Sector may be thought of as "departments" with relationships to other departments in a given governmental jurisdiction.

There are basically three configurations for organizing decision-making entities in government departments. (Figure 7.16 illustrates these three configurations.)

First, decision entities may be organized as autonomous departments under an executive authority. Normally, this executive authority is consistent with the area of jurisdiction over which each department has control. If no executive authority is designated for a department, the department may be considered executive authority over itself, as in the case of special districts.

Second, decision entities may be organized as General Administration, under the direct control of an executive authority. In this configuration, departments become line items in an administrative budget and are staff from a General Administration employment pool. This configuration permits governmental growth to allow autonomous departments in an evolutionary manner. As an example, an assessment department would have decision authority over assessments but for all other purposes be indistinguishable from General Administration, except as a line item on General Administration's budget. This configuration also implies that other sources, such as higher governmental authorities or consultants may be required to perform functions which the General Administration may not be capable of performing. An example would be a master planning study, or taxation study.

Third, decision entities may be formed as a combination of the first and second configurations. Thus, an executive authority may have both an expanded General Administration and autonomous

FIGURE 7.17
CONFIGURATIONS OF GOVERNMENT DECISION-MAKING ENTITIES

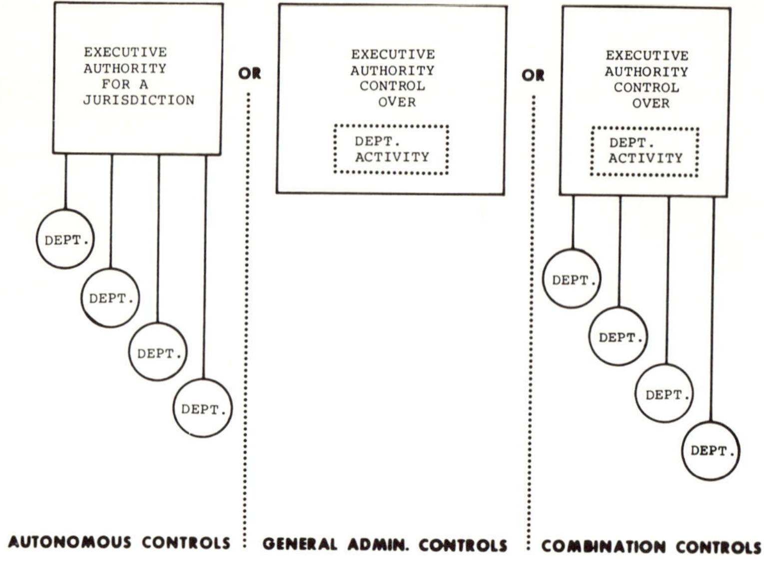

department or special districts. In this case, General Administration functions are funded as budget items and all income and expenditures are taken from a pool, while separate departments are funded by appropriation and employ independently[25] (Figure 7.17).

Functional Characteristics in the Government Sector

Assessment Department—The Assessment Department for each jurisdiction makes decisions relating to the taxation of privately owned property (land and developments) represented in the model. This department has the opportunity to operate selectively on the property assessment ratios. (See Table 7.6.)

Market Value—The market value of unowned land is calculated on the basis of existing values of surrounding parcels and characteristics such as proximity to highways, terminals, employment, residences and the existence of utilities and zoning. The market value of land will change for either of two reasons: (1) after construction of a new development or an additional level of development on a parcel, and (2) after the purchase of a parcel. The model assumes that the market value of a parcel is always updated by the actual purchase price of a parcel as long as that price is not less than the previously existing market value.

Developments—Once a new development appears on a parcel, the market value of land increases as a function of the Ratio of Land Development Value. To determine the market value of land with a new development on it, the model multiplies the New Development Value times the development level times the value ratio/100 times the Ratio of Land/Development Value. For example, if an HI1 (value ratio = 100), is upgraded to an HI2 (value ratio = 100), the market value of land for the parcel would be $105,000,000 times 2 times 1 times .30 or $63,000,000.

Assessed Value—The assessed value of land and development is determined by multiplying the assessment rate times the market value of land or development. In the case of land, the assessment rate is applied only to the market value of the portion of land which is privately owned.

Education Department—Schools hire teachers from the high and

TABLE 7.6
ASSESSMENT DEPARTMENT

Development Types	Market Values of New Level One Developments (millions of dollars)
Manufacturing	
HI – Heavy Industry	
FL – Furniture and lumber	300
SG – Stone and glass	240
MP – Primary metals	240
MF – Fabricated metals	320
NL – Nonelectrical machinery	150
EL – Electrical machinery	140
TE – Transportation equipment	180
LI – Light Industry	
FO – Food	230
TA – Textiles and apparel	120
PA – Paper	250
CR – Chemical, plastics and rubber	250
Non-Manufacturing businesses	
NS – National services	50
BG – Business goods	25
BS – Business services	30
PG – Personal goods	45
PS – Personal services	20
Residences	
RA – Single family	1
RB – Garden apartments	6
RC – High-rise apartments	25
Other Assessment Codes:	
Jurisdiction-Wide Assessment Ratios	
UL = Undeveloped land	
DL = Developed land	
FR = All farms	
Fn = Type of farm (F1, F2, . . .)	
Parcel Specific Assessment Ratios:	
AD = Developments	
AL = Land	
AF = Farms	
Parcel Specific Dollar Assessments:	
SD = Developments	
SL = Land	
SF = Farms	

middle income population units only. There are 120 teachers in a PH and 160 teachers in a PM. There is an optimal employment mix. This mix, however, does not determine output, but rather the number of students which a school can serve (i.e., design capacity).

The value ratio also affects capacity. For example, the design capacity of an SC1 with 1 PH teachers and 4 PM teachers is 17,460 students, but its effective capacity is determined by multiplying its design capacity times value ratio/100.

The use index of a school is a measure of the quality of school services within a school district. It is derived from the ratio of the school units demanded to the units supplied. Specifically, it is determined by dividing its use by its effective capacity and multiplying the result by 100. If the use index is greater than 100, the school is overcrowded and the quality declines. Overcrowded schools contribute to dissatisfaction and thus to migration in the Social Sector.

In sum the quantity and quality of local public school services is a function of the level of the school facility, its value ratio, the number of population units hired from high and middle skill levels and the facility crowding.

School Assignments–Students are assigned to schools. Middle- and high-income families have certain criteria for the school in their district. If the school fails to meet these criteria, these students will be assigned by the computer to private schools at the expense of the population unit they represent. For high-income students the school must have (1) a student/teacher ratio of at least one teacher per 18 students, (2) a value ratio above 80, and (3) at least 1 PH teacher unit for every PM teacher unit. Middle-income students will not attend public school unless there is (1) a student/teacher ratio no greater than 21-1, (2) a value ratio of 60 and (3) at least 3 PH teacher units to every 4 PM teacher units. Students of the low socio-economic class go to the public school in their district regardless of the high- and middle-class criteria, unless their residence location is excluded from a district. The costs of private education are $37,500 per PH (130 students), $25,000 per PM (140 students), and $12,500 per PL (100 students).

Adult Education–The School Department can offer courses in adult education on a jurisdictionwide basis. Thus, adult education is not tied to a particular location or school. The number of population

TABLE 7.7
SCHOOL DEPARTMENT

General Characteristics

	SC1
Construction Cost	$27,000,000
Land Requirements	6%
Annual Depreciation Rate	2%
BG and BS Requirements	
For 1% Maintenance	
BG	2 units
BS	.7 units
For Normal Operation	
BG	8 units
BS	3 units
Federal-State Aid	
Capital	$ for every local $1
Current (automatic)	$225 per student

Design Capacity (in Students) as a Function of the Number and Class of Population Units Assigned to Teach There

		PM 0	1	2	3	4	5	6
	0		2,520	4,140	6,840	9,900	12,240	13,140
	1	3,600	5,910	8,460	11,200	13,320	15,300	17,100
	2	7,200	9,900	12,600	15,500	17,460	19,440	21,240
PH	3	10,800	14,040	16,920	20,000[a]	21,960	23,760	25,560
	4	13,140	17,460	21,060	23,400	25,200	27,000	28,620
	5	17,100	20,700	23,400	26,640	28,440	30,000	31,500
	6	19,800	23,850	26,820	29,880	31,320	32,850	34,200

Population Unit Characteristics

Characteristics	PH	PM	PL
Number of students	130	140	100
Criteria for refusal to attend public schools value ratio (min.)	80	60	None
Student-teacher ratio (maximum)	18:1	22:1	None
Ratio of high to middle teachers (minimum)	1:1	3:4	None
Cost of private education (for students)	$39,000	$24,500	$12,500

Capital Federal-State Aid

1st request:	60% chance of acceptance
2nd request:	40% chance of acceptance
3rd request:	30% chance of acceptance

Adult Education

School Demand	School Supply
Ead time unit allocated to public adult education is a unit of demand.	Classes held in public school facilities—only additional cost is for part-time teachers.

One Unit of Time by P1 Hired	Provides Units of Adult Education
PH	15
PM	10

a. The least cost design capacity of an SC1

units hired from the PH and PM classes on part-time basis determines the capacity of the adult education program to serve population units who allocate time for free adult education.

All adult education teachers are part-time workers. The department indicates the number of time units to be hired from the high- and/or middle-population classes. One part-time employment unit of middle-income teachers supplies one adult teacher unit, while one part-time employment unit of high-income teachers supplies one-and-one-half adult teacher units. One adult teacher unit provides ten units of adult education.

Revenues—The School Department receives revenue to its current and capital accounts from various sources. These include:

(a) *Appropriations.* These are funds distributed to the current and/or capital account of the departments.

(b) *Federal-State Aid.* Current federal-state aid is automatically granted to the department in the amount of $225 for each student enrolled in public schools in the jurisdiction. Capital federal-state aid may be applied to the construction of new schools.

(c) *Bonds.* Current bonds are automatically floated by the computer if the current expenditures of the department exceed its current revenue. Current bonds have a duration of two years and the interest rate is set by the model. Capital bonds may also be floated for a department. Capital bonds have a duration of 25 years and interest rate is set by the model.

(d) *Miscellaneous.* These revenues include such items as cash transfers to the capital or current accounts of the department and income from the sale of land (capital account only).

Expenditures—(See Table 7.7) Schools must spend money on the following items:

(a) *Goods and Services.* The School Department must purchase business goods (BG) and business services (BS) for the normal operation of its schools and for the maintenance and/or renovation of its schools. BG ad BS may be purchased either from establishments owned by local economic decision makers (competitive prices usually range around $100,000 per unit) or from the outside system (i.e., the computer) at fixed prices of $130,000 per unit.

(b) *Full-Time Salaries.* The typical salary for a PH worker is $10,000, and the typical salary for a PM worker is $5,000. There are 120 workers (teachers) in a PH and 160 workers (teachers) in a PM.

(c) *Miscellaneous.* These expenditures include cash transfers from the capital or current accounts of the department to the Economic or Government Sector or from one account to another account.

(d) *Bond Payments.* These include payments on interest and principal of outstanding capital bonds and current bonds floated by the department.

(e) *Adult Education.* These are salaries for part-time workers for adult education. One PH part-time teacher unit costs $15,000 and supplies 15 units of adult education. One PM part-time teacher unit costs $10,000 and supplies 10 units of adult education.

(f) *School Construction.* This includes funds expended for the construction of a new school, the upgrading of an old one, or the demolition of a school. The typical cost of an SC1 is $27,000,000.

(g) *Land Purchase.* This includes expenditures for the purchase of land from Government or Economic Sector or the outside system.

Municipal Services Department (MS)–The function of the Municipal Services Department is to provide fire, police, sanitary and other general government services to the simulated area. This service is expressed in terms of MS units.

Employment and Capacity–The Municipal Services Department employs from the middle- and low-income-population units only. Like schools, the design capacity of an MS plant is determined by its employment mix.

Value ratio also affects the capacity of an MS plant. The effective capacity of an MS plant is determined by multiplying its design capacity times the value ratio/100.

The supply of municipal services for a district is therefore a function of the level of the plant, its value ratio, and the skill level of the population units hired.

Drain on Municipal Services–As in a real city, all private developments require municipal services. Each land user has a set drain of MS units and total demand is therefore a function of the number and type of residence units and business activity located in a district. The quality of MS service affects depreciation of economic land uses and Social Sector dissatisfaction. Quality of service deteriorates when an MS plant is drained of more units of service than its effective capacity. The factor by which land uses served by an MS plant depreciate is expressed in terms of the MS Use Index.

Income—The Municipal Services Department receives income for its current and capital accounts from various sources. These include:

(a) *Appropriations.* These are funds distributed to the current and/or capital accounts of the department.

(b) *Federal-State Aid.* Current federal-state aid is automatically granted to the department for welfare payments. Aid is granted on the basis of 2 federal-state dollars for each local dollar up to a maximum equivalent of $35 per resident of a jurisdiction. The Municipal Services Department is not eligible for capital federal-state aid.

(c) *Miscellaneous.* This income includes such items as cash transfers to the capital or current account of the department and income from the sale of land (capital account only).

(d) *Bonds.* Current bonds are automatically floated by the computer if the current expenditures of the department exceed its current revenue. Current bonds have a duration of two years and the interest rate is set by the computer. Capital bonds may be floated. They have a duration of 25 years and the interest rate is set by the computer.

Expenditures—(See Table 7.8.) The Municipal Services Department spends money on the following items:

(a) *Welfare Payments.* Welfare payments for unemployed workers are distributed from the current accounts of the Municipal Services Department.

(b) *Goods and Services.* The Municipal Services Department must purchase business goods (BG) and business services (BS) for the normal operation of its plants and for the provision of its service functions.

(c) *Miscellaneous.* These expenditures include cash transfers from the capital or current accounts of the department to the Government or Economic Sectors or from one account to another account.

(d) *Salaries.* The typical salary for one PM worker is $5,000 and the typical salary for one PL worker is $2,500.

(e) *Bond Payments.* These include payments on interest and principal of outstanding capital and current bonds floated by the department.

(f) *Construction.* This includes funds expended for the construction of a new MS plant or the demolition of an old one.

(g) *Land Purchase.* This includes expenditures for the purchase of land either from a Government or Economic Sector or from the Outside System.

TABLE 7.8
MUNICIPAL SERVICES DEPARTMENT

General Characteristics

Typical Construction Cost	$30,000,000
Land Requirement	6%
Annual Depreciation Rate	3.3%
BG and BS Requirements	
For 1% renovation or maintenance	
BG	2 units
BS	1 unit
For normal operation	
BG	7 units
BS	3 units

Design Capacity (MS units) as a Function of the Number and Class of Population Units Assigned to Work There

		PL 0	1	2	3	4	5	6
	0		140	230	380	500	680	730
	1	200	330	470	620	740	850	950
	2	400	550	700	860	970	1,080	1,180
PM	3	600	780	940	1,100*	1,220	1,320	1,420
	4	730	970	1,170	1,300	1,400	1,500	1,590
	5	950	1,150	1,300	1,480	1,580	1,670	1,750
	6	1,100	1,325	1,490	1,660	1,740	1,825	1,900

Effective capacity of an MS plant:

Effective capacity = design capacity x value ratio/100.

MS Use Index – affects depreciation of economic land uses and social sector dissatisfaction.

$$\text{MS Use Index} = \frac{\text{actual no. of MS units drained} \times 100}{\text{effective capacity of MS plant}}$$

MS Use Index above 100 means the plant is being overused and depreciation and dissatisfaction will be increased.

Federal-State Aid for Welfare Payments.

$2 Federal-State for each local dollar up to a maximum equivalent to $35 per resident of a jurisdiction.

Utility Department (UT)—The Utility Department is responsible for providing utilities such as sewer, water and electrical power to economic developments. Units of utility service are provided by utility plants. Utility plants have three possible levels of development A UT1 requires 20 percent of a square mile.

Installation of Service—When providing service to a parcel, the Utility Department installs levels of service. There may not be more than nine levels of service on a parcel. Each level of service provides a certain number of utility units. At least as many units must be provided as an economic activity requires for operation. The installation costs for providing levels of service are fixed and deducted from the financial accounts of the department by the computer.

There is no design capacity of a utility plant. In terms of operating cost, however, a UT1 has a least cost (per unit) capacity of 1500 units.[26] The variable cost function of a UT1 is given in the Master Sheet.

The units which a utility plant serves are the equivalent of the drain of utility units by the land uses which require utility service. These are fixed for each land use.

Revenues—Unlike other departments the Utility Department is a quasi-private company and does not receive income to its current or capital accounts from direct appropriations. The department can, however, receive income from any of the following sources:

(a) *Subsidies.* These are public subsidies to the current and capital accounts of the department.

(b) *Bonds.* Current bonds are automatically floated by the computer if the current expenditures of the department exceed its revenues. Current bonds have a duration of two years and the interest rate is set by the computer.

(c) *Miscellaneous.* These revenues include such items as cash transfers to the capital or current accounts of the department and income from the sales of land (capital account only).

(d) *Income from Users.* Since the Utility Department can set a price for its service, it earns income for every unit of service which is consumed by the Economic Sector land uses. The typical price charged by the department is $10,000 per unit of service. The computer deducts all utility charges from the accounts of the economic activities and credits income to the Utility Department.

TABLE 7.9
UTILITY DEPARTMENT

Level of Service	General Characteristics Installation Costs (millions)	Number of Utility Units Installed
1	2	100
2	4	200
3	5	300
4	6	400
5	8	500
6	11	600
7	14	700
8	18	900
9	35	2,500

Utility Units Served	Operating Costs for a UTI as a Function of the Number of Utility Units Served Per Unit Operating Costs	Total Operating Costs
300	$20,000	$ 6,000,000
600	13,333	8,000,000
900	9,630	8,666,667
1200	7,778	9,333,333
1500[a]	6,667[a]	10,000,000[a]
1800	7,407	13,333,333
2100	7,936	16,666,666
2200	8,080	17,777,778

a. The least cost design capacity of a UT1.

	Utility (unit)	Water (MG)		
Normal Price of Service	$10,000	a		
	Utility Plant	**Utility Level**	**Intake**	**Outflow**
Cost of Lowest Level Plant (millions)	$30	$2	$.1-4.5	$.1-4.5[b]
Capacity	2400	100		3 MGD
Typical Operating Cost Per Capacity Unit	$7000 to $8000		0-$600[c]	$25-300[b]
Land Requirement	6%	None	1%	1%

	Intake Treatment Costs per MG Water Quality Level								
	1	2	3	4	5	6	7	8	9
UT	5	60	80	100	180	300	450	600	NA

Annual cost to operate an ambient water quality sampling station	$50,000
Annual cost to operate a point source water quality sampling station	$25,000

a. Water prices may be set by type of user

b. Depending upon treatment type

c. Depending upon water quality

Expenditures—(See Table 7.9.) The Utility Department spends money on the following items:

(a) *Operating Costs.* Total operating costs were discussed earlier. Operating costs increase with the number of utility units served; but the per unit operating cost is least at 1500 units.

The methods for determining operating costs are outlined as follows:

Let X = the number of utility units drained. If X ≤ 600, cost = $4,000,000/600 (X) + $4,000,000. If 600 < X ≤ 1,500, cost = $2,000,000/900 (X − 600) + $8,000,000. If X > 1,500, cost = $10,000,000/900 (X − 1500) + $10,000,000.

(b) *Miscellaneous.* These expenditures include cash transfers from the capital or current accounts of the department to the Economic or Government Sector or from one account to another.

(c) *Bond Payments.* These include payments on interest and principal of any outstanding capital or current bonds floated by the department.

(d) *Plant Construction.* This includes funds expended for the construction of a new utility plant, the upgrading of an old one, or the demolition of an existing one.

(e) *Extension of Service.* These costs include installation costs for levels of service and redistricting costs.

(f) *Land Purchase.* This includes expenditures for the purchase of the land either from the Government or Economic Sector or from the outside system.

The Water and Sewer Office—This office is contained within the Utility Department, and it is charged with the responsibility of supplying the municipal water requirements within each of the utility districts. That is, the water and sewer districts are identical to the utility districts. Presently, GEM is being designed to include a full multi-media model which adds solid waste and air to the water module.

The water office supplies water for a district by building a certain level of intake treatment plant. It also has to find a source of water. It is assumed that the cost of treating a unit of water (an MGD) is directly related to the quality level of the water. That is, it costs more to treat a unit of 8 quality water than a unit of 3 quality water.

Intake treatment plants must be located within the jurisdiction that contains the utility district. The actual inflow point (the point at which water is withdrawn from a body of water) need not be in the same jurisdiction, however.

If the total demand for municipal water within a utility district is larger than the amount that can be supplied by the intake plant, the municipal water users are obliged to purchase the needed amount of water from the outside system.

The total amount of municipally supplied water must also be returned to the local water system. It is up to each utility district to determine the amount of its water effluent that will be treated and the type of treatment.

Effects of the Water Quality Index—(See Tables 7.10 to 7.15.) The Water Quality Index on a parcel of land has direct effects on the following factors:

(1) Treatment costs of water withdrawn from that parcel by the Water Department.

(2) Treatment cost of water withdrawn by an industrial surface water user on that parcel.

(3) The amount of personal consumption eminating from Major Recreation Areas located on that parcel.

The Pollution Index is a part of the Environmental Index which is used as a basis for determining the attractiveness of a residential parcel of land for potential inmigrants. A high Pollution Index also affects the probability of population units moving away from a residential parcel.

The Health Index for a parcel of land influences the amount of money spent by population units for health services. It also affects the Personal Index, which in turn influences the amount of dissatisfaction experienced by population units on a parcel. The Health Index for a parcel of land is based upon the concentration of coliform bacteria in the water. This is the only case in which a single component of the water quality index is handled separately.

Transportation Department

The Transportation Department is concerned with two types of developments: highways and terminals.

Highways—*Types.* There are three types of highways in the model: HY1, HY2, and HY3. An HY3 is the largest road.

The value ratio of a segment of highway will reduce its design capacity by a function of VR/100 times design capacity. The product is equivalent to effective capacity.

TABLE 7.10
WATER

Physical Characteristics	
	Location – parcel number
	Type – river or lake
	Volume flowing to next parcel – MGD
	Rate of flow – parcels per day.

Water Quality Rating	Quality of Water Comment
1	Drinkable – best quality water
2	Drinkable with minor treatment
3	Swimable – direct body contact possible
4	Boating and fishing – indirect body contact
5	Fair esthetic value
6	Poor esthetic value – treatable at moderate cost
7	No esthetic value – treatable at high cost
8	Negative esthetic value – treatable at very high cost
9	Nonusable water

Types of Pollution

Symbol	Name	Units of Measure
BOD	Biochemical oxygen demand	Pounds per million gallons of water
CL	Chlorides	Lbs/MG
NO_3	Nutrients	Lbs/MG
CO	Coliform bacteria	Parts per million gallons
T	Temperature deviation	Degrees (°)
OFS	Oil and floating solids	Yes or no
HLW	High level wastes	Yes or no

TABLE 7.11
ELIMINATION OF THREE POLLUTANTS DUE TO TIME IN THE WATER

Rate of Flow of the River (parcels per day)	Percentage of Original Pollutant Remaining at the End of a Flow Through a Parcel		
	BOD	Nutrients	Coliform
1	50	33	17
2 (sluggish)	75	67	58
4	89	83	79
6 (slow)	92	89	86
8	96	92	90
11 (average)	96	94	93
15	97	96	95
22 (fast)	97	97	96
30	98	98	97
44 (rapid)	99	99	98

TABLE 7.12

BIODEGREDATION OF POLLUTANTS

Eleven parcels per day is the typical normal rate of flow of water in the RIVER BASIN MODEL. The following table shows the percentage or amount of each pollutant if the water volume does not vary and the rate of flow of the river is eleven parcels per day.

Start Parcels Downstream	BOD 100%	Nutrients 100%	Coliform 100%	Temperature 10°	O&S HLW 1
1	96	94	93	10°	1
2	92	88	86	7°	1
3	88	83	80	4°	1
4	84	78	74	1°	1
5	81	73	69	0	1
6	78	69	64	0	0
7	75	65	60	0	0
8	72	61	56	0	0
9	69	57	52	0	0
10	66	54	48	0	0
11	63	52	45	0	0
12	60	49	42	0	0
13	58	46	39	0	0
14	56	43	36	0	0
15	54	40	33	0	0

TABLE 7.13

DEFINITION OF THE NINE COMPREHENSIVE WATER QUALITY LEVELS

	Water Quality Levels								
Pollutant Types (maximums)	1	2	3	4	5	6	7	8	9
BOD (Lbs/MG)	10	20	30	40	60	100	150	300	>300
Chlorides (Lbs/MG)	5	10	15	20	30	40	60	80	>80
Nutrients (Lbs/MG)	25	50	100	200	400	800	1600	3200	>3200
Coliform bacteria (parts per MG)	2	6	12	20	40	70	120	160	>160
Temperature	0	0	1	2	4	7	10	14	>14
Oil & floating solids	0	0	0	0	0	>0	>0	>0	>0
High level wastes	0	0	0	0	0	0	0	>0	>0

Explanation of the table:

In order to determine the water quality level or index of given amounts of water, take the concentrations of each of the seven pollutant categories and calculate the water quality level based upon each pollutant separately. For example, a BOD concentration of 25 Lbs/MG would yield an index of 3, coliform bacteria of 169 parts per MG would yield an index of 9, and the presence of oil and floating solids would allow the water quality to be no better than 6. The worst (highest) water quality index that was calculated using the pollutant types separately, is assigned to the given amount of water. If the water on parcel x had the three pollutants described above, it would be assigned a water quality Index of 9.

Looked at another way, water quality level 4 is attained when a body of water has concentrations of BOD that exceed 30 but fall below 41, coliform bacteria concentrations above 12 but below 21, etc.

TABLE 7.14
CHARACTERISTICS OF OUTFLOW TREATMENT PLANTS

	Level of Treatment Plant							
	1	2	3	4	5	6	7	8
Maximum Capacity (MGD)	3	8	16	26	40	60	90	200
Land Requirement (% of parcel)	1	2	3	4	5	6	7	8
Construction Costs (millions of dollars)								
CL	.1	.2	.4	.6	.8	1.0	1.2	1.6
PT	.5	1.0	2.0	3.0	4.0	5.0	6.0	8.0
ST	1.5	3.0	6.0	9.0	12.0	15.0	18.0	24.0
TT	4.5	9.0	18.0	27.0	36.0	45.0	54.0	72.0
Operating Costs (dollars per MG)								
CL	25	24	23	22	21	20	19	18
PT	100	95	90	85	80	75	70	65
ST	200	190	180	170	160	150	140	130
TT	300	285	270	255	240	225	210	195

Intake treatment plants have the same construction costs as ST outflow treatment plants.

	Percentage Pollution Removed by Treatment Types			
	CL	PT	ST	TT
BOD	0	50	80	99
Chlorides	0	0	60	99
Nutrients	0	0	50	70
Coliform	99	99	99	100
Temperature	0	0	0	100
Oil and Floating Solids	0	100	100	100
High Level Wastes	0	0	0	100

TABLE 7.15

POLLUTION CHARACTERISTICS OF ECONOMIC ACTIVITIES

	Water Consumption			Polution Generated						
				Pounds per MG			Parts per MG			
	MGD	Days per Year	MGY	BOD	CL	NU	COLI	Temper-ature	OFS	HLW
Surface Water Users										
FL	61	260	15,860	600	100	1000	20	9	1	0
MP	225	260	58,500	1000	170	500	20	6	1	0
FO	49	260	12,740	6000	400	10000	300	9	1	0
TA	17	260	4,420	6000	130	4000	20	18	1	1
PA	333	260	86,580	3000	380	3000	150	16	1	1
CR	31	260	8,060	2000	500	8000	50	4	1	1
Municipal Water Users										
Industries										
SG	10	260	2,600	500	100	1000	10	0	0	0
MF	9	260	2,340	500	150	700	30	0	1	0
NL	12	260	3,120	400	150	100	20	0	0	0
EL	5	260	1,300	800	200	200	20	0	0	0
TE	8	260	2,080	500	180	100	30	0	0	0
Commercial										
NS	.18	260	47	100	0	0	20	0	0	0
BG	.13	312	41	200	0	0	10	0	0	0
BS	.17	312	53	150	0	0	15	0	0	0
PG	.23	312	72	250	0	0	20	0	0	0
PS	.18	312	56	100	0	0	15	0	0	0
Residential										
HA	.08	364	29	1250	50	100	5	0	1	0
HB	.07	364	25	1250	50	100	5	0	1	0
HC	.06	364	22	1250	50	100	5	0	1	0
MA	.07	364	25	1100	40	80	5	0	1	0
MB	.05	364	18	1100	40	80	5	0	1	0
MC	.03	364	11	1100	40	80	5	0	1	0
LA	.03	364	11	1000	30	70	5	0	1	0
LB	.03	364	11	1000	30	70	5	0	1	0
LC	.02	364	7	1000	30	70	5	0	1	0

Roads are used by population units to travel to and from employment and shop locations and by basic industry and commercial establishments to transport products to terminals and to purchase the necessary goods and services for maintenance and normal operations. Population units travel to work during peak-hour travel only. Buses also consume road units during peak-hour.

Depreciation. Highways depreciate as a function of use. The annual depreciation rate of a mile segment of highway is 5.0Z where Z is the actual number of road units consumed divided by effective capacity of the road segment.

Congestion. Congestion occurs when the use index [(Actual Use/Effective Capacity) X 100] of a highway is greater than 100. Congestion is recorded only during peak-hour travel. When congestion occurs, it takes additional time for population units to travel on highways in the city. The amount of additional time is directly proportional to the amount of congestion on the highway. For example, if the peak-hour congestion is 110 percent, the time to travel a road is 10 percent greater than otherwise. Time consumed in transportation to and from work affects the allocation of leisure time in the Social Sector.

Terminals—Terminals (TM) are used by HI, LI, and BG. HI and LI use terminals to ship output to national demanders and BG receives goods from national suppliers. A TM1 supplies 10,000 capacity units; a TM2 supplies 20,000 capacity units; and a TM3 supplies 30,000 capacity units.

Revenues—The Transportation Department receives income to its current and capital accounts from various sources. These include:

(a) *Appropriations.* These are funds distributed to the current and/or capital accounts of the department.

(b) *Federal-State Aid.* The Transportation Department is eligible for capital federal-state aid for the construction of new highways or the upgrading of existing ones. The matching ratio of federal-state funds to local funds for a HY1 is 1 federal-state dollar to 9 local dollars; for a HY2, 1:1; and for an HY3, 2:1.

(c) *Bonds.* Current bonds are automatically floated by the computer if the current expenditures of the department exceed its current revenue. Current bonds have a duration of two years and the interest rate is set by the computer. Capital bonds may be floated and have a duration of 25 years. The interest rate is set by the computer.

TABLE 7.16
TRANSPORTATION DEPARTMENT
(Characteristics for Level One Unless Stated Otherwise)

Facility	Highways	Terminals
Location Requirements		
Percentage of parcel	(from both sides)	(from 4 corners)
Level 1	8	12
Level 2	12	16
Level 3	16	20
Construction Costs		
(Millions of dollars)	.8	14
Depreciation		
Due to use	5.0Z[a]	NA
Road Maintenance		
Purchases per 1% maintenance	\$20,000/segment	NA
Capacity Measures		
Design capacity (standardized units)	500/segment	10,000
Consumption by users (standardized units)		
P1	10	
BUS (level 1)	50	
BG		1 per CU sold
FL, NL, EL, TA		1000
MF, TE		2000
FO, PA, CR		3000
MP		6000
SG		10000

Federal-State Aid for Capital Construction

Road Type	Matching Federal	Matching Local	Probability of Receiving Aid
Level 1	\$1	\$9	80%
Level 2	\$1	\$1	50%
Level 3	\$2	\$1	30%

Limit on the number of road segments requested by a jurisdiction is 5.

a. Z = highway units used/effective capacity; and, effective capacity is the design capacity times the value ratio expressed as a percent.

(d) *Miscellaneous.* This income includes such items as cash transfers to the capital or current account of the department and income from the sale of land (capital account only).

Expenditures–(See Table 7.16.) The Transportation Department spends money on the following:

(a) *Road Maintenance.* The Transportation Department must purchase business goods and business services for the maintenance and/or renovation of its roads. BG and BS are purchased by the Transportation Department at fixed costs from the outside system. The goods and services cost per mile maintained for 1 percent renovation and/or maintenance are outlined as follows:

Road Type	BG	BS
HY1	$ 7,000	$1,000
HY2	14,000	2,000
HY3	21,000	3,000

(b) *Bond Payments.* These include payments on interest and principal of outstanding capital and current bonds floated by the department.

(c) *Miscellaneous.* These expenditures involve cash transfers from the capital or current accounts of the department to the Economic or Government Sector or from one account to another.

(d) *Road and Terminal Construction.* The Transportation Department can build, upgrade or demolish highways (HY) and terminals (TM).

(e) *Land Purchase.* This includes expenditures for the purchase of land either from the Government or Economic Sector or from the outside system.

(f) *Miscellaneous.* These expenditures involve cash transfers from the capital or current accounts of the department to the Government or Economic Sectors or from one account to another.

Bus and Rapid Rail

Although Bus and Rapid Rail are separate quasi-private areas, they will be treated in the same section due to the similarities between the two. Neither is limited to a single jurisdiction; both have interjurisdictional authority.

Bus and Rapid Rail provide additional modes of transportation (besides automobile) to the population units who live and work in the simulated area. Population units take bus or rail to work only; they do not use either mode of transportation for shopping.

Capacity—Bus and Rapid Rail have rolling stock with three possible levels of service (1, 2, and 3). Level of service indicates the actual number of buses or railroad cars which may serve a particular route.

The number of passengers (capacity that can be effectively serviced by a rail or bus route) is determined by its level of service. A bus route with a level of service of 1 has a design capacity of 3,000 passengers and a rail route with a level of service of 1 has a design capacity of 6,000 passengers. Like highways, the design capacity of a bus or rail route is not necessarily its effective capacity. Effective capacity is determined by multiplying the value ratio of equipment divided by 100 times the design capacity. Effective capacity can be further reduced by employment. If the Bus and Rapid Rail Company receive only a percentage of the employees which they requested, the actual effective capacity of that route is the percentage times the design capacity.

It must be noted, however, that effective capacity does not refer to the number of people who actually use a bus or rail. A bus or rail route may serve less or more people than its effective capacity. In such a case the model has decided for these people (see "The Employment Process") that, despite the overcrowding, it is still cheaper in terms of time and money to take a bus rather than another mode of transportation.

Equipment—Bus and Rapid Rail do not buy individual pieces of rolling stock. Rather, they purchase units of equipment for each mile of service. One unit of equipment costs $10,000. Forty units of equipment are required to operate a bus (level of service = 1) for one mile and 80 units of equipment are required to operate a rail (level of service = 1) for one mile.

Depreciation and Maintenance—Bus and Rail equipment which is used depreciates at an average rate of 3.5 percent per annum. The costs of 1 percent maintenance or renovation are $40 per equipment unit (goods) and $60 per equipment unit (services).

Employment—Bus and Rail employ workers from middle-income population units only. Fifty units of labor are required to operate a bus or rail for one mile. One PM of workers therefore serves 20 miles of a BUS1 or RAIL1.

Passenger Assignments—Passengers are assigned to travel to work by bus and/or rail by the computer. The basis upon which a population unit may or may not be assigned to bus or rail transportation is the dollar value of their time. Those population units with the lowest dollar value of time will take the cheapest but probably the longest route of transportation to work. Those population units with a high dollar value of time take a more expensive but quicker mode.

Routes—Buses travel along roads and trains go along tracks, as in the real world. The Bus Company must therefore specify routes only on existing highways, while the Rail Department can have routes wherever they build tracks, including on the diagonal across parcels and either overground or underground. Routes must begin and end at intersections. Further, although bus and rail transport workers to and from their places of employment, the direction of the route is specified in order to meet the residence to work demands. For example, assume that people live in the parcels above the line 15 and that most employment locations are at parcels 7018, 7020 and 7220. The routes that are specified are the morning routes that bring people to work. In this instance they are 7113 to 7119 (for bus) and 7713 to 7119 (for rail). A bus stops at every intersection but a rail will stop only where there are stations and there can be stations only at intersections. In the example on the preceding page, therefore, the rail has three stops: 7713, 7515, and 7119 (Figure 7.18).

Land Requirements—Although buses do not require land (they operate on highways), surface rail tracks, of course, do. All land must be purchased by the company prior to the construction of tracks. Underground rail tracks to not require land.

Revenues—Like the Utility Department, the Bus and Rapid Rail Companies are quasi-private departments and therefore do not receive direct appropriations. Both companies, however, can receive income from any of the following sources:

(a) *Subsidies.* These are public subsidies granted to the current or capital accounts of either company.

(b) *Bonds.* Current bonds are automatically floated by the computer if the current expenditures of either company exceed current revenues. Current bonds have a duration of two years and the

TABLE 7.17
BUS COMPANY AND RAIL

General Characteristics		
Characteristics	**Bus**	**Rail**
Land Development		
Typical development costs		
Underground tracks		$14,000,000/mi.
Surface tracks		4,000,000/mi.
Stations		1,000,000
Land requirements		4% surface tracks (for one side only)
Operating Expenses		
Fixed cost of equipment per mile	$400,000 (40 units)	$800,000 (80 units)
Employment[a]		
Typical cost of labor per mile	40,000	40,000
Units of labor required per mile	50	50
Depreciation and Maintenance of Equipment		
Average rate (annual)	3.5%	3.5%
BG and BS Requirements for 1% Renovation or Maintenance		
BG	$40/unit of equipment	$40/unit of equipment
BS	$60/unit of equipment	$60/unit of equipment
Passenger Capacity (people)		
When value ratio = 100		
Level 1 Route	3000	6000
Level 2 Route	6000	12000
Level 3 Route	9000	18000

Distance for Diagonal Rapid Rail Segments

		Horizontal Distance Between Stations				
		1	2	3	4	5
Vertical distance between stations	1	1.414	2.236	3.162	4.123	5.099
	2	2.236	2.828	3.606	4.472	5.385
	3	3.162	3.606	4.243	5.000	5.831
	4	4.123	4.472	5.000	5.657	6.403
	5	5.099	5.385	5.831	6.403	7.071

a. Bus and Rail hire middle income (PM) workers only. There are 160 workers in a PM. The typical salary per worker is $5000. One PM supplies 1000 units of labor and 50 units of labor are required to operate a bus (level 1) and rail (level 1) for one mile.

interest rate is set by the computer. Capital bonds may be floated for either company. Capital bonds have a duration of 25 years and the interest rate is determined by the computer.

(c) *Fares.* The primary source of income for the Bus Company and Rail Company is the fares which they charge to passengers who use their service. Fares are deducted by the computer from the accounts of population units represented by the social decision makers on the basis of 250 trips to and from work each year.

(d) *Miscellaneous.* These revenues include such items as cash transfers to the capital or current accounts of either company and income from the sale of land (capital account of Rail Company only).

Expenditures—(See Table 7.17.) Bus and Rail spend money on the following items:

(a) *Vehicle Maintenance.* This includes the cost of maintenance and renovation costs of vehicles owned by the companies. It involves purchases of goods and services at fixed prices from the outside system.

(b) *Salaries.* Since both companies hire middle-income workers, they must offer competitive salaries.

(c) *Bond Payments.* These include payments on interest and principal of any outstanding capital or current bonds floated by either company.

(d) *Miscellaneous.* These expenditures include cash transfers from the capital or current accounts of the company to the Economic or Government Sector, or from one account to another.

(e) *Vehicle Purchase.* This is a capital expenditure for the purchase of rolling stock. If any stock is sold, this item will subtract the selling price of stock which will be credited to the capital account of the company.

(f) *Station Construction.* (Rail Company only). This includes expenditures for the construction or upgrading of rail tracks. The cost of diagonal tracks is a function of the hypotenuse of the triangle formed by the rail segment. This relationship is explained as follows:

Distance for Diagonal Rapid Rail Segments

		Horizontal Distance Between Stations				
		1	2	3	4	5
Vertical	1	1.414	2.236	3.162	4.123	5.090
distance	2	2.236	2.828	3.606	4.472	5.385
between	3	3.162	3.606	4.243	5.000	5.831
stations	4	4.123	4.472	5.000	5.657	6.403
	5	5.099	5.385	5.831	6.403	7.071

In other words, a segment of surface track crossing a single (one square mile) parcel diagonally does not cost $4,000,000, but 1.414 times 4,000,000 or $5,656,000.

(g) *Land Purchase.* This item includes expenditures for land purchased from the Government or Economic Sectors or from the outside system.

Transportation Allocator—The transportation system in the model is being redesigned to allow intraparcel travel (wholly within a parcel) and interparcel travel (between parcels). The parameters and characteristics of different modes of transportation in the real world (time and dollar cost of use, cost of construction and maintenance, congestion, etc.) are represented in the model by a weighted sum to produce a corresponding set of characteristics for inter- and intraparcel travel. Since origins and destinations do not have specific locations within parcels, each parcel will have a use capacity (for congestion) and an accessibility index (a measure of time and dollar cost of use) for intraparcel travel. Interparcel travel takes place on interparcel links which also have a capacity and a time and dollar cost of use. Transportation users in the model consist of population units (traveling to work, shop, recreation, etc.) and businesses (distribution of goods and services). Use is also broken down into peak and off-peak times. Population units traveling to full-time employment are assumed to be peak, while population units traveling to part-time employment are split, most business use is also split between peak and off-peak.

Intraparcel—Each parcel would have a General Parcel Accessibility; this index is calculated as follows: a set combination of land used and capital expenditures will yield a given number of transportation units; the number of units times a value ratio will yield the number of effective units (and hend a capacity); the number of effective units divided by the area of the parcel will yield the General Parcel Accessibility. Each activity (residences, commercial, industry, terminals, etc.) will have an activity index which will be a function of activity type and the number of levels of development of that type on a parcel; the activity index times the GPA will yield the Activity Access Index. Intraparcel travel costs, both time and dollar are determined by summing the AAI of the origin and destination, and by considering congestion (a function of effective units and use—passenger or commercial, peak or off-peak).

Each transportation unit has a given capital cost and consumes a given amount of land; the unit has a value ratio which indicates the quality of the transportation units on the parcel (and thus yields its effective capacity). The value ratio will be affected by depreciation (function of use, etc.). Maintenance (ad through it the value ratio) can be influenced by a player and constitute a current expenditure. The transportation unit also has a design capacity for use and each user (population units going to employment or to commercial and movement of goods by businesses) consumes part of the capacity; the consumption for an O-D trip is a function of the AAI's involved.

Interparcel—Each parcel is to contain what is conceptually called a node, assumed (for convenience only) to be located at the center of the parcel. Interparcel links (again representing a weighted sum of all nodes) allows access between parcel nodes; these links represent the sum of all transportation access between parcels and thus interparcel travel may only take place on interparcel links. There can be links between the nodes of any two parcels which share a common boundary (a necessary condition for creation of interparcel links). Each interparcel link consists of a number of link levels which have a design capacity.

Routing—When both origin and destination of a trip are on the same parcel, only the intraparcel parameters are used in calculating the time and dollar cost of the trip. If a trip involves interparcel travel, (i.e., a worker living on parcel A and employed on parcel B) the initial routing is done as follows:

The time and dollar cost of the trip from the residence to the parcel node are determined by using the Activity Accessibility Index for the residence on the parcel, considering congestion and peak or off-peak travel.

Node to Node: A matrix showing all links between the nodes of all adjacent parcels are available, a modified Moore algorithm approach is used to find the least time path between nodes of parcels A and B (influence of congestion and mode choice is explained later). The assumption of least time (especially in the absence of a specific modal split) is in agreement with Department of Transportation studies stating that, in general, most people will attempt to take the least time path from origin to destination. Since there may not be direct link from parcel A to parcel B (there will not be one if A and B are not adjacent), the traveler must go via interparcel links through

FIGURE 7.18
TRANSPORTATION PROCESS

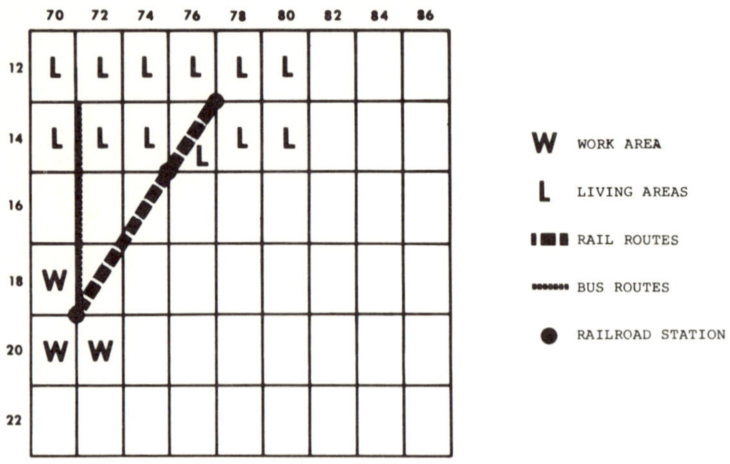

FIGURE 7.19
TERMINALS ALLOCATION PROCESS

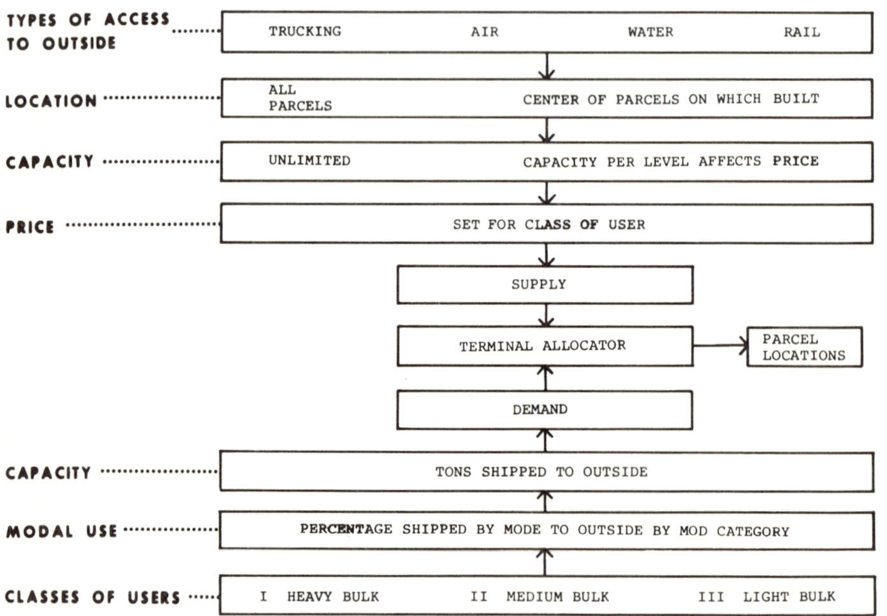

other parcels. The interparcel link route will yield a time and dollar cost.

Once at the node of parcel B, the Activity Accessibility Index of the employment location on parcel B is used to determine the time and dollar cost of the final intraparcel journey. The total time and dollar cost to the consumer of the trip (residence to work) is the sum of the three individual calculations.

Terminals—Three types of terminals are considered in the model: air, water, and rail. Trucking via highway is the only mode by which goods can be shipped within the local system, and trucking also serves as a mode of transport to the outside markets, along with the other three modes associated with the terminals. The business activities that use terminals are divided into transportation classes depending upon the bulk of their output. Each transportation class has a price per ton shipped and each MOD type a specified percentage of its output that should be shipped via the four modes.

Levels of terminals have a design capacity (in number of tons shipped). This capacity, when exceeded, forces the price charged per ton of output by class to rise. (Figure 7.19 on the following page illustrates the terminal allocation process.)

Planning and Zoning Department (PZ)—The Planning and Zoning Department is responsible for zoning, the acquisition of parkland and the creation and demolition of public institutional land.

Planning and Zoning—As the name of the department implies, the powers of this department go somewhat beyond zoning. This department is assumed to have the powers at its disposal to develop a master plan for the city for future redevelopment. It may regulate at its discretion the location of all private construction by enforcing zoning codes to which private developers must conform.

Parkland and Public Institutional Land—The Planning and Zoning Department also has responsibility for two types of public land uses: parkland and public institutional land. Parkland is equivalent to open space recreational areas and is used by the Social Sector model when it allocates time to recreation. Public institutional land is equivalent to parkland with developments; it represents such things as museums, zoos, libraries, and public golf courses.

TABLE 7.18
ZONING

Code	Allowable Uses										
	HI[a]	LI[b]	NS	BG	BS	PG	PS	RA	RB	RC	Park Land
—	X	X	X	X	X	X	X	X	X	X	
00	X	X	X	X	X	X	X	X	X	X	
10	X	X	X	X	X	X	X				
20	X	X									
21	X										
22		X									
30			X	X	X	X	X				
31			X								
32				X							
33					X						
34						X					
35							X				
40								X	X	X	
41								X			
42									X		
43										X	
50											X

a. HI includes FL, SG, MP, MF, NL, EL, TE
b. LI includes FO, TA, PA, CR

TABLE 7.19
PARKS

Demand for Recreational Space

One PH, PM, or PL is equal to
500 units of recreational demand.

Supply of Recreational Space

One percent of a land parcel devoted to parkland provides
250 units of recreation supply.

One percent of a land parcel devoted to public institutional land provides
500 units of recreation supply.

Park Use Index (for a parcel with either or both types of parks) =

$$\frac{\text{units of recreation demand}}{\text{units of recreation supply}}$$

Revenues—The Planning and Zoning Department receives income from various sources. These include:

(a) *Appropriations.* These are funds distributed to the department.

(b) *Bonds.* Capital bonds may be floated for the department. Capital bonds have a duration of 25 years and the interest rate is set by the computer.

(c) *Federal-State Aid.* The Planning and Zoning Department is eligible for capital federal-state aid for the purchase of parkland, which may later be developed as public institutional land use.

(d) *Miscellaneous.* This income includes such items as cash transfers to the capital account of the department and income from the sale of land.

Expenditures—(See Tables 7.18 and 7.19.) *The Planning and Zoning Department spends money* on the following items:

(a) *Bond Payments.* This includes payments on interest and principal of outstanding capital bonds floated by the department.

(b) *Land Purchase.* This involves purchases of undeveloped land from the Government or Economic Sector or the Outside System for the purpose of providing parkland.

(c) *Public Institutional.* This is an expenditure for the development of parkland into public institutional use. Demolition of public institutional uses is included in this item.

(d) *Miscellaneous.* These expenditures involve cash transfers from the capital account of the department to the Economic and Government Sectors.

Resources in the Government Sector—Overview—The Government Sector performs several primary functions: it allocates money in the form of operating and capital expenditures, it controls activities in its own and other sectors through enforced regulations, and it wields political power resulting from its electoral mandate to develop and implement policy. As part of the Government Sector functions, these resources are allocated based upon supply and demand consideration, using inputs that flow through relationships that have been interpreted and designed from real world phenomena.

Figure 7.20 illustrates relationships between supply, demand, and resources in the Government Sector.

Money, as a resource, is allocated to either land, buildings, materials and equipment, or people. Money can be used to expand a

FIGURE 7.20
SUPPLY AND DEMAND RELATIONSHIPS IN THE GOVERNMENT SECTOR

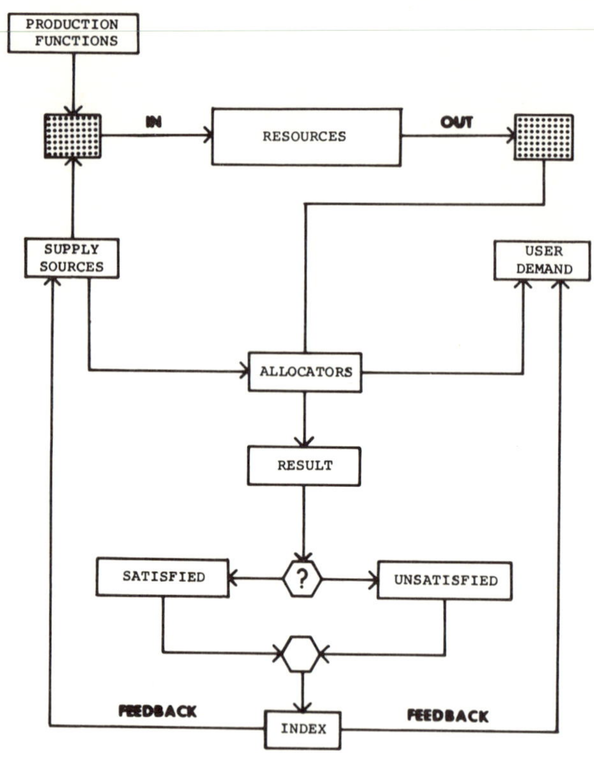

government's capital web or in providing services to its constituent population.

Decision-making entities perform numerous activities (make decisions) to carry out the collection and distribution of government resources. These activities can be described according to a set of relationships which essentially balance supply and demand of resources in the Government Sector. Activities primary to the Government Sector include revenue generation and expenditure, provision of services, and instituting and enforcing legislation. In the model, some of these activities may be placed in the Outside System, which would fix their relationships with the system under study, or in the local system.

Within a defined system, Government Sector relationships are defined and expressed according to the structure and hierarchy determined by the executive routines.

Sources of Income—Aside from appropriations and bonding, there are two other sources of revenue for most governmental departments. These sources are federal-state aid and miscellaneous income.

Federal-state aid is available to Schools, Highways and Planning and Zoning for capital expenses on federally approved projects. School and highway aid is for construction at approved sites; Planning and Zoning is for purchases of parkland and is not restricted to specific locations. If capital aid is granted to Schools or Highways, it is in the form of a fixed ratio of aid to local funds spent. Current federal-state aid is also available until spent, limited only to whatever location and level restrictions that are imposed by the granting agency.

All public departments may receive income from miscellaneous sources, such as the sale of land they own or cash transfers from other departments or decision makers in other sectors. Sources of revenue such as this have great potential for a variety of uses (Figure 7.21).

Regulation—A health department may have the power to regulate the condition of housing or equipment used by a business. In the case of housing, deficiencies may come from the social decision makers or by the department's own investigations. Depending on local laws, the department may impose a fine on offenders or even, in the case of businesses, force them to cease production. For example, if a department has authority to regulate pollution emission, it could use its powers to enforce anti-pollution laws.

FIGURE 7.21
GOVERNMENT REVENUE FLOW

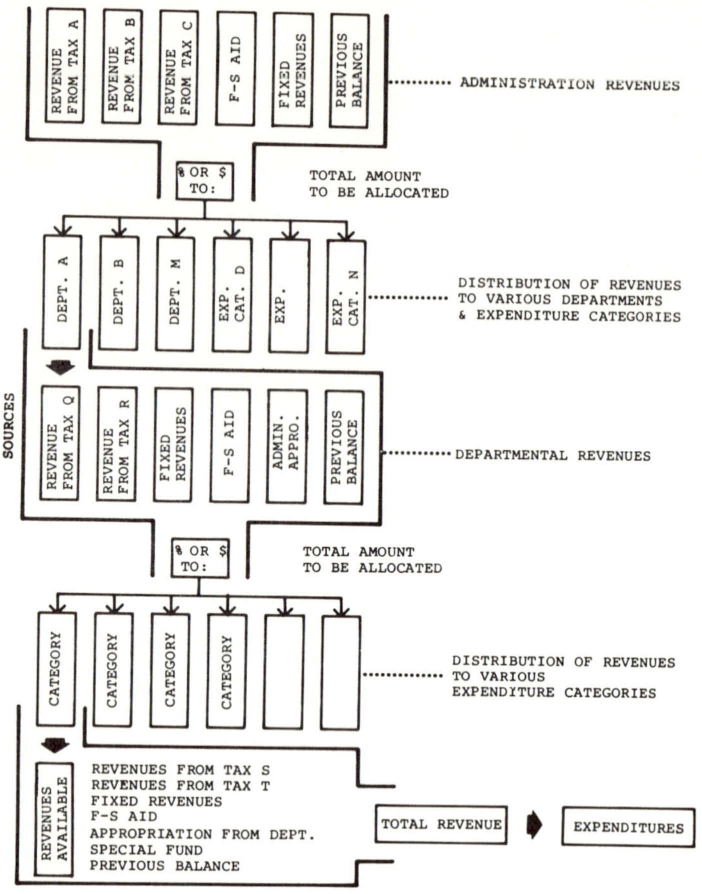

Measurement of Government Services—The present discussion has centered around what the Government Sector can do—what decisions it can make and what resources it has. Other sectors of the model require government services. The adequacy of those services affects such things as the quality of the physical environment; the amount of damage to lives and buildings due to fire; crime and natural disasters; the attractiveness of an area to business and residential development; and the dissatisfaction of those businesses and people already occupying an area.

Government service adequacy is measured for each government function as an index (see Figure 7.22). After establishing the amount of service to be provided, there is a capital cost as well as an increased operating cost for land, building and equipment associated with an increase in service. For the measure of adequacy, the amount of service is adjusted by a measure of the quality of service. Quality of service is derived from the amount and skill of labor and the quantity and quality of space and equipment. For some government functions, such as fire protection, old or poorly maintained equipment is a major limitation on performance. Labor which is above average in skill adds to performance.

The quantity and quality of service for each government function is related to the need for those functions in the calculations of the adequacy index. The determination of need is performed differently for each function. An index is the supply of services, in terms of quantity and quality, divided by the need for those services. Thus, an index of 1.00 would indicate that a function is being adequately performed.

The effects of these indexes on other parts of the model will vary. Potential in-migrants look at the local school indexes; Businessmen concerned about property protection look at the police and fire indexes. The other sectors select only those indexes which are relevant to their concerns.

For those departments which set levels of service (those which set salaries and own equipment but do not own land at specific locations), the general production function described in the Economic Sector is used to measure the quality of services. The quantity of a department's services is equal to the number of service levels. The quantity and quality of service is related to the demand for that service in the final index calculation.

The general production function uses a department's total employment, building and equipment quality and quantity in order

FIGURE 7.22
INDICATORS OF GOVERNMENT SERVICE

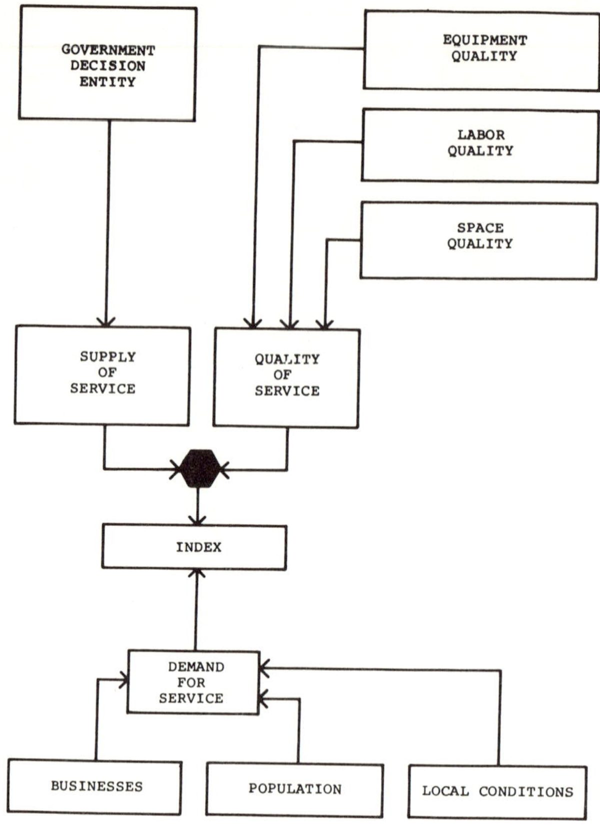

to derive an output index for the department. This output index is a measure of quality of service. Just as the equation's weights and exponents can vary by industrial category, they can vary by department type. For example, equipment quality might be a much more important measure of a fire department than of a General Administration department.

The output index of a department (1.00 is normal) is multiplied by the number of service levels at which the department is attempting to operate. The result is the effective level, or the supply of that service. Thus, better-than-average employee skills or modern equipment could raise a department's effective level of service above that of a department with the same number of employees who are poorly skilled or who are using obsolete equipment.

The demand for a department's services are expressed as a number of levels of service requested, or needed. A department's index is its effective level divided by the need for its services. An index of 1.00 indicates that a department's services are adequate.

Summary

In summary, the Government Sector provides the public service functions for the area under consideration. It allocates, through its various departments, the resources of capital and power, providing a viable business environment and a place for its citizens to live. The next section, the Social Sector, describes the people base of the community.

SOCIAL SECTOR

Functional Characteristics

People, or their behavior, and the ways in which they allocate their time are resources to an environmental system, and it is these factors which delineate the domain of the Social Sector. The range of the relationships includes decision-making opportunities to represent behavioral vagaries and the management of human resources, money and activity. Relationships other than user options include social functions such as voting, recognizable behavior patterns in personal consumption and transportation, and time allocation.

To enable operations and relationships which require differential

FIGURE 7.23
DECISION SCHEMA

DECISIONS / DEPARTMENT TYPE	Education	Highways	Public Welfare	Hospitals	Health	Police	Fire	Parks & Recreation	Planning & Zoning	Sewerage	Other Sanitation	Natural Resources	Housing & Renewal	Assessment	Water Transport & Terminals	Utilities	General Administration
Regulate					●		●		●								●
Assess																	●
Allocate Revenues	●	●	●	●	●	●	●	●	●	●	●	●	●		●	●	●
Set Prices				●	●			●		●	●		●		●	●	
Recieve Grant FS Aid	●	●	●	●	●	●	●	●				●	●				●
Reorganize	●	●	●	●	●	●	●	●	●	●	●	●	●	●	●	●	●
Annex																	●
Set Welfare Policies			●														
Float Bonds	●	●	●	●	●	●	●	●		●	●	●	●		●	●	●
Purchase & Sell Equipment	●	●		●	●	●	●	●		●	●		●		●	●	●
Set Mainten-ance Levels	●	●		●	●	●	●	●		●	●		●		●	●	●
Set Salaries	●	●		●	●	●	●	●		●	●		●		●	●	●
Change Levels of Service	●			●	●	●	●			●	●					●	●
Buy & Sell Land		●						●				●	●			●	

population characteristics, both as functional variables and decision-making resources, equal numbers of households have been aggregated into basic units (the population unit, P1). Each population unit possesses a number of fixed and variable characteristics which permit different operational patterns (at both decision and function levels). It is assumed that households which are composed of a specific poplation unit have identical characteristics. The fixed characteristics are always retained (i.e., 500 persons per population unit, class characteristics) and variable ones (i.e., transportation, employment) may be changed dynamically as a unit. Thus, the population unit is the smallest functional entity in the Social Sector.

Decision-Making Entities

Figure 7.23 depicts the population unit whose characteristics will likely be dependent and/or independent variables of functional relationships within the model. The decision-making entities are responsible for the management of human resources. The fundamental split in such entities is based on location. Thus exists the first order of separation which yields location-specific and non-location specific decision-making entities. In other words, decision control over some but not all areas of population is tied very closely to geographic units.

Resources in the Social Sector

The primary human resources are the potentials for spending money and for structuring activity systems. In providing demand for numerous economic and governmental goods and services, the recycling of money to those sectors insures and fulfills a great number of system relationships. By managing the time and energy available for activities, the population sector can further structure the demand for goods and services and influence the allocation of the resources of the other sectors, such as power and policy in the Government Sector and labor productivity in the Economic Sector. Perhaps the most important aspect of the population activities is that they reflect the stability, prominence, and even viability of that sector in its relationship to the total environmental system (Figure 7.24).

Population resources are presented through the description of the individual population unit characteristics as they are equivalent to or imply the existence of the primary resources.

FIGURE 7.24
SOCIAL SECTOR

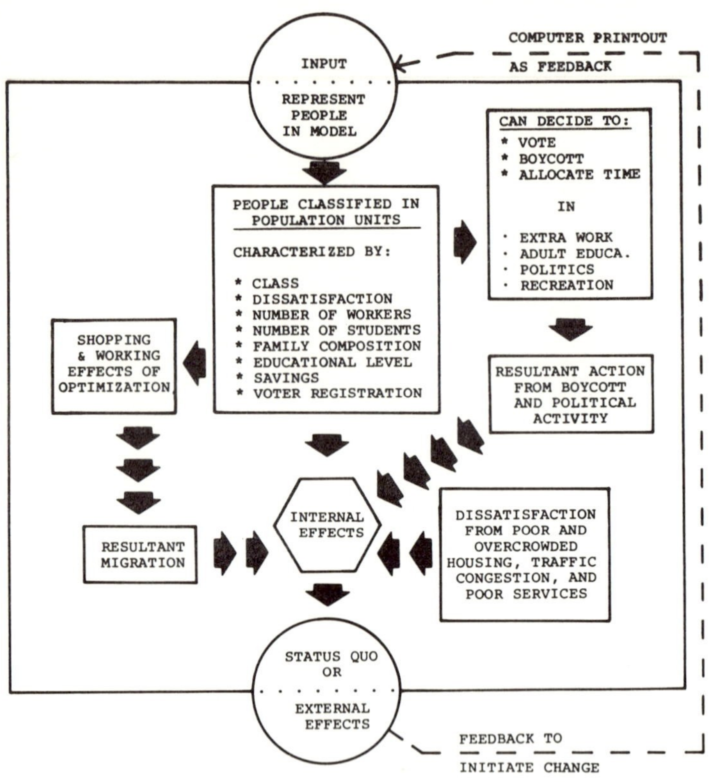

A specific Social Sector represents people who live and work in the simulated area. These people perform several different activities: they vote, boycott, save and spend money, and they allocate time to such activities as extra education, part-time employment, politics, and recreation.

People—People in the model are divided into population units (P1's) of 500 persons each. In addition, population units are divided into three socio-economic classes: high, middle, and low.

Migration

Migration is a phenomenon inherent to all urban areas. People are continually moving within, into or out of a city. In GEM, population units may migrate in three ways: within the system, out of the system, and into the system. The model chooses a certain percentage of the local population units with the highest total dissatisfaction indices for migration. In addition, the computer randomly selects a percentage of population units from the local system to move, regardless of their dissatisfaction indices (Figure 7.25).

Internal Migration—Each of the population units chosen to migrate looks for vacant housing which has a lower housing dissatisfaction index than the housing vacated. If the population unit can find one or several residences with a lower housing dissatisfaction index, it moves into the residence with the lowest housing dissatisfaction index.

Out-Migration—In each round there are a certain number of migrating population units unable to find better housing. This group is selected randomly by the computer from the total population. Population units which are unable to find better housing will out-migrate, leaving the city for the Outside System.

In-Migration—In each round, population units are moved into the simulated urban system. These people are called in-migrants. The total number of in-migrants will average 5 percent of the total local population, plus or minus the effect of the attractive or repulsive qualities of the system as a whole. The computer moves people into the system on the basis of the attractiveness of the area as measured by the relative salary, available housing, job opening, overall school and municipal services conditions and tax rates.

FIGURE 7.25
THE P1 GENERATOR PROCESS

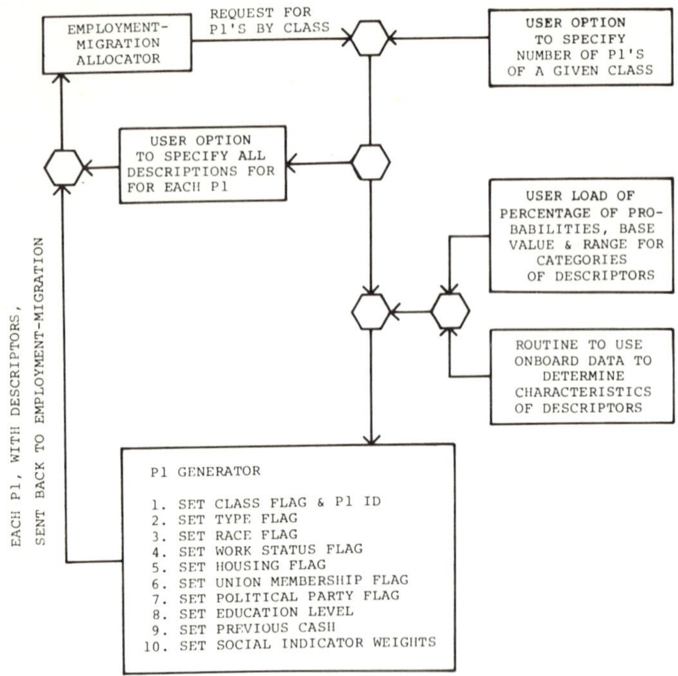

FIGURE 7.26
MIGRATION ALLOCATOR

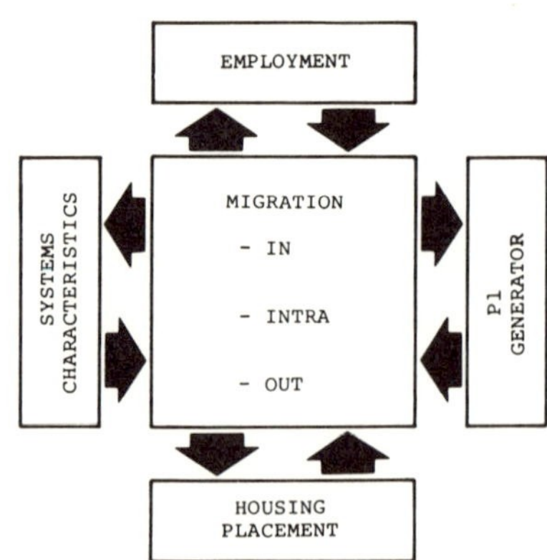

If people can afford it, they are apt to move away from poorly maintained housing in bad neighborhoods which may be tying them to second-rate jobs. By the same token, there is a certain percentage of any population which will grow tired of a particular location and leave for no apparent reason. There will also be people from other areas who find jobs in the city and move from the Outside System into the local system. These are the migratory patterns that GEM takes into account.

Dissatisfaction Index—The people in the simulated area will react to any decisions which affect them. The computer calculates the amount of dissatisfaction which a population unit experiences. Dissatisfaction is measured in terms of a population unit's dissatisfaction with its residence, housing dissatisfaction, and its personal situation in the community. Housing dissatisfaction is determined by quality index, school quality, municipal service quality, taxes, and rent. Personal dissatisfaction is determined by the employment status of the population units involved and the amount of time which they were not able to spend in an activity that had been allocated for. The population units with the highest dissatisfaction index will then be the most likely to migrate.

Migration Allocator: Summary of General Process—The Migration Allocator is an Operational Program which moves population units (people) into, around, and out of the simulated area. The allocator categorizes why people move (i.e., what they move in response to) and in what magnitudes. It uses in-system characteristics (and their comparisons to national and/or regional data) in order to establish the migration climate of the area and thus influence the number and type of in-migrants. The Migration Allocator interacts closely with the Employment Allocator as the movement of the population unit may involve both work location and housing location; in addition, the success or failure of a population unit in either its employment or housing match strongly influences its potential for migration (Figure 7.26).

Migration is one of the first processes to be carried out in a given round. The inputs to the round are processed and among these would be any changes affecting the data needed for the Migration-Employment—Residence Placement Allocators.

The Migration Allocator begins by considering candidates for direct out-migration. These categories are the unemployed, P1's finding a better job outside and some random moves. Next, candidates for intramigration are considered. These are P1's which are presently in the system and are searching to better their housing or employment; those which are successful take the new job or housing and those failing are candidates for out-migration.

Migration is run separately for each class in order of high, middle, low. P1's categorized as immigrants in either of the two versions assume certain characteristics as described below.

When a P1 moves into a residence, its characteristics are averaged with those of the inhabitants in its class and it takes the same preferred allocation as the previous residents. If a P1 moves into a residence which was previously unoccupied by its class, its characteristics and preferred time allocation are the same as they were at the previous residence location, or, in the case of new in-migrants, the characteristics and preferred time allocations shown in the table below.

If more than one P1 moves into a housing unit previously unoccupied by that class and the P1's have different characteristics (coming from different locations), the characteristics of the P1's comprising a plurality of the in-migrating P1's are assumed for all the P1's. If two groups of P1's tie for being the most numerous, a random choice is made as to which group's characteristics are assumed to hold for all the P1's on the parcel of that class.

A P1 which moves within the system from one place to another keeps its previous job location. Although its previous job may not turn out to be its best job after the move, there is a bias toward retaining the previous job.

There are five groups of people looking for housing:

(1) *Most dissatisfied in the System.* A randomly selected half of the 20 percent most personally dissatisfied P1's living on the board move out of their previous housing. The random selection is not made P1 by P1, but by employment group (all of a class on a parcel who work at one place).

(2) *Randomly Chosen in the System.* Of the other 80 percent, a random 1 percent of PL's, 5 percent of PM's and 7 percent of PH's will leave their current housing.

(3) *Natural Population Growth.* One-and-one-half percent of the total population of each class is added to the in-migrant pool in order to represent natural population growth.

(4) *In-Migrants.* The number of in-migrants in any class is 5 percent of the number in the class in the local system plus a number

equal to the number of jobs in that class which were not filled last round.

(5) *Displaced People.* All people who lived on parcels on which all residences have been demolished look for new housing. Those who cannot find housing below their previous dissatisfaction index will out-migrate. The residents on a parcel on which only some of the housing has been demolished are not specifically selected to look for new housing.

The list of P1's looking for housing is randomly ordered. Each P1 takes the best (lowest housing dissatisfaction) acceptable available housing. If the best housing would be over 120 percent crowded if the P1 were to move in, the P1 cannot find housing which meets its criteria, it will out-migrate (Figure 7.27).

Time Allocation–The Social Sector allocates the leisure time for population units in each jurisdiction of the simulated metropolitan area. Hours or minutes are converted to units in the model. There are 100 units of leisure time available to workers in each population unit. However, this leisure time is decreased by the amount of time which it takes workers to travel to and from their place of employment. Therefore, the actual amount of time which can be allocated by social decision makers is 100 units minus time spent traveling to and from work.

Extra Work. The ability to augment income by working longer hours or at more than one job. There are only select areas which offer part-time employment opportunities; the School Department in the Government Sector and a few in the Economic Sector. Workers are paid in proportion to the amount of time they are able to work and in direct proportion to their salary.

If there is no part-time position available, population units will not gain extra employment. The unfulfilled requested time becomes involuntary leisure and adds to personal dissatisfaction.

Education. Education in the model represents not only formal education but training (on the job and elsewhere). It is assumed that unless a certain amount of time is spent in keeping up skills and learning new techniques and information, the education-skill level of the population units declines relative to other population units. It is the level of this skill that largely determines the ability of population units to get better jobs–in fact, it may determine the ability to get a job at all.

To provide for formal training, there is adult education. This

FIGURE 7.27
MIGRATION CYCLE

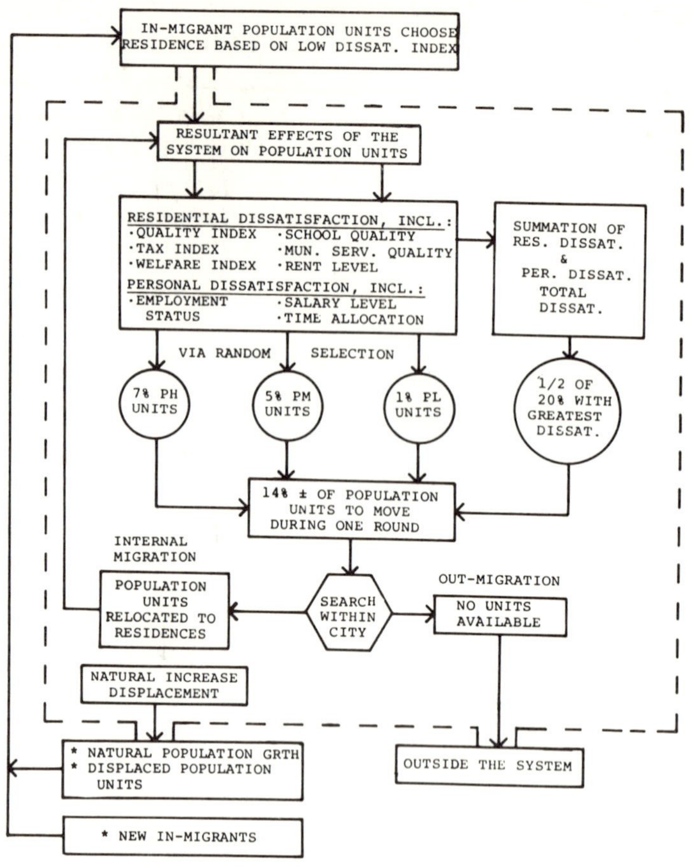

education can be provided both on the public and private sector. The public education is free (the private, of course, is not).

If there is no adult education or not enough made available by the School Department, the time allocated to this use will be assigned to involuntary leisure time and add to personal dissatisfaction.

Politics. The number of voters turning out for the election of a particular candidate, a poll, or a referenda, is normally determined as a random percentage of a population unit (varied by socio-economic class). This percentage can be positively influenced by the expenditure of greater amounts of time in political action. The influence is specific, in that the class of the population units which experience the increased turnout is the one which assigns the time to politics (Figure 7.28).

Recreation. The amount of leisure time available positively affects the dissatisfaction of the population units. However, a decision to spend time in this fashion requires the expenditure not only of time units but also the purchase of goods and services from PG and PS establishments.

Money

Income—The major source of personal income for P1's is wages earned from full and part-time employment. P1's have one of four possible job types: full-time only; full and part-time; part-time only; none. P1's classified with either of the first three job types can earn income from wages.

Closely associated with wages, and the potential for earning wages, are governmental and interest group subsidies dependent upon secondary classifications. Both apply only to those P1's who are members of the full-time labor market.

Government subsidies in this category are in the form of unemployment benefits. That is, all full-time P1's who are unemployed receive compensation enabling them to obtain a minimum standard of living. This situation occurs even in the case of underemployment (full-time workers accepting part-time jobs in lieu of full-time jobs), where the compensation is reduced but still allows the minimum level.

Expenditures—The expenditures of the Social Sector have been alluded to in the previous sections. They include the computer determined cost of goods and services, education costs, recreation

FIGURE 7.28
THE VOTING PROCESS

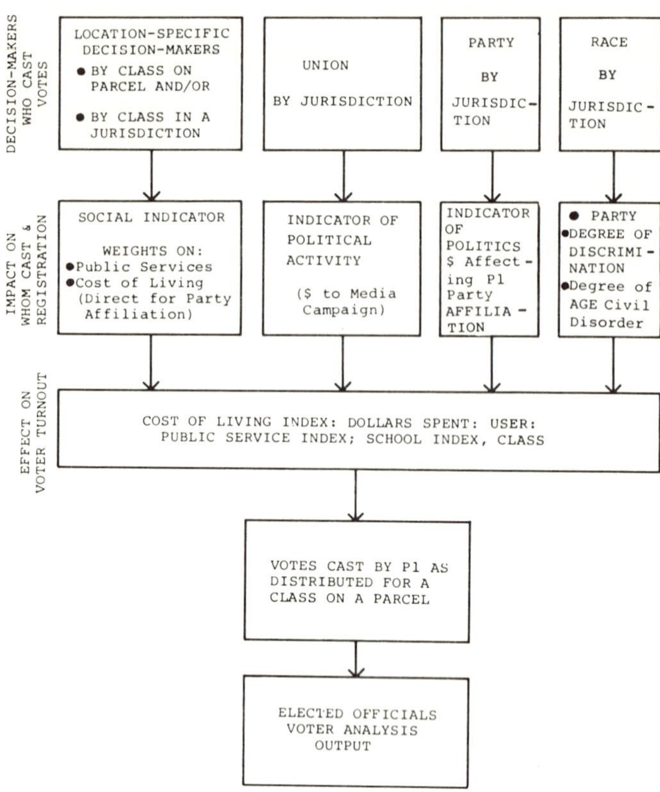

charges, taxes, rent, transportation, health, and other miscellaneous charges. (See Tables 7.20 and 7.21.)

Setting the Dollar Value of Time—The computer assigns all population units to modes of transportation to and from work on the basis of least cost. Least cost includes transportation charges per mile (which differ according to mode of transportation, type of road and amount of congestion) as well as the dollar value of time spent traveling. The model is able to indicate the dollar value of one time unit consumed traveling to and from work for each of the classes which a P1 represents. As the dollar value of a time unit spent traveling increases, the chances are that the computer will assign a more expensive but quicker mode of transportation to work (in almost all cases, via automobile).

Social Sector Indicators and Their Weights—The social indicator serves two functions. The first is the provision of indices that provide summary output for the government departments and are illustrative for various groups within the community. In addition, the indices yield criteria for migration and other automatic system operations.

The functions appropriate for each index have the same general form. They are composed of the user set weight, a weight or function dependent on the type and/or class of a P1, and the straight value of the index.

The straight value of the index is derived from calculations usually done in other function levels, as in the case of the School Index. The data used for each index calculation may vary on four levels: by jurisdiction, by parcel, by residence or employment group, by P1. Each value is based on a scale of 0-100; as such, indices become relative measures. The higher the value index (closer to 100), the worse the situation and greater the dissatisfaction.

The primary characteristic of the weights is that they may be adjusted by class, per parcel. Theoretically, the weights hover around a certain designed value based on socio-economic behavior for each of the classes (see Figure 7.29).

(1) *Level of Aggregation.* Indicates the level at which the index varies. That is, the value is the same for all of the P1's in each grouping of this level.

(2) *Where Calculated.* The operating program or sector where the index is calculated. The main independent variables composing the index are listed in parentheses.

TABLE 7.20
POPULATION UNIT

	PH	PM	PL
General Characteristics			
Population	500	500	500
Workers	120	160	200
Students	130	140	100
Education range	70-99	40-69	0-39
Registered voters	200	140	100
Mobility Characteristics			
Selection of movers			
Random movers	7%	5%	1%
Most dissatisfied	(Half of the 20% with highest quality of life index)		
Percentage of unemployed	33	25	15
Percentage of underemployed	33	25	NA
Selection of housing criteria			
Housing QI range considered	71-100	40-100	20-70
Maximum occupancy considered	120%	120%	120%
Environment index	(Lowest index value is most preferred)		
Characteristics of in-migrants from outside			
Education level	85	55	15
Voter registration	200	140	100
Previous saving	0	0	0
Time allocation			
Extra job	20	30	40
Public adult education	0	30	20
Private adult education	20	5	0
Politics	40	20	10
Recreation	10	10	20
Income Characteristics			
Workers per P1	120	160	200
Full employment salary	(Salary per worker times number of workers)		
Part-time salary	(80 time units provides full-time salary)		
Welfare	(Local jurisdiction payment per worker times the number of unemployed workers)		
Miscellaneous	(Cash transfers from other accounts)		
Expenditure Characteristics			
Rent			
Rent paid factor	2.00	1.33	1.00
Space units consumed	2	1.5	1
Transportation			
Maximum percentage of salary willing to be spent to get a job.			
Costs per worker for job	10%	15%	25%
Auto			
Base auto cost	$210	$190	$140
Cost per HY link (uncongested)			
HY3	$100	$ 87	$ 75
HY2	$125	$112	$100
HY1	$150	$137	$125

TABLE 7.20 (Continued)

	PH	PM	PL
Public transit	(Fare set by transit authority)		
Maximum P1's per RR1	50	40	30
Maximum P1's per BUS 1	25	20	15
Unit public transit consumed	2	2.5	3.3
Travel to PG (and to PS)			
Base cost per CU	$50	$50	$50
Cost per CU consumed (along HY3)	$125	$125	$125
(Along HY2 is twice as much and along HY1 is three times as much)	(There commercial transportation costs are only incurred if purchases are made from local suppliers).		
Normal PG consumption (CU's)	34	28	21
Additional CU's of PG for each time unit in recreation	.1	.05	.025
Normal PS consumption (CU's)	16	11	7
Additional CU's of PS for each time unit in recreation	.075	.05	.0
Schooling of children			
Criteria for attending public school			
Minimum school value ratio	80	60	None
Maximum ratio of students/teacher	18	22	None
Minimum ratio of PH teachers to PM	1.0	.75	None
Cost of private education (per full P1)	$39,000	$24,500	$12,500
Cost per student	$300	$175	$125
Schooling of adults			
Cost per time unit allocated to private adult education	$3000	$3000	N/A
Health expenditures (per P1)			
Base amount	$8000	$4000	$2000
Coliform PARTS/MG greater than 100	$400/part	$200/part	$100/part
Coliform PARTS/MG less than 100	$160/part	$80/part	$40/part
Taxes			
Sales Tax			
State	(3% of the dollar amount of PG and PS purchases)		
Local	(Depends upon the rates set by the local jurisdiction of PG and PS separately)		
Income Tax			
Federal (on salaries)	8%	4%	1%
Local	(Set by the local jurisdictions)		
Automobile taxes	(Depends upon rates levied—jurisdiction of residence and/or work)		
Miscellaneous expenses	(Cash transfers to other accounts in the social, economic, or government sectors)		
Time allocation (total time units)	100	100	100
Auto transportation (uncongested)			
Per link HY3	2.5	2.5	2.5
Per link HY2	5.0	5.0	5.0
Per link HY1	7.5	7.5	7.5

TABLE 7.20 (Continued)

		PH	PM	PL
Bus transportation				
Waiting		1	1	1
Along HY3		5.0	5.0	5.0
Along HY2		7.5	7.5	7.5
Along HY1		10.0	10.0	10.0
Rapid rail trasportation		2.5	2.5	2.5
Waiting		1	1	1
Walking		2.5	2.5	2.5
Illness		(Health index for the parcel on which the P1's residence is located divided by 10)		
Extra job		(80 units of part-time work is equivalent to a full-time job)		
Education				
Time units required to maintain the highest level		32	24	30
Time units required to maintain the education level specified in the parenthesis		16(80)	12(50)	12(10)
		24(90)	18(60)	18(20)
		32(99)	24(69)	24(30)
Typical decline in educational level if no time is allocated for adult schooling		2	2	2
Allocation typically needed for stay at present level		16	12	18
Politics—units of time required to increase voter registration:		(Increases in voter registrations last for only one round)		
7%		10	10	10
10%		50	50	50
15%		60	60	60
Water consumption (MG)				
Daily if living in:	RA	.08	.07	.03
	RB	.07	.05	.03
	RC	.06	.03	.02
Annually if living in:	RA	29	25	11
	RB	25	18	11
	RC	22	11	7

Congested roads at peak-hours (all to work trips) cause an increase in the dollar and time costs of automobile usage. For example, a road that is 25% congested (utilized 125%) will cost 25% more in both money and time for those workers who use it.

TABLE 7.21
QUALITY OF LIFE FACTORS FOR POPULATION UNITS

	PH	PM	PL
Health Index			
Maximum value	100	100	100
Poor MS	(MS use index – 100) ÷ 4; maximum = 25		
Residence crowding	(% occupancy – 100) ÷ .8; maximum = 25		
Coliform index	PARTS/MG ÷ 4; maximum = 50		
Time Index			
Transportation time consumed			
Auto – waiting	0	0	0
HY3	2.5	2.5	2.5
HY2	5.0	5.0	5.0
HY1	7.5	7.5	7.5
Bus – waiting	1	1	1
HY3	5.0	5.0	5.0
HY2	7.5	7.5	7.5
HY1	10.0	10.0	10.0
Rail – waiting, any level, walking (per segment)	1	1	1
Recreation	(Maximum = 0, minimum = –100)		
Involuntary	(Desired time in extra job and public adult education minus actual time in extra job and public adult education); maximum = 100.		
Pollution Index	Value printed for that parcel of land on which the residence is located; maximum = +166; minimum = –16.		
Neighborhood Index			
QI of housing	100-QI	90-QI	70-QI
Rent	(Rent–$330,000)2(Rent–$200,000) 3(Rent–$140,000)		
MS use index	MS use index – 100; maximum = 100		
School use index	School use index – 100; maximum = 100		
Tax rates in local jurisdiction			None
Each mil on resident income	.25	.25	
Each mil on goods	.25	.25	None
Each mil on services	.25	.25	None
Each mil on land	.125	.125	None
Each mil developments	.125	.125	
Welfare payment			
For each $100 below $2000	None	None	4

Health Index + Time Index = Personal Index

Pollution Index = Neighborhood Index = Environment Index

Personal Index = Environment Index = Quality of LIfe Index

INDEX	LEVEL OF AGGREGATION	WHERE CALCULATED (MAJOR COMPONENTS IN PARENTHESES)	INTERPRETATION OF INDEX
JOB **1**	Full-time typed Population Unit; differs for each employer location by class hired	Employment (salary; rate of return; transportation; value ratio)	Indicates satisfaction derived from full-time job
HOUSING **2**	Population Unit; differs for each residence location	Migration; Residence Placement (value ratio, cost, socio-economic mix, parcel accessibility)	Indicates physical characteristics of residences. Does not include level of public services on parcel
SCHOOL **3**	District (one or more parcels)	Government function (quality and quantity vs. demand)	Measure of adequacy of service to Pl's with children
PUBLIC SERVICES **4**	Jurisdiction (one or more parcels)	Government function (quality and quantity vs. demand)	Measure of adequacy of municipal services
HEALTH **5**	Pl for demand, jurisdiction for supply (see next box)	Function pairing public supply (quality and quantity of services) with Pl demand (type and VR of employer; pollution index on residence parcel; feed from natural disaster simulator; other standards; total medical expenditures)	Reasons for level of medical expenditures
POLLUTION **6**	Parcel	Function (emission simulator; climate; topography)	Composite indicator of pollution emission and controls
COST OF LIVING **7**	System	Function (prices; rents; business cycle; average standard of living)	Permits comparison over time of relative cost to maintain normal standard of living. Inflation indicator
STANDARD OF LIVING **8**	Pl	Function (goods and services; units purchased; health; school; housing; indices; savings)	Quality of life indicator
RECREATION/ AMENITIES **9**	Parcel	Function (Park Index [from government]; public investments; tourism/amusements capacity)	Availability of leisure time entertainment; indicates strength of tourism industry

INTERPRETATION OF WEIGHTS	SECONDARY FACTOR A FUNCTION OF:	WHERE WEIGHTS FEED	WHERE INDEX FEEDS
Indicates emphasis which job satisfaction has to Pl; high means Pl's want best possible. High weight here and high S-O-L (#8) weight puts Pl in part-time job market.	Pl class; Pl job type; farm/non-farm	Full and part-time employment; union membership. Strike vote. OJT enrollment.	Employment, strike success. Dissatisfaction.
Relative degree of importance of abode as quality of life indicator.	Pl class; home or rent flag; Farm/non-farm	Dissatisfaction; candidate for migration; success of housing programs	Criterion for residence placement;-standard of living
Degree of concern; high weight causes greater demand to school authorities	Pl class; Pl demographic type	Vote turnout; migration; dissatisfaction; government function	Vote direction; dissatisfaction; migration; standard of living
Degree of concern and involvement in local government	Pl class	Interest group activity; vote turnout; dissatisfaction; government function	Vote direction; dissatisfaction; migration; standard of living
Degree of concern; high means more expense but better standard of living results	Pl class; Pl demographic type	Dissatisfaction; government response; personal consumption	Personal consumption; dissatisfaction; vote direction; standard of living
Degree of concern. Higher indicates civic action to oppose it. High standard of living weight will override this weight	None	Dissatisfaction; government response; voter turnout; (higher weight means more people)	Dissatisfaction
Propensity to consume (savings preference); high also indicates desire for part-time job	Pl class	Vote direction; personal consumption; dissatisfaction; employment	Health index; migration; dissatisfaction
Degree of emphasis on material well-being	Pl class; Pl demographic type	Cost of living; pollution weights; voter turnout; interest group activity; dissatisfaction	Dissatisfaction; vote direction cost of living function
Degree of importance	Pl class; Pl demographic type	Dissatisfaction; government response; personal consumption; interest; group activity; pollution weight	In-migration; dissatisfaction

Figure 7.29: SOCIAL INDICATORS

(3) *Interpretation of Index.* Indicates meaning of the index to the social decision maker.

(4) *Interpretation of Weights.* Indicates the implication and machine interpretation of the weights. All references are made in relative terms, both in regard to the individual weight and to all the weights viewed together.

(5) *Secondary Factor a Function of:* The secondary factor is that adjustment required by the variability in composition of P1's (class, etc.). This column lists the main independent variables accounting for the sector. The variables are all fixed characteristics of P1's.

(6) *Where Weights Feed.* The weights are parameter inputs to a number of system relationships. This column lists the relationships where there is a significant effect.

(7) *Where Index Feeds.* The index either independent of or in combination with the corresponding weight, also provides data for several operating programs and their component functions. The areas which are fed are listed.

As an illustration, look at the sixth index, Pollution. Reading across, one can determine the following information:

(1) The index is calculated for each parcel from column 1.

(2) The effects of pollution are the same for all P1's living on the same parcel (column 1), regardless of any other P1 characteristics (column 5).

(3) The index is calculated as a unique operating program (column 2).

(4) Its value is a function of total emissions, climate and topography (column 2).

(5) The effectiveness of controls and regulations are also represented (column 3).

(6) The weight stands for degree of concern of the local population (column 4).

(7) The standard of living weight can counteract the pollution weight (column 4).

(8) The weight feeds into dissatisfaction accounting, government response (the success of regulatory action), and voter turnout (column 6).

(9) The index feeds into the Health Index.

(10) The index contributed to P1 dissatisfaction and as such is a factor in migration (column 7).

General Summary

The chapter has described, in general, GEM-CITY. For those who are programmers, the experience has been frustrating as the algorithms are not sufficiently detailed for direct computer application. However, the purpose of the chapter has been to describe a model building theory not to document a specific model. Reference manuals available with CITY, as well as the code itself, will provide the necessary information for those so inclined.

In addition to all of the other possible disagreements with the former presentation, there is the almost glaring addition of the resource structures of each of the sectors. There is little argument in the use of money as a resource. Although newly rediscovered, time is still a discrete parameter, but what of power? Further, what is the transfer function which relates them to each other? It was not seen as the principal function of the design of GEM to solve these problems but to build a model as if they were already solved. We have found that others have begun to relate time and money to each other, but have also found little agreement on the real value of money. Further, there are certainly numerous well-founded disagreements with the data bases and other parameter values chosen, as they were merely illustrative and can be changed easily. These very knotty problems will still have to be solved by continuing to build models so that the value of the resources in real terms is determined by the users of the model. It has also been suggested in this book that general, holistic models of the environment will have to be man-machine simulations, at least in the foreseeable future.

NOTES

1. References to the "model" unspecified, unless otherwise noted, refer to GEM.

2. In fact, the contracts from the federal government and the business community explicitly required that the model be transportable to other locales and be versatile enough for a wide variety of people. This resulted in much of our research being influenced to satisfy that goal.

3. The CITY version of GEM is, as noted in the preface, a work of a number of people. This group was organized into a non-profit company called Envirometrics of which I was the president.

4. The last contribution of modeling to a research effort suggests some very important elements of good model-building research strategy. The first of these elements involves assembling a preliminary version of a model as rapidly as is reasonable during the early parts of a research program. Then, observations of how model output responds to systematic changes in the values of parameters, and in the form of the relationships themselves, will provide valuable guidance as to where further research effort is needed. This approach indicates that the research should be what might be termed 'balanced and iterative' in nature. 'Balance' will be obtained by allocating research effort to the segments of an overall program in relation to their importance.

"The research program will proceed in an 'iterative' fashion because the first model will suggest further research resulting in a modified model, which may, in turn, indicate the need for additional effort along new paths. This iterative process will continue, within the practicalities of research resource limitations, until a model that is judged satisfactory for its intended uses is developed." [Hamilton et al., 1969].

5. It is not necessary to detail the structure actually adapted except to say that it was an extensive of matrix forms whereby each sector was specified in such a fashion that only non-zero values were stored. The file handling procedure was designed so that instead of having to reference each specific parameter, the executive routines only had to call sectors, which had been designed in a known and standard fashion.

6. Recent innovations in computer hardware and software (not to mention in mathematics itself) has led to the concept of "real time" modeling. However, actual implementation of this concept still rests far into the future because of the amount of data needed and the absolutely perfect knowledge of the system which will be required for true real-time modeling.

7. The concept of model and the use of a model to interrelate a specific data base has been so confused that some models have only been identified with one use rather than with their intrinsic forms. CITY is a model; the use of CITY to represent Washington, D.C. (one of the Data Bases available) is a path through the model and represents only one of many.

8. The complete documentation of these programs is now available from numerous sources, including the Environmental Protection Agency.

9. There are numerous other universal models of this form, suggesting that many of our model builders, after numerous studies into specific designs, recognized one or more general theories that could be harnessed to save time and reduce the seeming "magic" of the professional systems analyst. It should be noted, however, that not all professionals believe that any form of general model can be developed—and suggest instead that each problem is unique and requires individual and unique solution. This latter opinion has been recently expressed by Shubik of the Rand Corporation in research which reviewed the state-of-the-art of simulations.

10. As Catanese and Steiss (1969) define a system, "A system may be defined as any entity, physical or conceptual, which is composed of interrelated parts, united by some form of regular interaction of interdependence."

11. The need for describing a total system is obvious to a mathematician or theoretician but has often been neglected by social scientists as they are forced to study various action-oriented problems. The search for a study population whereby all of the actions and reactions of the study group are accounted for is referred to as closure. The reminder that such a concept is noted as drastically portrayed in Boulding and Fuller's concept of "Spaceship Earth." The interest in environmental pollution problems has reminded us that earth itself is a closed system, hence a spaceship.

12. The quantity of people or people-time is, of course, not a constant homogeneous asset. Differing amounts of education or skill make one group of people more efficient or valuable in a particular job than another.

13. The maintenance level is the means by which the landlord controls the quality index (QI) of each residence. The quality index describes the physical condition of the residence. For each income class there is a specific range of housing QI which delimits for each class acceptable residences.

14. This is presently available. For example, the scale could be changed to one-ninth of a square mile with say, as few as 50 people in P1 units.

15. The concept of periods is misleading. No research has been done on balancing the time component in the model. Therefore, although the decisions were made over four rounds, in reality the feedbacks and outcome of specific portions might be significantly in error.

The research technique used, on the other hand, mitigates the comparative effects of this weakness. The model is run for four iterations. Then it is run again with the change of one parameter. This technique places question on the results obtained in the first run but not the second.

16. Lindblom has immortalized this practice in his concept of real world decision-making which he has labeled as "muddling through."

17. Of course, if model results are to be used, it is often necessary for the model-builder to impart his faith in the model to others who must take action.

18. This construct is meant to represent the rate of return from investments made outside the local system.

19. See note 18.

20. In a sense, the city's economic activity provides a rationale for its existence and its dynamic growth and future development. In the GEM model, therefore, the Economic Sector is not only concerned with maximizing its own profit, but is also a sector whose decisions, biases and judgments will greatly influence and change the simulated area.

21. The later model added 11 specific heavy or light industry uses, including FL–Furniture and Lumber, SG–Stone, Clay, and Glass, MP–Primary Metals, MF–Fabricated Metals, NL–Nonelectrical Machinery, EL–Electrical Machinery, TE–Transportation Equipment, FO–Food, TL–Textiles, Apparel, and Leather, PA–Paper, CR–Chemical, Plastics and Rubber.

22. The development level for a particular land use represents the size and the number of buildings which make up a certain industrial, commercial or residential development. Development levels range from 1 to 3 for all land uses except residences which have 8 potential development levels. Development level is included as the characteristic of economic land uses because the number representing a development level is a multiplier by which to determine other numbers throughout the model. For example, suppose that an HI1 occupies 28 percent of a square mile parcel. To determine how much land an HI3 occupies, multiply 28 percent times 3. The same holds true for other numbers, such as those representing employees required, typical construction costs, purchases of goods and services, design capacity, etc.

23. Municipal Services (MS) is a governmental department in the model. Its main function is to provide services such as police and fire protection to the community. The quality of services which the MS Department provides influences the rate at which the value ratio of a development declines over time.

24. They will therefore not be reported again in detail here.

25. Provision is also made for a government decision entity to perform an Economic Sector role, such as engaging in some form of business. It would be possible for such an entity to act as an independent department and be either a non-profit or profit activity. Further, any portion of the net income of any entity in the model to be transferred to any other entity in the model is provided for. Thus, a maximum degree of flexibility exists in terms of allowing management and control over a given decision entity. For example, a portion of the income from a housing project owned by a government department could be entered in the revenues for that department. The geographic area of authority for any given department may range in size from one parcel up to an entire area.

26. If 1500 units is the least cost capacity of a UT1, this means that if the per unit operating cost is above $6,667, the plant is not operating at its optimum production level. Maximum profit also occurs at 1500 units served.)

REFERENCES

ABT Associates, INC. (1968) The Northeast Corridor Transportation Game I, Planning Simulation and Administrator's Manual (prepared for the Department of Commerce, National Bureau of Standards).

--- (n.d.) Survey of the State of the Art: Social, Political, and Economic Models and Simulations. Cambridge.

ACKOFF, R. L. (1968) "Toward a behavioral theory of communication," in W. Buckley (ed.) Modern Systems Research for the Behavioral Scientist. Chicago: Aldine.

ADRIAN, C. R. (1969) "The quality of urban leadership," pp. 375-393 in Schmandt and Bloomberg, The Quality of Urban Life. Beverly Hills, Calif.: Sage Publications.

ALONSO, W. (1968) "Predicting best with imperfect data." J. of the American Institute of Planners 34 (July): 248-255.

ANDREWS, R. B. (1954) "Mechanics of the urban economic base: historical development of the bast concept." Land Economics 30 (May): 164-172.

ARNOLD, C. C. (1969) Toward Building a General Urban Systems Theory: Persona. Washington, D.C.: Envirometrics, Inc.

ASHBY, W. R. (1968) "Regulation and control," in W. Buckley (ed.) Modern Systems Research for the Behavioral Scientist. Chicago: Aldine.

ASIMOV, I. (1951) Foundation. New York: Doubleday.

BARCLAY, G. W. (1958) Techniques of Population Analysis. New York: John Wiley.

BARNES, C. P. and F. J. MARSCHNER (1958) "Our wealth of land resources," in U.S. Department of Agriculture's (ed.) Land; The Yearbook of Agriculture, 1958. Washington, D.C.: Government Printing Office.

Battelle Memorial Institute. (n.d.) A Dynamic Model of the Economy of the Susquehanna River Basin.

BAUER, R. A. [ed.] (1966) Social Indicators. Cambridge: MIT Press.

BEAUJEU-GARNIER, J. and G. CHABOT (1967) Urban Geography. New York: John Wiley.

BEAVER, J. (1968) Population Density. Cornell: MRP thesis.

BECKMAN, M. J. (n.d.) City Hierarchies and the Distribution of City Size. Bobbs-Merrill (reprint).

BERRIEN, F. K. (1968) General and Social Systems. New Brunswick, N.J.: Rutgers University Press.

BERRY, B.J.L. (1964) "Cities as systems within systems of cities," pp. 116-137 in J. Friedman and W. Alonzo (eds.) Regional Development and Planning. Cambridge: MIT Press.

——— (n.d.) City-Size Distribution and Economic Development. Bobbs-Merrill Reprint Series, S-340.

BLALOCK, H. and A. A. BLALOCK (1959) "Towards a clarification of system analysis in the social sciences." Philosophy of Science 26.

BLAU, P. M. and W. R. SCOTT (1963) Formal Organizations. New Castle, N.H.: Chandler.

BLUMBERG, D. F. (n.d.) The City as a System. Decision Sciences Corp.

BLUMENFELD, H. (1949) "On the concentric circle theory of urban growth." Land Economics 25 (May): 209-212.

BOGUE, D. J. (1950) The Structure of the Metropolitan Community. Ann Arbor: University of Michigan (chs. 1 and 3).

BOLLENS, J. C. and H. J. SCHMANDT (1965) "Nature and dimensions of the metropolitan community," pp. 32-57 in the Metropolis; Its People, Politics, and Economic Life. New York: Harper & Row.

BOSKOFF, A. (1962) The Sociology of Urban Regions (chs. 15-16, pp. 297-325). New York: Appelton-Century Crofts.

BOULDING, K. E. (1968) "General systems theory—the skeleton of science," pp. 3-10 in W. Buckley (ed.) Modern Research for the Behavioral Scientist. Chicago: Aldine.

——— (1962) A Reconstruction of Economics. Science Editors, Inc., John Wiley.

——— (1965a) The Image. Ann Arbor, Michigan: University of Michigan Press.

——— (1965b) "Toward a general theory of growth," pp. 109-124 in J. Spengler and O. Duncan (eds.) Population Theory and Policy: Selected Readings. New York: Free Press.

——— (1955) The Malthusian model as a general system." Social and Economic Studies 4 (September).

BRILLOUIN, L. (1968) "Thermodynamics and information theory," in W. Buckley (ed.) Modern Systems Research for the Behavioral Scientist. Chicago: Aldine.

BROWN, H. (1954) The Challenge of Man's Future. New York: Viking Press.

BUCK, G. and A. JACOBS (1968) "Social evolution and structural-functional analysis." American Sociology Rev. 33 (June): 343-355.

BUCKLEY, W. [ed.] (1968) Modern Systems Research for the Behavioral Scientists. Chicago: Aldine.

——— (1967) Sociology and Modern Systems Theory. Englewood Cliffs, N.J.: Prentice-Hall.

BURD, G. (1969) "The mass media in urban society," pp. 293-321 in Schmandt and Bloomberg, The Quality of Urban Life. Beverly Hills, Calif.: Sage Publications.

BURGESS, E. W. (n.d.) "The determination of gradients in the growth of the city," pp. 178-184 in Publications of the American Sociological Society 21.

CAILLOIS, R. [M. Barash, trans.] (1961) Man, Play and Games. New York: Free Press.

CARROTHERS, G.A.P. (1956) "A historical review of the gravity and potential concepts of human interaction." J. of the American Institute of Planners 20: 94-102.

CATANESE, A. J. and A. W. STEISS (1969) "The search for a systems approach to the planning of complex urban systems." Plan (April): 13 pp.

Center for Real Estate and Urban Economics (1968) Jobs, People and Land–Bay Area Simulation Study (BAAS). Berkeley: University of California.

CHAPIN, F. S., Jr. (1968) "Activity systems and urban structure: a working schema." J. of the American Institute of Planners 34 (January): 11-18.

––– and S. F. WEISS (n.d.) Factors Influencing Land Development. North Carolina.

CLARK, C. (1945) "The economic functions of a city in relation to its size." Econometrics 13 (April): 97-113.

COHEN, K. J., W. R. DILL, A. A. KUEHN, and P. R. WINTERS (1964) The Carnegie Tech Management Game–An Experiment in Business Education. Homewood, Illinois: Richard D. Irwin.

COLEMAN, J. S. (n.d.) "Games as vehicles for social theory." American Behavioral Scientist.

COLLEY, C. H. (1930) "The theory of transportation." Sociological Theory and Social Research. New York: Henry Holt.

COTTRELL, W. F. (1939) "Of time and the railroader." Amer. Soc. Rev. (April): 190-198.

COWGILL, D. O. (1956) "The theory of population growth cycles," pp. 125-134 in J. J. Spengler and O. D. Duncan (eds.) Population Theory and Policy. New York: Free Press.

CRECINE, J. P. (n.d.) "Computer simulation in urban research." Public Administration Rev.: 66-69.

CRESSEY, P. F. (n.d.) Population Succession in Chicago: 1898-1930. Bobbs-Merril Reprint.

CUTRIGHT, P. (1963) "National political development: measurement and analysis." Amer. Soc. Rev. 28: 253-264.

DAVIE, M. R. (1961) "The pattern of urban growth," pp. 77-92 in G. A. Theodorson's (ed.) Studies in Human Ecology. New York: Harper & Row.

DEUTSCH, K. (1961) "On social communication and the metropolis," in L. Rodwin (ed.) The Future Metropolis. New York: George Braziller.

DEWEY, R. (1956) "The neighborhood, urban ecology, and city planners," pp. 783-790 in P. K. Hatt and A. J. Reiss (eds.) Cities and Society. New York: Free Press.

DICKINSON, R. E. (1961) "The metropolitan regions of the United States," pp. 538-547 in G. A. Theodorson (ed.) Studies in Human Ecology. Evanston, Illinois: Row, Peterson.

DONNELLY, T. (n.d.) A Probabilistic Model for Residential Growth. North Carolina.

DUNCAN, OTIS D. (1961) "From social systems to ecosystems." Sociological Inquiry 31 (Spring): 140-149.

--- (1960) Metropolis and Region. Baltimore: Johns Hopkins Press for Resources for the Future. (ch. 3).

--- (1957) "Optimum size of cities," pp. 759-772 in P. K. Hatt and A. J. Reiss (eds.) Cities and Societies. New York: Free Press.

--- and L. SCHNORE (1959) "Cultural, behavioral and ecological perspectives in the study of social organization." American J. of Sociology 65: 132-153.

DUNCAN, O. D. and B. DUNCAN (1957) "Residential distribution and occupational stratification," pp. 283-296 in P. K. Hatt and A. J. Reiss (eds.) Cities and Societies. New York: Free Press.

DUKE, R. (1968) Apex: A Gaming Simulation for Air Pollution Experience in a Simulated Metropolitan Environment.

DYCKMAN, J. (1971) "New normative styles in urban studies." Public Administration Rev. 3 (May/June): 327-334.

--- (1966) "Transportation in cities." Cities: A Scientific American Book. New York: A. A. Knopf.

--- (1965) "Transportation in cities." Scientific American CCXIII (September): 162-177.

EASTON, D. (1965) A Systems Analysis of Political Life. New York: John Wiley.

EMSHOFF, J. R. and R. L. SISSON (1970) Design and Use of Computer Simulation Models. Macmillan.

ENZER, S., T. J. GORDON, R. ROCHBERG and R. BUCHELE (1969) A Simulation Game for the Study of State Policies. Middletown, Conn.: The Institute for the Future.

Federal Reserve Bank of Kansas City (1952) "The employment multiplier in Wichita." Monthly Rev. 37 (September).

FEIBLEMANN, J. and J. W. FRIEND (1945) "The structure and function of organization." Philosophical Rev. 54 (January): 19-44.

FELDT, A. G. (1966) "Operational gaming in planning education." J. of the American Institute of Planners (January).

--- (n.d.) Some Thoughts and Speculations on the Development and Use of Games in Teaching and Research.

--- and R. WELLER (1965) "The balance of economic, demographic and social change in Puerto Rico: 1950-1960." Demography 2 (September): 474-489.

FIREY, W. (1961) "Sentiment and symbolism as ecological variables," in G. A. Theodorson (ed.) Studies in Human Ecology. Evanston, Ill.: Row, Peterson.

FITCH, L. C. (1964) Urban Transportation and Public Policy. San Francisco: Chandler.

FLEISHER, A. (1961) "The influence of technology on urban forms," pp. 64-79 in L. Rodwin (ed.) The Future Metropolis. New York: George Braziller.

FOLEY, D. (1957) "The use of local facilities in a metropolis," pp. 607-616 in P. K. Hatt and A. J. Reiss (eds.) Cities and Societies. New York: Free Press.

FORM, W. (1961) "The compatibility of alternative approaches to the delimitation of urban sub-areas," pp. 176-187 in J. P. Gibbs, Urban Research Methods. New York: Van Nostrand Reinhold.

——— (1954) "The place of social structure in the determination of land use." Social Forces 32 (May): 317-323.

FORRESTER, J. W. (1971) "Counterintuitive behavior of social science." Technology Rev. (January): 53-60.

——— (1968a) "Notes on complex systems." Urban Dynamics. Cambridge: MIT Press.

——— (1968b) Urban Dynamics. Cambridge: MIT Press.

FRASER, D. and J. MILTON (1966) Future Environments of North America. National History Press.

FRASER, H. W. (n.d.) Simulation and Game Approach to the Teaching of Economic Principles, A Preliminary Report. Washington University.

FREEMAN, L. and R. WINCH (1957) "Social complexity: an empirical test of a typology of societies." American J. of Sociology 62: 461-466.

FRIEDMAN, J. and W. ALONZO [eds.] (1964) Regional Development and Planning: A Reader. Cambridge: MIT Press.

GAMSON, W. A. (1969) SIMSOC–Simulated Society. New York: Free Press.

GAKENHEIMER, R. A. (1967) "Urban transportation planning: an overview" pp. 392-411 in H. W. Eldredge (ed.) Taming Megalopolis I: What Is and What Could Be. Garden City, N.Y.: Doubleday.

GEORGE, T. A. (1955) "What is a population?" Philosophy of Science 22: 272-279.

GIBBS, J. P. (1961) "Some Measures of Spatial Distribution . . . " in J. P. Gibbs Urban Research Methods. New York: Van Nostrand Reinhold.

GIBBS, J. P. and W. T. MARTIN (1959) "Toward a theoretical system of human ecology." Pacific Sociology Rev. 2: 29-36.

——— (1958) "Urbanization and natural resources: a study in organizational ecology," Amer. Soc. Rev. 23 (June): 266-277.

GILMAN, R. H. (1967) "Terminal planning," pp. 383-392 in H. W. Eldredge (ed.) Taming Megalopolis I: What Is and What Could Be. Garden City, N.Y.: Doubleday.

GIST, N. P. and L. A. HALBERT (1963) Urban Society (Fourth Edition): 3-15.

GOLDNER, W. (1971) "The lowry model heritage." J. of the American Institute of Planners 37 (March): 100-110.

GREER, S. (n.d.) "Urbanization and social character," pp. 95-126 in Schmandt and Bloomberg, The Quality of Urban Life.

GROSS, B. M. (1966) "The state of the nation's social systems accounting," in R. A. Bauer (ed.) Social Indicators. Cambridge: MIT Press.

——— (n.d.) The City of Man: A Social Systems Reckoning.

GEUTZKOW, H. [ed.] (1962) Simulation in Social Science: Readings. Englewood Cliffs, N.J.: Prentice-Hall.

HADDEN, J. and E. F. BORGATTA (1965) American Cities: Their Social Characteristics. Chicago: Rand McNally.

HAGGETT, P. (1965) Locational Analysis in Human Geography. London: Edward Arnold.

HALL, A. D. and R. E. FAGAN (1968) "Definition of system," pp. 81-92 in W. Buckley (ed.) Modern Systems Research for the Behavioral Scientist. Chicago: Aldine.

HALLIDAY, D. and R. RESNICK (1962) "Entropy and the second law of thermodynamics." Physics for Students of Science and Engineering. New York: John Wiley.

HAMILTON, H. R., S. E. GOLDSTONE, J. W. MILLIMAN, A. L. PUGH III, E. B. ROBERTS, and A. ZELLNER (1969) Systems Simulation for Regional Analysis: An Application to River-Basin Planning. Cambridge: MIT Press.

HAMILTON, W. F. II and D. K. NANCE (1969) "Systems analysis of urban transportation." Scientific American 221 (July).

HANDLIN, O. (1951) The Uprooted. Grosset & Dunlap.

HANSEN, W. L. and C. M. TIEBOUT (1963) "An intersectoral flows analysis of the California economy." Rev. of Economics and Statistics 45 (November).

HARDIN, G. (n.d.) The Cybernetics of Competition: A Biologist's View of Society.

HARRIS, C. C. and E. L. ULLMAN (1957) "The nature of cities," pp. 237-247 in P. K. Hatt and A. J. Reiss (eds.) Cities and Society. New York: Free Press.

HARRIS, B. (1966) "The uses of theory in the simulation of urban phenomena." J. of the American Institute of Planners (September).

HATT, P. K. and A. J. REISS [eds.] (1957) Cities and Society. New York: Free Press.

HAUSER, P. M. (1965) "Urbanization: an overview," pp. 1-5 in P. Hauser and L. F. Schnore (eds.) The Study of Urbanization. New York: John Wiley.

--- and L. F. SCHNORE [eds.] (1965) The Study of Urbanization. New York: John Wiley.

HAWLEY, A. (1950) Human Ecology. New York: Ronald Press.

HEMMENS, G. C. (1966) The Structure of Urban Activity Linkages. Chapel Hill, N.C.: Institute for Research in Social Science, University of North Carolina.

Highway Research Board (1967) Special Report 97: Urban Development Models. Washington, D.C.: National Academy of Sciences.

HILL, A. V. (1955) "The effects of scientific progress on metropolitan communities," pp. 253-274 in R. M. Fisher (ed.) The Metropolis in Modern Life. New York: Russell & Russell.

HIRSCH, W. Z. (1963) Urban Life and Form. Holt.

HOOVER, E., Jr. (1948) "Land use competition," pp. 90-102 in Hoover, Location of Economic Activity. New York: McGraw-Hill.

HOUSE, P. and P. PATTERSON (1972) An Environmental Laboratory for the Social Sciences, Washington, D.C.: Environmental Protection Agency.

--- (1969 "An environmental gaming simulation laboratory." J. of the American Institute of Planners. (November)

HUGHES, J. and L. MANN (1969) "Systems and planning theory." J. of the American Institute of Planners 35 (September): 330-333.

ISARD, W. (1956) Location and Space–Economy. Cambridge: MIT Press.

——— and R. KAVISH (1954) "Economic structural interrelationships of metropolitan regions." American J. of Sociology 9 (September): 152-162.

ISARD, W., T. E. SMITH, P. ISARD, T. HSIUNG TUNG, and M. DACEY (1969) General Theory: Social, Political, Economic, and Regional with Particular Reference to Decision-Making Analysis. Cambridge: MIT Press.

KAIN, J. F. and J. R. MEYER (1968) "Computer simulations, physio-economic systems, and intra-regional models." American Economic Rev. (May).

——— (1961) A First Approximation to a RAND Model for Study of Urban Transportation. Rand Corporation Memorandum RM-2978-FF.

KALTER, R. J. (1968) An Interindustry Analysis of the Central New York Region. Ithaca: Department of Agricultural Economics, Cornell University.

KELLER, S. (1968) The Urban Neighborhood. New York: Random House.

KEYFITZ, N. (1965) "Political-economic aspects of urbanization in south and southeast Asia," pp. 270-274 in P. Hauser and L. F. Schnore (eds.) The Study of Urbanization. New York: John Wiley.

KILBRIDGE, M. D., R. O'BLOCK, and P. TEPLITZ (1968) A Conceptual Framework for Urban Planning Models. Boston: Graduate School of Business Administration, Harvard University (January).

KINDLEBERGER, C. P. (1968) International Economics. (chs. 5, 6, 7) Homewood, Ill.: Richard D. Irwin.

KLAUSNER, S. Z. [ed.] (1967) The Study of Total Societies. Garden City, N.J.: Doubleday.

KROEBER, A. L. (1917) "The superorganic." American Anthropology 19. Bobbs-Merrill Reprint.

KUNKEL, J. (1967) "Some behavioral aspects of ecological approach to social organization." American J. of Sociology 73: 12-29.

LANSING, J. B. (1966) pp. 167-400 in Transportation and Economic Policy. New York: Macmillan.

LAWSON, B. (1969) New Town–An Urban Land Use and Development Game, Instruction Booklet.

LITTLE, A. D., Inc. (n.d.) San Francisco Community Renewal Program.

LONG, N. (1958) "The local community as an ecology of games." American J. of Sociology 64 (November): 251-261.

LOWRY, I. S. (1967) Seven Models of Urban Development: A Structural Comparison. Santa Monica, Calif.: Rand Corporation.

——— (1965) "A short course in model design." J. of the American Institute of Planners 31 (May): 158-166.

LYNCH, K. (1965) "The city as environment." Scientific American CCXIII (September): 209-219.

——— (1961) "The pattern of the metropolis," pp. 103-128 in L. Rodwin's (ed.) The Future Metropolis. New York: George Braziller.

——— (1960) Image of the City. Cambridge: MIT Press.

MADDEN, C. H. (1956) "Some spatial aspects of urban growth in the United States." Economic Trends and Cultural Change 4 (July): 371-387.

MARTIN W. T. (1962) "Urbanization and natural power to requisition resources." Pol. Sci. Rev. 5: 93-97.

——— and J. P. GIBBS (1962) "Urbanization, technology and the division of labor: international patterns." Amer. Soc. Rev. 27 (October): 667-677.

MARTINDALE, D. (1966) Institutions, Organizations and Mass Society. Boston: Houghton Mifflin.

MARUYAMA, M. (1963) "The second cybernetics: deviation-amplifying mutual causal processes." American Scientist 51: 164-179.

MATTILA, J. M. and W. R. THOMPSON (1961) "The measurement of the economic base of the metropolitan area," pp. 329-348 in J. P. Gibbs, Urban Research Methods. New York: Van Nostrand Reinhold.

McKELVEY, B. (1963) The Urbanization of America (1860-1915). New Brunswick: Rutgers University Press.

McKENSIE, R. D. (1927) "Spatial distance and community organization." American J. of Sociology 33: 28-42.

McLOUGHLIN, B. J. (n.d.) Pp. 157-162 in Urban and Regional Planning: A Systems Approach. New York: Frederick A. Praeger.

McLUHAN, M. (1964) Understanding Media: The Extension of Man. New York: McGraw-Hill.

MEADOWS, P. (1957) "The city, technology and history." Social Forces (December): 141-147.

MEGGERS, B. T. "Environmental limitations on the development of culture." American Anthropologist 56: 801-824.

MEIER, R. L. (1963) "Living with the coming urban technology," pp. 59-70 in E. Geen, J. R. Lowe, and K. Walker (eds.) Man and the Modern City. Pittsburgh: University of Pittsburg Press.

——— (1962) A Communication Theory of Urban Growth. Cambridge: MIT Press.

——— (1961) "The evolving metropolis and new technology," ch. 2 in Harvey Perloff (ed.) Planning and the Urban Community. Pittsburgh, Pa.: University of Pittsburgh Press.

——— (1959a) "Explorations in the realm of organization theory III: decision making, planning, and the steady state." Behavioral Science (July): 235-244.

——— (1959b) "Human time allocation." J. of the American Institute of Planners 25: 27-33.

——— and R. D. DUKE (1966) "Gaming simulation for urban planning." J. of the American Institute of Planners.

MEYER, J. (n.d.) "Regional economics: a survey." American Economics Review.

MILLER, G. A. (1968) "What is information measurement?" in W. Buckley (ed.) Modern Systems Research for the Behavioral Scientist. Chicago: Aldine.

MILLER, J. G. (1965) "Living systems: structure and process; and cross-level hypotheses." Behavioral Science 10 (October): 337-379, 380-411.

——— (1955) "Toward a general theory for the behavioral sciences." American Psychologist (September).

MILLS, R. W. (1969) Review of Systems Analysis and Policy Planning: Applications in Defense by E. S. Quade and W. I. Boucher. J. of the American Institute of Planners 35 (September): 352-353.

MITCHELL, R. B. and C. RAPKIN (1954) Urban Traffic: A Function of Land Use. New York: Columbia University Press.

MOORE, W. E. (1957) "Utilization of human resources through industrialization," pp. 518-531 in J. J. Spengler and O. D. Duncan (eds.) Demographic Analysis. New York: Free Press.

MOWITZ, R. J. and D. S. WRIGHT (1962) Profile of a Metropolis. Detroit: Wayne State University Press.

MYERS, J. K. (1961) "Assimilation to the ecological and social systems of a community," in G. A. Theodorson (ed.) Studies in Human Ecology. Evanston, Ill.: Row, Peterson.

National Commission on Technology, Automation, and Economic Progress (1966) Applying Technology to Unmet Needs. Washington, D.C.: Government Printing Office.

National Resources Committee (1957) "The problems of urban America," pp. 743-758 in P. K. Hatt and A. J. Reiss (eds.) Cities and Society. New York: Free Press.

National Resources, School of (1968) Annual Report to the Ford Foundation, December, 1968, Computer Equipment for Urban Research and Training –The M.E.T.R.O. Project. Ann Arbor, Mich.: University of Michigan.

NELSON, R. R., M. J. PECK, and E. D. KALACHEK (1967) Technology, Economic Growth, and Public Policy. Washington, D.C.: Brookings Institution.

NIEBERG, H. I. (1969) "The tech-fix and the city," pp. 211-242 in Schmandt and Bloomberg, The Quality of Urban Life. Beverly Hills, Calif.: Sage Publications.

OGBURN, W. F. (1957) "Cultural lag as theory." Sociology and Social Research 41: 167-174.

——— (1956a) "Technology as environment." Sociology and Social Research 41: 3-9.

——— (1956b) "On the social aspects of population changes," pp. 435-440 in J. J. Spengler and O. D. Duncan (eds.) Population Theory and Policy. New York: Free Press.

——— (1956c) "Population, private ownership, technology, and the standard of living," pp. 152-158 in J. J. Spengler and O. D. Duncan (eds.) Population Theory and Policy. New York: Free Press.

ORCUTT, G. H., M. GREENBERGER, J. KORBEL, and A. M. RIVLIN (n.d.) Microanalysis of Socioeconomic Systems–A Simulation Study. New York: Harper & Brothers.

OWEN, W. (1959) Cities in the Motor Age. New York: Viking Press.

——— (1957) "Transportation." Annals of the American Academy of Political and Social Science 314 (November): 30-38.

PARK, R. (1961) "Human ecology," pp. 22-29 in G. A. Theodorson (ed.) Studies in Human Ecology. Evanston, Ill.: Row, Peterson.

PARSONS, T. (1960) Structure and Process in Modern Society. New York: Free Press.

——— (1959) "The principle structures of community," pp. 250-279 in T. Parsons (ed.) Structure and Process in Modern Society. New York: Free Press.

——— (1949) The Structure of Social Action II. New York: Free Press.

——— and N. SMELSER (1965) pp. 13-28 in Economy and Society. Free Press.

PARSONS, T. and E. A. SHILLS (1951) Toward a General Theory of Action. Cambridge: Harvard University Press.

PERLOFF, H. S. (n.d.) "Common goals and the linking of physical and social planning," pp. 346-359 in Frieden and Morris, Urban Planning and Social Policy.

——— and L. WINGO, Jr. [eds.] (1968) Issues in Urban Economics. Baltimore: Johns Hopkins Press.

——— (1964) "Natural resource endowment and regional economic growth," pp. 215-239 in J. Friedmann and W. Alonso (eds.) Regional Development and Planning. Cambridge: MIT Press.

PETERSEN, W. (1958) "A general typology of migration." Amer. Soc. Rev. 23 (June): 256-266.

QUINN, J. A. (n.d.) "The Burgess zonal hypothesis and its critics." Bobbs-Merrill Reprint Series, S-480.

RAMSOY, O. (1963) Social Groups as Systems and Subsystems. New York: Free Press.

RASER, J. R. (1969) Simulation and Society—An Exploration of Scientific Gaming. Boston: Allyn & Bacon.

RAPOPORT, A. and W. HORVATH (1968) "Thoughts on organization theory," pp. 71-75 in W. Buckley (ed.) Modern Systems Research for the Behavioral Scientist. Chicago: Aldine.

RAUSCH, E. (1968) The Community. Chicago: Science Research Associates.

RAYMOND, R. C. (1968) "Communication, entropy and life," in W. Buckley (ed.) Modern Systems Research for the Behavioral Scientist. Chicago: Aldine.

REISS, A. J., Jr. (1956) "Functional specialization of cities," pp. 555-575 in P. K. Hatt and A. J. Reiss (eds.) Cities and Society. New York: Free Press.

——— (n.d.) "The sociological study of communities." Bobbs-Merrill Reprint Series, S-233.

ROBINSON, W. A. (1961) "Ecological correlations and the behavior of individuals," pp. 115-120 in G. A. Theodorson (ed.) Studies in Human Ecology. Evanston, Ill.: Row, Peterson.

ROBSON, B. T. (1969) Urban Analysis: A Study of City Structure With Special Reference to Sunderland. Cambridge: The University Press.

ROSS, E. A. (1968) "The location of industries." Q. J. of Economics 10 (April): 247-268.

SAMPSON, R. J. and M. FARRIS (1966) Pts. 1, 2; ch. 14, pt. 4 in Domestic Transportation, Practice, Theory, and Policy. Boston: Houghton Mifflin.

SAUNDERS, H. W. (1956) "Human migration and social equilibrium," pp. 219-229 in J. J. Spengler and O. D. Duncan (eds.) Population Theory and Policy. New York: Free Press.

SCHLETTLER, C. (1943) "Relation of city-size to economic services." Amer. Soc. Rev. 8: 60-62.

SCHNEIDER, J. B. (1971) "Solving urban location problems: human intuition versus the computer." J. of the American Institute of Planners (March): 95-99.

SCHNORE, L. (1965) "On the spatial structure of cities in the two Americas," in Hauser and Schnore (eds.) The Study of Urbanization. Wiley and Sons.

--- (1961) "The myth of human ecology." Sociological Inquiry 31: 128-139.

--- (1958) "Social morphology and human ecology." American J. of Sociology 63: 620-634.

SCHRODINGER, E. (1968) "Order, disorder and entrophy" in W. Buckley (ed.) Modern Systems Research for the Behavioral Scientist. Chicago: Aldine.

SHEVKY, E. and W. BELL (1961) "Social area analysis," pp. 226-235 in G. A. Theodorson (ed.) Studies in Human Ecology. Evanston, Ill.: Row, Peterson.

SHILS, E. (1969) "The theory of mass society," pp. 298-316 in Minar and Greer, The Concept of Community. Chicago: Aldine.

SIEGEL, A. I. and J. J. WOLF (1969) Man-Machine Simulation Models. New York: John Wiley.

Simulation Games for the Social Studies Classroom (n.d.) New Dimensions, An FPA School Services Publication for Teachers.

SJOBERG, G. (1965) "Theory and research in urban sociology," pp. 170-171 in P. Hauser and L. F. Schnore (eds.) The Study of Urbanization: New York: John Wiley.

SMELSER, N. (n.d.) "The economy and other social sub-systems," pp. 36-38 in The Sociology of Economic Life.

STANISLAWSKI, D. (1961) "The origin and spread of the grid-pattern town," pp. 294-303 in G. A. Theodorson (ed.) Studies in Human Ecology. New York: Harper & Row.

STEGER, W. (n.d.) The Pittsburgh Urban Renewal Simulation Model.

STRAND, S. (1971) "Models and ethics." J. of the American Institute of Planners 37 (January): 42-44.

SWANSON, C. V. and R. L. WALDMANN (1970) "A simulation model of economic growth dynamics." J. of the American Institute of Planners 36 (September): 314-322.

TAUBER, C. (1965) "Taking an inventory of 180 million people: the U.S. Censuses," pp. 84-99 in R. Freedman (ed.) Population: The Vital Revolution. New York: Anchor.

TAYLOR, J. L. and K. R. CARTER (n.d.) Instructional Simulation in Urban Development: A Preliminary Report.

TEMPLE, V. E. (1971) SIMSTATE, A Computer Simulation Game for State Governments I. Duke University.

TERRIEN, F. W. and D. L. MILLS (1955) "The effect of changing size upon the internal structure of organizations," Amer. Soc. Rev. 20 (February): 11-13.

THOMAS, W. L. (n.d.) Pp. 453-469 in Man's Role in Changing the Force of the Earth.

THOMPSON, L. (1961) "The relationship of men, animals, and plants in an island community," pp. 462-470 in G. A. Theodorson (ed.) Studies in Human Ecology. Evanston, Ill.: Row, Peterson.

THOMPSON, W. S. (1930) Population Problems. New York: McGraw-Hill.

THOMPSON, W. R. (1965) A Preface to Urban Economics: Toward a Conceptual Framework for Study and Research. Baltimore: Johns Hopkins Press for Resources for the Future.

THORELLI, H. B. and R. L. GRAVES (1964) International Operations Simulation. New York: Free Press.

––– and L. T. HOWELLS (1963) INTOP Players Manual, "International Operations Simulation." New York: Free Press.

TIEBOUT, C. M. (1962) The Community Economic Base Study. Supp. paper 16, New York: Committee for Economic Development.

––– (1956) "The urban economic base reconsidered." Land Economics 32 (February): 95-99.

TJERSLAND, T. (1969) Regional Inter-Industry Economics: The Economic Structure of Metropolitan San Diego, 1968. La Jolla: Western Behavioral Sciences Institute.

U.S. Department of Health, Education and Welfare (1967) Today and Tomorrow in Air Pollution. Washington, D.C.: Government Printing Office.

ULLMAN, E. L. (1962) Presidential Address: The Nature of Cities Reconsidered. Papers and Proceedings of the Regional Science Association, Vol. 9: 7-23.

––– (1956) "A theory of location for cities," pp. 227-236 in P. K. Hatt and A. J. Reiss (eds.) Cities and Society. New York: Free Press.

VANCE, R. B. and S. SMITH (1957) "Metropolitan dominance and integration," pp. 189-200 in P. K. Hatt and A. J. Reiss (eds.) Cities and Society. New York: Free Press.

VAPNARSKY, C. (1969) "On rank-size distribution of cities: an ecological approach." Economic Development and Cultural Change 17: 584-595.

VERNON, R. (1959) The Changing Economic Function of the Central City. New York: Committee on Economic Development.

VINING, R. (1955) "A description of certain spatial aspects of an economic system." Economic Development and Cultural Change 3: 147-195.

VON BERTALANFFY, L. (1962) "General system theory–a critical review." General Systems 7: 1-20.

——— (1956) "General systems theory." Yearbook of the Society for General Systems Research Volume I: 1-10.

WARREN, R. (1963) "The community's horizontal pattern: the relation of local units to each other," ch. 9 in Warren, The Community in America. Chicago: Rand McNally.

——— (n.d.) "Community action and community development," ch. 10, pp. 303-339 in The Community in America.

WATT, K.E.F. (1966) Systems Analysis in Ecology. New York: Academic Press.

WEBBER, M. M. (1967) "The roles of intelligence systems in urban-systems planning," pp. 644-666 in H. W. Eldredge (ed.) Taming Megalopolis II. Garden City, N.Y.: Doubleday.

——— (1964a) Exploration into Urban Structure. Philadelphia: University of Pennsylvania Press.

——— (1964b) "The urban place and the nonplace urban realm," pp. 79-153 in M. M. Webber (ed.) Explorations into Urban Structure. Philadelphia: University of Pennsylvania Press.

——— (1963) Explorations into Urban Structure. Philadelphia: University of Pennsylvania Press.

WHITE, L. (1943) "Energy and the evolution of culture." American Anthropology 45: 335-356.

WEINER, N. (1968) "Cybernetics in history," pp. 31-36 in W. Buckley (ed.) Modern Systems Research for the Behavioral Scientist. Chicago: Aldine.

WINGO, L., Jr. (1961) Transportation and Urban Land. Washington, D.C.: Resources for the Future.

WIRTH, L. (1938) "Urbanism as a way of life." American J. of Sociology (July): 1-24.

WOLMAN, A. (1965) "The metabolism of cities," Scientific American CCXIII (September): 178-190.

——— (1956) "Disposal of man's wastes," pp. 807-815 in W. L. Thomas, Jr. (ed.) Man's Role in Changing the Face of the Earth. Chicago: University of Chicago Press.

WOLPERT, J. and D. ZILLMAN (1969) "The sequential expansion of a decision model in a spatial context." Environment and Planning (April): 91-104.

WRONG, D. (1967) Population and Society. New York: Random House.

ZARBAUGH, H. W. (1961) "The natural areas of the city," in G. A. Theodorson (ed.) Studies in Human Ecology. New York: Harper & Row. A. Theodorson (ed.) Studies in Human Ecology. New York: Harper & Row.

APPENDIX

MACRO RESOURCE ALLOCATION

MACRO-EQUATIONS RELATING BOTH MAN AND MACHINE DECISION STRUCTURES IN THE CITY MODEL

(RBN Version)

I. THE MODEL DEFINED

GEM-CITY is a descriptive, resource allocation model which is presented here in a discrete, static form. The salient feature of the model is that it sets forth a method of relating a wide variety of resources to one another in a highly interactive manner. The equations as presented are generally not ones which are descriptive of the actual computer algorithms but are an attempt to represent the combined decisions of the human user and these algorithms. Consequently, the equations are, at best, estimations of behavior. (See Appendix II for a list of the conventions used in notation, III for the standard subscripts, and V for a complete glossary of the variables.)

Throughout this discussion, presentation of the model will take the form of definition of the resources to be allocated or the receptors to handle the resource (usually balanced by a matching function using supply and demand relationships) and a description of the rationale for the allocation of the resources. The objective in the allocation of resources is to maximize the total resource base of the system.

$$RC = \alpha \sum_{i=1}^{NH} PLC_i + \beta \sum_{j=1}^{NJ} \sum_{g=1}^{NG_j} GLC_{gj} + jT + \sigma P \tag{I.1}$$

where: RC is total readily allocatable resources; PLC_i is the liquid capital of some private economic entity; NH is the number of private economic entities; GLC_{gj} is the liquid capital of a governmental department in a jurisdiction; NG_j is the number of governmental departments in jurisdiction j; NJ is the number of jurisdictions; T is total available time; P is the sum of all public and private power; α, β, j, and σ are weighting coefficients.

Private Capital Allocation

$$MY = \sum_{i=1}^{NH} \left[SV_i + DIV_i + \sum_{m=1}^{NSR_i} (BW_{im} - CBW_{im}) \right] \tag{I.2}$$

where: MY is the total money available for investment; SV_i is the savings of entity i; DIV_i is the discounted value of present investments of actor i; BW_{im} is the amount of money borrowed from source m by actor i; CBW_{im} is the cost to i to borrow money from source m; NSR_i is the number of sources from which i has borrowed money.

The total money available for investment by economic actors is the sum of the private liquid capital of each actor plus the potential amount of money which the actor may borrow less the cost of borrowing. For each actor, the amount of liquid and semi-liquid capital is the sum of savings and the discounted value of present investments, or

(I.3) $$PLC_i = SV_i + DIV_i$$

where: PLC_i is the private liquid capital of economic actor i.

The amount of money which may be borrowed is not unlimited but must be less than or equal to a percentage of the actor's liquid capital plus his fixed assets (buildings, land, equipment) less the actor's current debt.

(I.4) $$\sum_{m=1}^{NSR_i} BW_{im} \leqslant a(PLC_i + FA_i - DBT_i),\ a < 1$$

where: FA_i is the total of all fixed assets of actor i; DBT_i is the current debt of i.

The cost of borrowing money is the interest rate times the amount borrowed from the Source, or

(I.5) $$CBW_{im} = BW_{im} \cdot LR_m$$

where: LR_m is the interest rate charged by source m.

Choice of Investment

An actor is faced with a large number of alternative investments when deciding how to use his money. A decision to invest in a specific activity x is based on five criteria:

(1) the total amount of money available to be invested,
(2) the cost of investing in an activity,
(3) the interest rate on the money borrowed to invest,
(4) the rate of return on the type of the activity,
(5) the cost of obtaining investment information.

No actor will invest in an activity x if the rate of return on $x(R_x)$

is less than the interest rate charged by source m(LR_m). Since each investment made decreases an actor's supply of available funds,

(I.6) $$MY_{ix} = PLC_i + \sum_{m=1}^{NSR_i} [BW_{im} - CBW_{im}] - \sum_{y=1}^{x-1} [K_y + CII_y]$$

where: MY_{ix} is the amount of money available for i to invest in activity x; K_y is the cost of investment y; CII is the cost of investment information for investment y.

In other words, the amount of money available to i for investment in activity x is the sum of the liquid capital of i and the net amount of money borrowed minus the amount of money already invested.

No investment will be made in an activity x if the cost of the investment is greater than the amount of money available to the actor. Consequently, the following relations must be true in order for actor i to invest money in activity x:

(I.7) $$R_x \geqslant LR_m$$

(I.8) $$MY_{ix} \geqslant K_x + CII_x$$

As long as the amount of money is large relative to the cost of any potential investment, very little will be taken into account in deciding the investment other than the relationships expressed in I.7 and I.8. However, as variable funds shrink and the cost of investment begins to approach the amount of available money, the actor will tend to rank investments and choose that one which will give him the greatest possible return, and the probability that the investment chosen is the one with the highest net rate of return approaches 1.00.

(I.9) $$P(IC) \rightarrow 1$$

if: $x \in RN_x$;

$K_x + CII_x \rightarrow MX_{ix}$;

$RN_x/MY_i > RN_y/MY_i$

and kN, $x \geqslant 0$; $MY_i \neq 0$

where: IC is the investment chosen; RN_x is the net rate of return on activity x.

And for any investment x, the net rate of return is defined as the differences between the rate of return on activity x and the interest rate on the money borrowed.

(I.10) $$RN_x = R_x - LR_m$$

Rationally, all possible investment choices would be ordered so that:

(I.11) $$\max RN \geqslant RN_x$$

Since all liquid capital is assumed to earn a rate of return at least equal to the current rate of interest paid on savings, it is assumed that a rational actor would order investments so that the first capital to be used would be borrowed as long as $R_x > LR_m$.

Once borrowing becomes unprofitable; i.e., $LR_m > R_x$, savings and invested capital will be used so long as the rate of return from the new investment is greater than the expected rate of return on current savings and investments.

Private capital may be invested in three general types of activities–residential, commercial, and industrial. Although each general type of activity is further subdivided into specific activities, the determination of rate of return for all activities within a general type is identical.

For any property, the rate of return is defined as the ratio of the profits from the property (income less expenditures) to the capital value of the property, or

(I.12) $$R_p = \frac{Y_p - EX_p}{V_p}$$

where: Y_p is the income at p; EX_p is the expenditures at p; V_p is the capital value of p; R_p is the rate of return on p,

and the rate of return on a specific type of property is defined as the average rate of return on all properties of that type:

(I.13) $$\bar{R}_x = \frac{\sum_{p=1}^{NP_x} Y_p - \sum_{p=1}^{NP_x} EX_p}{\sum_{p=1}^{NP_x} V_p}$$

where: $\bar{R}_x$ is the average rate of return on activity x; NP_x is the number of properties of type x.

Prior to describing the rate of return equations for each of the general types, let us first describe V_p, since it is determined in the same manner for all types of activity.

The value of a property is defined as the sum of the value structure and the value of the land occupied by the structure, or:

$$V_p = LND_p + IMP_p \tag{I.14}$$

where: LND is the value of the land occupied; IMP is the value of the improvements; V_p is the value of a property.

The improvements value for a given property p is the original cost of a level 1 of the activity, x, at p multiplied by the value ratio of the structure, times the number of levels:

$$IMP_p = OSC_x \cdot VR_p \cdot LV_p \tag{I.15}$$

where: OSC_x is the original cost of a level 1 structure for activity x; VR_p is the value ratio of the structure; LV_p number of levels.

The value of the land occupied is the product of the unit value of land at p, the number of levels, and the number of units of space required for a level 1 of activity x;

$$LND_p = SPX_x \cdot LV_p \cdot UVL_p \tag{I.16}$$

where: SPX_p is the amount of land space required for a level 1 of activity x; UVL_p is the unit value of land at p.

Combining I.15 and I.16 and summing over all properties of type x, we have

$$\sum_{p=1}^{NP_x} V_p = \left[SPX_x \cdot \sum_{p=1}^{NP_x} LV_p \cdot UVL_p \right] + \left[OSC_x \cdot \sum_{p=1}^{NP_x} LV_p \cdot VR_p \right] \tag{I.17}$$

Residential Rates of Return

Income. The income for a residential property is the product of the rent per space unit and the amount of space occupied;

(I.18) $$Y_p = RNT_p \cdot SPO_p,$$

where: RNT_p is rent per space unit at p; SPO_p is amount of space occupied at p; Y is the income at p.

and the amount of space occupied is the sum over all classes living at p of the population of the class times the amount of space required per population unit for each class:

(I.19) $$SPO_p = \sum_{k=1}^{NK} POP_{pk} \cdot SPK_k.$$

where: POP_{pk} is the number of population units of class k at p; SPO_k is the number of space units occupied.

Substituting in 2:

(I.20) $$Y_p = RNT_p \cdot \left[\sum_{k=1}^{NK} POP_{pk} \cdot SPK_p \right]$$

Summing over all parcels:

(I.21) $$\sum_{p=1}^{NP_x} Y_p = \sum_{p=1}^{NP} RNT_p \cdot \left[\sum_{k=1}^{NK} POP_{pk} \cdot SPK_k \right]$$

Expenditures. Expenditures for a residential property are given by:

(I.22) $$EX_p = CU_p + TX_p + MT_p + WTR_p$$

where: CU_p is the cost of utility service at p; TX_p is the total taxes paid on p; MT_p is the cost of maintenance at p; WTR_p is the cost of water at p; EX_p is the expenditure at p.

Substituting I.20, I.22, and I.17 in I.13 and summing over all properties p of residential type x, we have:

(I.23)

$$R_x = \frac{\sum_{p=1}^{NP_x} RNT_p \cdot \left[\sum_{k=1}^{NK} (POP_{pk} \cdot SPK_k)\right] - \sum_{p=1}^{NP_x} [CU_p + TX_p + MT_p + WTR_p]}{\left[SPX_x \cdot \sum_{p=1}^{NP_x} (LV_p \cdot UVL_p)\right] + \left[OSC_x \cdot \sum_{p=1}^{NP_x} (LV_p \cdot VR_p)\right]}$$

Industrial Rates of Return

Income. The income of any industrial property is the product of the units produced and the price per unit (type specific) paid for the products.

(I.24) $$Y_p = PU_x \cdot UP_p$$

where: PU_x is the industry specific price per unit paid for products from activity x; UP_p is the number of units produced at p.

Expenditures. Expenditures for an industrial property is given by

(I.25) $$EX_p = CU_p + TX_p + MT_p + WTR_p + TR_p + SL_p + GS_p + TM_p + PTN_p$$

where: TR_p is transportation costs for goods and services; SL_p is the amount of salaries paid; GS_p is cost of goods and services; TM_p is costs associated with use of shipping terminals; PTN_p is costs connected with pollution control.

Substituting I.23 and I.24 in I.13, the rate of return on industrial type x is

(I.26)

$$R_x = \frac{\sum_{p=1}^{NP_x} [PU_x \cdot UP_p] \quad \left[\sum_{p=1}^{NP_x} [CU_p + TX_p + MT_p + WTR_p + TR_p + SL_p + GS_p + TM_p + PTN_p]\right]}{\left[SPX_x \cdot \sum_{p=1}^{NP_x} (LV_p \cdot UVL_p)\right] + \left[OSC_x \cdot \sum_{p=1}^{NP_x} (LV_p \cdot VR_p)\right]}$$

Commercial Rates of Return

Income. Income for a commercial property is the product of the number of units sold and the price per unit.

(I.27) $$Y_p = PPU_p \cdot US_p$$

where: PPU_p is the price per unit charged at p; US_p is the number of units sold at p.

Expenditures. Expenditures for a commercial property are given by:

(I.28) $$EX_p = CU_p + TX_p + MT_p + WTR_p + TR_p + SL_p\ GS_p$$

Substituting in I.13 and summing over all parcels p of commercial type x, the rate of return for commercial activity x is

(I.29)

$$R_x = \frac{\left[\sum_{p=1}^{NP_x} (US_p \cdot PPU_p)\right] - \left[\sum_{p=1}^{NP_x} [CU_p + TX_p + MT_p + WTR_p + TR_p + SL_p + GS_p]\right]}{\left[OSC_x \cdot \sum_{p=1}^{NP_x} (LV_p \cdot VR_p)\right] + \left[SPX_x \cdot \sum_{p=1}^{NP_x} (LV_p \cdot UVL)\right]}$$

The Government Budget

The total amount of money available to a jurisdiction is:

(I.30) $$MYG_j = TAX_j + SVC_j + BND_j + CT_j$$

where: MY_j is the total money available to jurisdiction; TAX_j is total tax income for jurisdiction; SVC_j is total of all service charges in jurisdiction; BND_j is bond income; CT_j is cash transfers to the government.

Aid from federal and state sources is not treated as income but as a reduction in the cost of local projects which they support.

Departmental Performance Indices

The performance of governmental departments in providing necessary services is measured by the departmental performance index.

There exists, for each department, an I_{gj} which is the ratio of demand to supply for services provided by department d, or:

$$I_{gj} = \frac{D_{gj}}{S_{gj}} \tag{I.31}$$

where: D_{gj} is the demand for services of department g in jurisdiction j; S_{gj} is the supply of services by department g in jurisdiction j.

The objective for department d is to bring I_{gj} to 1.00 from either side, since

If $I_{gj} > 1.00$ $D_{gj} > S_{gj}$ and there is not sufficient supply of services from department g.

If $I_{gj} < 1.00$ $D_{gj} < S_{gj}$ and there is excess capacity and, consequently, waste.

School Department

$$I_{SC_j} = \frac{\sum_{d=1}^{ND_j} \sum_{p=1}^{NP_d} \sum_{k=1}^{NK} POP_{pk} \cdot STP_k}{\sum_{d=1}^{ND_j} LV_d \cdot VR_d \cdot TCM(HW_d, MW_d)} \tag{I.32}$$

where: STP_k is the number of students per population unit in class k; TCM is a function giving student capacity from teacher mix; HW_d is the number of high income teachers in district d; MW_d is number of middle income teachers in district d; ND_j is the number of departments in jurisdiction j.

Adult Education

(I.33) $$I_{AE_j} = \frac{\sum_{p=1}^{NP_j} \sum_{k=1}^{NK} TAE_{pk}}{PH_j + PM_j}$$

where: TAE_{pk} is the amount of time allocated to adult education by class k at parcel p; PH_j is the number of part-time high income teachers in jurisdiction j; PM_j is the number of part-time middle income teachers in jurisdiction j.

Welfare

(I.34) $$I_{WL_j} = \frac{\widehat{WLP_j}}{WLP_j}$$

where: WLP_j is the total welfare payment in jurisdiction i; $\widehat{WLP_j}$ is the total welfare required to cover minimum living costs.

Municipal Services

(I.35) $$I_{MS_j} = \frac{\sum_{d=1}^{ND_j} \sum_{p=1}^{NP_d} LV_p \cdot UTR(LU_p)}{\sum_{d=1}^{ND_j} LV_d \cdot VR_d \cdot MSC(MW_d, LW_d)}$$

where: LU_p is land use at parcel p; MSR is municipal service requirements function; MSC is municipal services capacity from employment function; LW_d is number of low income workers in district d; UTR is a utility requirement by land use function.

Utility Department

(I.36)
$$I_{VT_j} = \frac{\sum_{d=1}^{ND_j} \sum_{p=1}^{NP_d} LV_p \cdot UTR(LU_p)}{LCC \cdot \sum_{d=1}^{ND_j} LV_d}$$

where: LCC is the least cost design capacity of a level 1 utility plant.

Budget Allocation

If we assume that the overall government performance index is a function of the departmental performance indices, then:

(I.37)
$$IX_j = \frac{\sum_{g=1}^{NG_j} W_{gj} \cdot I_{gj}}{\sum_{g=1}^{NG_j} W_{gj}}$$

where: IX_j is the overall government performance index; W_{gj} are weights assigned to each of the departmental performance indices (I_{gj}).

Consequently, the decision objective in allocating funds among departments is to improve the department ratios in order to bring IX_j as close to 1.00 as possible.

Time Allocation

$$\text{(I.38)} \qquad TTM = \sum_{p=1}^{NP} \sum_{k=1}^{NK} \sum_{a=1}^{NA} POP_{pk} \cdot TVL_{pka} \cdot TAC_{pka}$$

where: TTM is the value of all time in the model; TVL_{pk} is the value of one time unit for class k at location p in activity a; TAC_{pka} is the time allocated by one population unit of class k at p in activity a.

The amount of time which a population unit may allocate is the difference in the total amount of time (constant) and the sum of the time committed to work and traveling and that lost to illness.

$$\text{(I.39)} \qquad TAL_{pk} = TMT - (TWK_{pk} + TIL_{pk} + TTR_{pk})$$

where: TAL_{pk} is the total time which may be allocated; TMT_{pk} is the total time in a day, year, etc.; TWK_{pk} is the time spent at work; TIL_{pk} is time lost due to illness; TTR_{pk} is time spent in traveling to work.

TAL may be distributed among various activities; viz, recreation, political activity, part-time work, free education and training programs, or education and training programs for which a fee is charged. Any allocation of time to an activity which is unsatisfied is added to involuntary time, as in any unallocated time.

$$\text{(I.40)} \qquad TIN_{pk} = TUA_{pk} + \sum_{a=1}^{NA} [TAC_{pka} - TSA_{pka}]$$

where: TIN_{pk} is total involuntary time; TUA_{pk} is unallocated time; TSA_{pka} is time actually spent in activity a, and TUA_{pk} is defined by:

$$\text{(I.41)} \qquad TUA_{pk} = TAL_{pk} - \sum_{z=1}^{NA} TAC_{pka}$$

reducing I.41 to:

(I.42)
$$TIN_{pk} = TAL_{pk} - \sum_{a=1}^{NA} TSA_{pka}$$

The only pursuits which result in an improvement of the resources of a population unit are political activity, free education, pay education and part-time work.

(I.43)
$$TRI_{pk} = TEF_{pk} + TEP_{pk} + TPL_{pk} + TPW_{pk}$$

where: TRI_{pk} is the total time spent which improves resources; TEF_{pk} is time spent in free education and training programs; TEP_{pk} is time spent in pay education and training programs; TPL_{pk} is time spent in political activity; TPW_{pk} is time spent in a part-time job,

and where TEF_{pk}, TEP_{pk}, TPL_{pk}, and TPW_{pk} are all elements of the set of TSA_{pka}.

Associated with each activity which results in an improvement in the resources of a population unit is a rate of return on time allocation

$$\left(\frac{TVL_{pka}}{\sum_{a=1}^{NA} TVL_{pka}} \right)$$

(a) Part-time Work. The rate of return on allocation of time to part-time work is the ratio of the income from the work and the value of the time allocated to it.

(I.44)
$$RTA_{PW,pk} = \frac{ICM_{pk}}{TPW_{pk} \cdot TVL_{pk}}$$

where: RTA is the rate of return on the allocation of time; ICM_{pk} is the income earned by class k at location p.

(b) Political Activity. The rate of return on allocation of time to political activity is the ratio of the increase in voter registration to the amount of time spent.

(I.45) $$RTA_{PL,pk} = \frac{\Delta VTR_{pk}}{TPL_{pk}}$$

where: ΔVTR is the rate of change in voter registration.

(c) Free Education. The rate of return on free education is the ratio of the change in the education level of a population unit to the amount of time spent.

(I.46) $$RTA_{EF,pk} = \frac{\Delta EDL_{pk}}{TEF_{pk}}$$

where: ΔEDL_{pk} is the rate of change in the education level of a population unit.

(d) Pay Education.

(I.47) $$RTA_{EP,pk} = \frac{\Delta EDL_{pk}}{TEP_{pk} \cdot CEP}$$

where: CEP is the cost per time unit for pay education.

Time will be allocated by population units in a manner which is likely to produce the greatest improvement in the resources of the population unit.

Assuming the existence of a factor, a_a, for each activity which translates the rates of returns for activities into commensurate units, the total benefit from the allocation of time can be expressed as:

(I.48) $$BEN_{pk} = \sum_{z=1}^{NA} a_a \cdot RTA_{a,pk} \cdot TSA_{pka}$$

where: BEN is the total benefit from the allocation of time.

Salaries

The salary to be offered by an employer at a specific location is a function of transportation costs, the unemployment rate, and salaries offered at other locations.

(I.49) $$SOF_{sk} = \overline{SPW}_k \cdot UEM_k \cdot \left[\frac{\overline{TCS}_{sk}}{\overline{TCW}_k}\right]$$

where: SOF_{sk} is the salary to be offered to workers of class k at location s; $\overline{SPW}_k$ is the average salary paid to workers in class k; UEM_k is the unemployment rate for class k; $\overline{TCS}_{sk}$ is the average transportation cost for workers in class k to get from their residence to location s; $\overline{TCW}_k$ is the average transportation cost for workers in class k to get from their residence to the site at which they are currently employed

and:

(I.50)
$$\overline{SPW}_k = \frac{\sum_{s=1}^{NS} SPW_{sk} \cdot WKR_{sk}}{\sum_{s=1}^{NS} WKR_{sk}}$$

where: SPW_{sk} is the salary per worker paid to workers of class k at location s; WKR_{sk} is the number of workers in class k at location s.

(I.51)
$$UEM_k = \frac{\sum_{s=1}^{NS} WKR_{sk}}{\sum_{p=1}^{NP} POP_{pk} \cdot WPU_k}$$

where: WPU_k is the number of workers per population unit in class k.

(I.52)
$$\overline{TCS}_{sk} = \frac{\sum_{p=1}^{NP} POP_{pk} \cdot TCS_{pks}}{\sum_{p=1}^{NP} POP_{pk}}$$

where: TCS_{pks} is the cost for workers of class k to get from residence location p to work location s.

(I.53)
$$\overline{TCW}_k = \frac{\sum_{p=1}^{NP} POP_{pk} \cdot TCW_{pk}}{\sum_{p=1}^{NP} POP_{pk}}$$

Rent

The rent for a particular dwelling can be calculated from the average rent in the system, the average quality and environmental indices, the occupancy rate, and the quality and environmental indices for dwelling.

(I.54)
$$RNT_s = \overline{RNT} \cdot \frac{\overline{QI}}{QI_s} \cdot \frac{\overline{EI}}{EI_s} \cdot OCR$$

where: $\overline{RNT}$ is average rent per space unit; $\overline{QI}$ is average quality index; $\overline{EI}$ is average environmental index; OCR is occupancy rate; QI_s is quality index at s; EI_s is environmental index at s,

and:

(I.55)
$$\overline{RNT} = \frac{\sum_{p=1}^{NP} RNT_p \cdot SPO_p}{\sum_{p=1}^{NP} SPO_p}$$

(I.56)
$$OCR = \frac{\sum_{p=1}^{NP} SPO_p}{\sum_{p=1}^{NP} SPT_p}$$

where: SPT is the total space at p.

(I.57)
$$\overline{QI} = \frac{\sum_{p=1}^{NP} QI_p \cdot SPT_p}{\sum_{p=1}^{NP} SPT_p}$$

(I.58)
$$\overline{EI} = \frac{\sum_{p=1}^{NP} EI_p \cdot SPT_p}{\sum_{p=1}^{NP} SPT_p}$$

Value of Structures and Capital Equipment

The value of a structure at the beginning of a time interval in the model is the value ratio of the structure times the product of the original cost of a level 1 structure and the number of levels.

(I.59)
$$IMP_p, t_0 = OSC(LU_p) \cdot LV_p \cdot VR_p$$

At the end of the time interval the value will be reduced by the amount of depreciation which has occurred.

(I.60)
$$IMP_p, t_1 = OSC(LU_p) \cdot LV_p \cdot [VR_p - DEP_p]$$

Money expended on maintenance does not increase the value of the structure but merely offsets the effects of depreciation. If MTL_p is the maintenance level of the structure then the value of the structure is given by equation I.60. Adjusting this to include maintenance:

(I.61)
$$NV_p = (VR_p - DEP_p + MTL_p)$$

(I.62)
$$IMP_p, ts = OSC(LU_p) \cdot LV_p \cdot NV_p$$

where: NV_p is the net value of the structure at location p.

Municipal Services

Municipal Services in the model is an aggregate of police, fire, and health services. Municipal services are provided on a district basis with one MS facility serving each district which will contain one or more contiguous parcels.

The demand for municipal services in each district is a function of the land use mix in the district, since each land use has a specific MS requirement.

(I.63) $$MSD_d = \sum_{p=1}^{NP_d} MSR(LU_p) \cdot LV_p$$

where: MSD_d is the demand for municipal services; MSR is the requirement for municipal services of specific land uses.

The supply of municipal services is a function of the size and age of the facility and the employment mix.

(I.64) $$SMS_d = LV_d \cdot VR_d \cdot MSE(MW_d, LW_d)$$

where: SMS_d is the supply of municipal services; $MSE(MW_d, LW_d)$ is the employment mix (middle and low income) of a municipal service.

The MS use index is the ratio of MSD_d to SMS_d and as the index exceeds 1.0 the quality of municipal services declines.

(I.65) $$I_{MS,d} = \frac{MSD_d}{SMS_d} = \frac{\sum_{p=1}^{NP_d} MSR(LU_p) \cdot LV_p}{LV_d \cdot VR_d \cdot MSE(NW_d, LW_d)}$$

Utilities

Utility demand in a district is a function of the various land uses on the parcels in the district.

(I.66) $$UTD_d = \sum_{p=1}^{NP_d} UTR(LU_p) \cdot LV_p$$

where: UTD_d is the demand for utility services; UTR is the utility requirements of specific land uses.

The supply of utilities in a district is a function of the level of utility service installed on each parcel in the district.

$$SUT_d = \sum_{p=1}^{NP_d} UTI(LUS_p) \tag{I.67}$$

where: LUS_p is the level of utility service installed at p; UTI is the utility service by level of installation function; SUT_d is the supply of utility service.

The utility use index is then:

$$I_{UT,d} = \frac{UTD_d}{SUT_d} = \frac{\sum_{p=1}^{NP_d} LV_p \cdot UTR(LU_p)}{\sum_{p=1}^{NP_d} UTI(LUS_p)} \tag{I.68}$$

However: SUT_d will almost always be greater than UTD_d with the consequence that $I_{UT,d}$ will be less than 1.00, since there is no limit on the amount of utilities which may be installed. There exists, however, for utility plants a least cost capacity at which the cost per unit is minimized. Use of this measure would result in a more meaningful measure of the performance of a utility plant.

$$I_{UT,d} = \frac{\sum_{p=1}^{NP_d} LV_p \cdot UTR(LU_p)}{LV_d LCC} \tag{I.69}$$

where: LCC is the least cost capacity of a level 1 utility plant.

Depreciation

Depreciation of structures is a function of several factors; viz., age, land use, susceptability to flooding, fire damage, and deterioration due to greater than normal use.

$$\text{(I.70)} \qquad DEP_p = [I_{MS} - 1] \cdot MSD(LU_p) + AGE_p \cdot DDA(LU_p) + FSI_p \cdot DFL(LU_p) + \frac{US_p}{DC_p} \cdot DOC(LU_p) + \frac{WTO_d}{WTN_d} \cdot FRD(LU_p)$$

where: AGE_p is the age of the structure at p; FSI_p is the flood severity index for p; WTO_d is the water obtained by the utility district in which p is located; WTN_d is the amount of water needed by the district; MSD depreciation due to inadequate municipal services; DDA depreciation due to age and obsolescence; DFL depreciation due to flood damage; DOC depreciation due to use exceeding capacity; FRD depreciation due to fire damage;

and

$$1 \leqslant 1_{MS} \leqslant 2$$

$$1 \leqslant \frac{US_p}{DC_p} \leqslant 2$$

$$1 \leqslant \frac{WTO_d}{WTN_d} \leqslant 2$$

Commercial

Personal Goods and Services. In the commercial sector the total demand for personal goods or personal services is a function of the demand from the population and demand as a result of maintenance of residences. Demand from population results from regular demand for goods/services necessary to support daily activities and demand from the allocation of time to activities which require purchase of additional goods/services.

$$\text{(I.71)} \qquad PDP = \sum_{p=1}^{NP} \sum_{k=1}^{NK} PDK_k \cdot POP_{pk} \sum_{a=1}^{NA} PDA_{ka} \cdot TSA_{pka}$$

where: PDP is the population demand for personal goods/services; PDK_k is the normal demand factor by class; PDA_{ka} is demand resulting from the allocation of time by class k to activity a.

Demand resulting from maintenance of residences is given by:

$$RDP = \sum_{p=1}^{NP} DRD(LU_p) \cdot LV_p \cdot [MTL_p + DEP_p - VR_p] \tag{I.72}$$

where: RDP is residence demand for personal goods/services; DRD is demand resulting from 1 percent depreciation of a residence and is equal to either $PGD(LU_p)$ for goods demand or $PSD(LU_p)$ for service demand.

(NOTE: see equation IV.2)

Business Goods and Services. Total demand for business goods/services has four (4) components:

(1) Demand from industry for goods/services necessary for production.

(2) Demand resulting from sales of personal goods and services.

(3) Demand resulting from structural maintenance.

(4) Government contracts for business goods/services.

$$TBD = DIP + DDS + BDD + DGV \tag{I.73}$$

where: TBD is total demand for business goods/services; DIP is demand from industrial production; DDS is demand from sales of personal goods/services; BDD is demand from maintenance of deteriorating structures; DGV is demand from government contracts.

Demand from industrial production is a function of the industrial land use mix in the system:

$$DIP = \sum_{p=1}^{NP} DGS(LU_p) \cdot LV_p \tag{I.74}$$

where: DGS is goods and services demand function for a level 1 industry and equals $DBG(LU_p)$, demand for business goods, or $DBS(LU_p)$, demand for business services.

Demand for business goods/services from sales of personal goods/services is a function of the sales of PG and PS in the system.

$$DDS = DPS \cdot \sum_{p=1}^{NP} UPS_p + DPG \cdot \sum_{p=1}^{NP} UPG \tag{I.75}$$

where: DPS is demand per unit from sales of personal service and equals either GPS (goods demand) or SPS (services demand); DPG is demand per unit from sales of personal goods and equals either GPG (goods demand) or SPG (services demand); UPS_p is the units of personal services sold at p; UPG_p is the units of personal goods sold at p.

$$BDD = [MTL_p + DEP_p - VR_p] \cdot DDD(LU_p) \tag{I.76}$$

where: DDD is demand function by depreciation of land use and equals $BGD(LU_p)$ for goods demand or $BGS(LU_p)$ for services demand.

(NOTE: see equations IV.2 and IV.3)

Total supply of business goods/services is a function of design capacity of each establishment, number of levels, value ratio, and number of employees.

$$TS = DC \cdot \sum_{s=1}^{NS} \left[LV_s \cdot VR_s \cdot \left(1 - \frac{\sum_{k=1}^{NK} WKR_{sk}}{WRR_s} \right) \right] \tag{I.77}$$

where: WRR is the number of workers required at location s; DC is the design capacity.

Power

Power is easily the most difficult resource to allocate because of measurement problems. However, a few basic statements can be made.

(I.78) $$\text{PWR} = \sum_{i=1}^{NI} \text{PRI}_i + \sum_{j=1}^{NJ} \sum_{g=1}^{NG_j} \text{PUB}_{gj}$$

where: PWR is the total power in the system; PRI_i is the power of an economic entity; PUB_{gj} is the power of a government department.

Public Power. Public power is not easily expressed in a simple equation. However, it is a function of several factors:

(1) the ability to achieve its ends through legal action in the courts;
(2) the relative economic status in the system;
(3) the use of simple force; and
(4) persuasion of incumbent office holders.

(I.79) $$\text{PUB}_{gj} = f\left(\frac{\text{LAS}_{gj}}{\text{LAT}_{gj}}, \frac{\text{GMY}_{gh}}{\text{TMY}}, \text{FRC}_{gj}, \text{PSW}_{gj}\right)$$

where: LAS_{gj} is the number of successful litigations; LAT_{gj} is the total number of litigations; GMY_{gj} is money available to the department; TMY is total money in system; FRC_{gj} is force available; PSW_{gj} is persuasion.

Private Power. Private power can take a large number of forms; it is most commonly considered in the area of voting.

(I.80) $$\text{VTE} = \sum_{p=1}^{NP} \sum_{k=1}^{NK} \text{POP}_{pk} \cdot [\text{AV}_k + \text{RDV}_{pk}]$$

where: VTE is total votes costs; AV_k is the average number of voters/P1; RDV_{pk} is a random deviation (+ or –) from AV_k for each location and class.

Employment

The employment process matches the people who are looking for jobs with employers who are trying to find workers with specific skill levels.

Supply of Jobs. The supply of jobs is a function of the industrial/commercial mix of land uses in the system plus the number of workers requested by municipal services and teachers requested by the school system.

$$(I.81)\quad SJ_k = \sum_{p=1}^{NP} EMR(k,LU_p) \cdot LV_p + \sum_{j=1}^{NJ} \sum_{d=1}^{NMS_j} WR_{jdk} + \sum_{j=1}^{NJ} \sum_{d=1}^{NSC_j} TR_{jdk}$$

where: SJ_k is the supply of jobs in class k; EMR is a function giving employees required by class for each land use; WR_{jdk} is the number of MS workers in class k in MS district d in jurisdiction j; TR_{jdk} is the number of teachers requested in school district d in jurisdiction j.

Demand for Jobs. The demand for jobs is simply the total number of workers in a given class in the system.

$$(I.82)\quad DJ_k = \sum_{p=1}^{NP} POP_{pk} \cdot WKP_k$$

where: DJ_k is demand for jobs; WKP_k is the number of workers per population unit in class k.

Matching. The process of matching supply and demand for workers is accomplished by ranking workers in the order of skill or educational levels. The worker with the highest ranking then finds the job which maximizes his net income, and the technique is repeated until all workers are placed or all jobs are filled.

This process is also used to fill part-time jobs with workers who desire them.

Migration. Population movement into, out of, and within a system is dependent on conditions as they exist in the system.

The number of persons who are potential emigrees from the system includes fixed percentages of the most dissatisfied, the unemployed and underemployed and those persons who have been displaced due to demolition of their residences.

$$MOV_k = \alpha \sum_{p=1}^{NP} POP_{pk} + \beta UE_k + DPL_k \tag{I.83}$$

where: MOV_k is the number of migrants of class k in the system; UE_k is unemployed and underemployed; DPL_k is number of displaced persons in class k; $\alpha,\beta < 1.0$.

The number of out-migrants from the system is the potential emigrees less the number who find acceptable housing within the system. A migrant will stay within the system if and only if he can find available housing which has an environmental index (EI) less than the EI of his current residence. STA will denote the number of migrants who stay within the system. Thus:

$$OUT_k = MOV_k - STA_k \tag{I.84}$$

Transportation

Transportation uses a concept of ecological distance which measures both the time and money costs of travel. There are two approaches to the problem of transport, both of which seek to minimize the ecological distance between two points. The first solution, used by workers going to their places of employment, the object is to find the combination of routes and modes of transportation which minimize both the time required and the out of pocket costs of travel. The minimization sought is not absolute but is relative between time and money, since each population unit may value its travel time differently.

The cost, to a population, to traverse a single link in the transportation system is the product cost of the mode chosen and the level of the link. Added to these direct costs is the cost in time required to traverse link. The time required will vary as a function of the mode chosen, the level of the link, and the congestion on the link. Consequently, the cost to traverse a single link is:

(I.85) $LC_{l \cdot kps} = LV_l \cdot MDC(k, MOD_{kpsl}) + TVL_{pk} \cdot TUM(k, MOD_{kpsl}, COG_l)$

where: $LC_{l \cdot kps}$ is the cost (time and money) for class k to traverse link l on the optimum route from residence location p to work location s; MOD_{kpsl} is the mode chosen to traverse link l; COG_l is congestion on link l; MDC is the modal cost function for class and modal choice; TUM is the time consumption function for class, mode, and congestion.

For all other travel; i.e., non-work related, the optimum route is the one which minimizes the direct cost of transportation since time is considered only in work-related trips.

II. A LIST OF CONVENTIONS

The following basic conventions will hold throughout the discussion which follows:

(1) All variables in the model will be one to three letters in length and will be in capital letters; e.g., NP is the number of parcels in the model.

(2) All subscripts are lower case single letters; e.g., d is the subscript denoting district and NP_d is the number of parcels in some district d. (See the List of Standard Subscripts which follows.)

(3) To avoid confusion multiplication will be noted by the inclusion of a dot (·) between two variable names; e.g., $XX_p \cdot YY_p$ instead of $XX_p YY_p$ or $(XX_p)(YY_p)$.

(4) Variables will be defined on their first occurence but not subsequently. There is also a glossary of variables (Appendix V).

III. STANDARD SUBSCRIPTS

d	district	u	land use
j	jurisdiction	g	government departments
k	class	a	activity to which time may be allocated
p	parcel		
s	site or specific location	i	actor

IV. DEFINITION OF EXPENDITURES

Utility Costs

(IV.1) $$CU_p = UTR(LU_p) \cdot UTC_{pj} \cdot LV_p$$

where: UTR is a utility requirements function for level 1 of a land use type; UTC is the utility charge function by jurisdiction; LV_p is the number of levels of the land use at p.

Maintenance Cost

Commercial and Industrial

(IV.2) $$MT_p = LV_p \cdot [MTL_p + DEP_p - VR_p] \cdot [PBG_p \cdot BGD(LU_p) + PBS_p \cdot BSD(LU_p)]$$

Residential

(IV.3) $$MT_p = LV_p \cdot [MTL_p + DEP_p - VR_p] \cdot [PBG_p \cdot BGD(LU_p) + PBS_p \cdot BSD(LU_p) + PPG_p \cdot PGD(LU_p) + PPS_p \cdot PSD(LV_p)]$$

where: BGD is a function for business goods demand from 1 percent depreciation of a land use; BSD is a function for business service demand from 1 percent depreciation of a land use; PGD is a function for personal goods demand from 1 percent depreciation of a land use; PSD is a function for personal services demand from 1 percent depreciation of a land use; PBG_p is the price paid per unit for business goods; PBS_p is the price paid per unit for business services; PPG_p is the price paid per unit for personal goods; PPS_p is the price paid per unit for personal services.

Taxes

There are three types of taxes paid on residential properties—income, property, and sales.

(IV.4) $$TX_p = IT_p + PTX_p + STX_p$$

where: TX is the total taxes of parcel p; IT is the tax on income; PTX is the property tax; STX is the sales tax.

Income Taxes

Residential

(IV.5) $$ITX_p = TXR_{j_p} \cdot \sum_{k=1}^{NK} POP_{pk} \cdot SPK_k$$

where: TXR is a function relating the tax rate in a jurisdiction.

Commercial

(IV.6) $$ITX_p = TXR_{j_p} \cdot \quad PPU_p \cdot US_p$$

Industrial

(IV.7) $$ITX_p = TXR_{j_p} \cdot \quad PU(LU_p) \cdot UP_p$$

Property Taxes

(IV.8) $$PTX_p = ASR(J_p,LU_p) \cdot TXR_{j_p} \quad LV_p \cdot [SPX(LU_p) \cdot UVL_p + OSC(LU_p) \cdot VR_p]$$

where: ASR is a function giving assessment ratio from jurisdiction and land use.

Sales Taxes

(IV.9) $$STX_p = TXR_{j_p} \cdot MT_p$$

Salary Costs

(IV.10) $$SL_p = \sum_{k=1}^{NK} SPW_{pk} \cdot WKR_{pk}$$

where: WKR_{pk} is the number of workers of class k at p; SPW_{pk} is the salary offered per worker of class k at p.

Water Costs

Commercial and Industrial

(IV.11) $$WTR_p = WCR(LU_p) \cdot WC_j(LU_p)$$

where: WCR is water consumption requirements function for land uses; WC is water charge per unit function by jurisdiction and land use; WTR is the total water costs for parcel p.

Residential

(IV.12) $$WTR_p = \sum_{k=1}^{NK} POP_{pk} \cdot WCR(RT_p) \cdot WC_j(RT_p)$$

where: $RT_p = f(LU_p,k)$. RT_p is a residence type at p and is a function of the residential land use at p and the class k.

Pollution Costs

(IV.13) $$PTN_p = MGD_p \cdot [SWT(WQ_p) + EFT(LT_p)]$$

where: MGD_p is the amount of surface water required at p; SWT is a function relating cost per gallon to treat water at p to a usable level of quality; WQ_p is the existing water quality at p; EFT is a function relating cost of effluent treatment and level of treatment; LT_p is the level of treatment to which effluent is subjected.

V. GLOSSARY OF VARIABLES (as they appear)

1. RC = total allocatable assets.
2. NH = number of private economic entities.
3. PLC = liquid capital of a private economic entity.
4. NJ = number of jurisdictions.
5. NG = number of governmental departments.
6. GLC = liquid capital of a government department.
7. T = total allocatable time.
8. P = sum of all public and private power.
9. SV = savings
10. MY = total money available for investment.
11. DIV = discounted value of present investments.
12. BIM = amount of money borrowed.
13. CBW = cost to borrow money.
14. NSR = number of sources from which to borrow money.
15. FA = total of all fixed assets.
16. DBT = current debt.
17. LR = interest rate.
18. R = rate of return.
19. K = cost of investment.
20. CII = cost of investment information.
21. BW = amount of money borrowed.
22. IC = investment chosen.
23. RN = net rate of return.
24. Y = income.
25. EX = expenditure.
26. V = capital value.
27. R = rate of return.
28. LND = value of the land occupied.
29. IMP = value of the improvements.
30. OSC = original cost of a level 1 structure.
31. VR = value ratio of the structure.
32. LV = number of levels.
33. SPX = amount of space required for a level 1 activity.
34. UVL = unit value of land.
35. RNT = rental space per unit.
36. SPO = amount of space occupied.
37. POP = number of population units.
38. SPX = number of space units required.
39. EX = expenditures for residential property.
40. CU = cost of utility services.
41. TX = total taxes paid.
42. MT = cost of maintanence.

43. WTR = cost of water.
44. PU = industry specific price per unit paid for products.
45. UP = number of units produced.
46. TR = transportation costs for goods and services.
47. SL = amount of salaries paid.
48. GS = costs of goods and services.
49. TM = costs associated with the use of shipping terminals.
50. PTN = costs associated with pollution control.
51. PPU = price per unit charged.
52. US = number of units sold.
53. MY = money available.
54. TAX = total tax income.
55. SVC = total of all service charges.
56. BND = bond income.
57. CT = cash transfer.
58. I = ratio of demand to supply of services proved by a department.
59. D = demand for services by department.
60. S = supply of services of department.
61. STP = number of students per population unit.
62. TCM = function giving student capacity from teacher mix.
63. HM = number of high income teachers.
64. MM = number of middle income teachers.
65. ND = number of departments.
66. TAE = amount of time allocated to adult education by class.
67. PH = number of part-time high income teachers.
68. PM = number of part-time middle income teachers.
69. WLP = total welfare payments.
70. WLP = total welfare payments required to cover minimum living costs.
71. LU = land use.
72. MSR = municipal service requirements.
73. MSC = municipal service capacity from employment functions.
74. LW = number of low income workers.
75. UTR = utility requirement by land use function.
76. LCC = least cost design capacity of level 1.
77. IX = overall government performance index.
78. W = weight assigned to government performance index.
79. TTM = value of all time in the model.
80. TVL = value of one time unit.
81. TAX = time allocated by one population unit.
82. NA = number of activities.
83. TAL = total time which may be allocated.
84. TMT = total time in a day, year, etc.
85. TWK = time spent at work.
86. TIL = time lost due to illness.

87. TTR = time spent traveling to work.
88. TIN = total involuntary time.
89. TUA = unallocated time.
90. TSA = time actually spent in an activity.
91. TRI = total time spent which improves resources.
92. TEF = time spent in free education and training programs.
93. TEP = time spent in paid education and training programs.
94. TPL = time spent in political activity.
95. TPW = time spent in part-time work.
96. RTA = rate of return of allocation of time.
97. ICM = income from work.
98. Δ VTR = rate of increase in voter registration.
99. Δ EDL = rate of change in the education level of a population unit.
100. CEP = cost per time unit for pay education.
101. BEN = total benefit from the allocation of time.
102. SOF = salary offered to workers.
103. $\overline{SPW}$ = average salary paid to workers.
104. UEM = unemployment rate.
105. $\overline{TCS}$ = average transportation cost for workers.
106. $\overline{TCW}$ = average transportation cost for workers to get from residence to site where currently employed.
107. WPU = number of workers per population unit.
108. TCS = cost for worker to get from residence to work.
109. $\overline{RNT}$ = average rent per space unit.
110. $\overline{QI}$ = average quality index.
111. $\overline{EI}$ = average environmental index.
112. OCR = occupancy rate.
113. SPT = total space available.
114. MTL = maintenance level of the structure.
115. NV = net value of the structure.
116. MSD = municipal service demand.
117. MSR = municipal service requirement.
118. MSE = municipal service employment mix.
119. SMS = supply of municipal services.
120. UTD = utility demand.
121. UTR = utility requirement.
122. SUT = supply of utility services.
123. LUS = level of utility service installed.
124. LCC = least cost capacity of a level 1 utility plant.
125. AGE = age of the structure.
126. FSI = flood severity index.
127. WTO = water obtained by the utility district.
128. WTN = amount of water needed by a district.
129. MSD = depreciation due to inadequate municipal services.
130. DDA = depreciation due to age and obselesence.

131. DFL = depreciation due to flood damage.
132. DOC = depreciation due to exceeding capacity.
133. FRD = depreciation due to fire damage.
134. PDP = population demand for personal goods/services.
135. PDK = normal demand factor.
136. PDA = demand resulting from the allocation of time.
137. RDP = residence demand for personal goods/services.
138. DRD = demand resulting from 1 percent depreciation of residence.
139. PGD = a function of personal goods demanded from a 1 percent depreciation of a land use.
140. PSD = a function of personal service demand from a 1 percent depreciation of a land use.
141. TBD = total demand for business goods and services.
142. DIP = demand from industry for business goods and services.
143. DDS = demand from the sale of personal goods and services.
144. BDD = demand generated by structural maintanence.
145. DGV = demand generated from government contracts.
146. DGS = goods and service demand as a function of a level 1 industry.
147. DPS = demand per unit from sales of personal services.
148. DPG = demand per unit from sales of personal goods.
149. UPS = units of personal services sold.
150. UPG = units of personal goods sold.
151. DDD = demand function by depreciation of land use.
152. DC = design capacity.
153. WRR = number of workers required.
154. WKR = number of workers.
155. PWR = total power in the system.
156. PRI = power of an economic entity.
157. PUB = power of a government department.
158. LAS = number of successful litigations.
159. LAT = total number of litigations.
160. GMY = money available to a department.
161. TMY = total money in the system.
162. FRC = force available.
163. PSW = persuasion.
164. VTE = total votes cast.
165. AV = average number of votes per population unit.
166. RDV = random deviation from AV.
167. SJ = supply of jobs.
168. EMR = employees required by class for each land use.
169. WR = number of MS workers.
170. TR = number of teachers requested.
171. DJ = demand for jobs.
172. WKP = number of workers per population unit.

173. MOV = number of migrants.
174. UE = unemployment.
175. DPL = number of displaced.
176. STA = emigrants which stay within the system.
177. Lcl = cost (time and money) to traverse link 1 on the optimum route from residence location to work location by class.
178. MOD = mode choice to traverse link 1.
179. COG1 = congestion in link 1.
180. MDC = modal cost function.
181. TUM = time consumption function.
182. UTR = utility requirements for a level 1 by land use.
183. UTC = utility charge functions by jurisdiction.
184. BGD = a function for business goods demand from a 1 percent depreciation in land use.
185. BSD = a function for business service demand from a 1 percent depreciation of land use.
186. PBG = price paid per unit for business goods.
187. PBS = price paid per unit for business services.
188. PPS = price paid per unit for personal services.
190. TX = total taxes.
191. IT = income tax.
192. PTX = property tax.
193. STX = sales tax.
194. TXR = tax rate.
195. WKR = number of workers.
196. SPW = salary offered per worker.
197. WCR = water consumption rates by land use.
198. WTR = total water costs.
199. WC = water charge.
200. RT = residence type.
201. MGD = amount of surface water required.
202. SWT = function relating cost per gallon to treat water to a useable level of quality.
203. WQ = existing water quality.
204. EFT = function relating the cost of effluent treatment and the level of treatment.
205. LT = level of treatment to which effluent is subjected.

ABOUT THE AUTHOR

PETER W. HOUSE received his doctorate at Cornell University in the area of public administration. His previous training was in the areas of economics and sociology. Dr. House's interest in holistic approaches to problems of the urban and environmental areas drifted toward modeling; particularly gaming and man-machine simulation. He resigned as a Research Economist at USDA and became the Director of Urban Systems Simulations at the Washington Center for Metropolitan Studies. From there, he became President of a non-profit company, Envirometrics, Inc. At present, he is the Director of the Environmental Studies Division of The Environmental Protection Agency.